Praise for *Without Concealment, Without Compromise*

"Jill L. Newmark fills a significant gap in scholarship on Civil War medicine with her deeply researched and detailed exploration of the Black military surgeons of the Civil War. In each biographical exploration, Newmark reminds us of the important work that Black surgeons performed, not only in the medical tent, but in claiming and advancing the work of civil rights."

—**Sarah Handley-Cousins**, author of *Bodies in Blue: Disability in the Civil War North*

"A magnificent accomplishment! This volume reconstructs the lives of 14 Black Civil War–era physicians through meticulous and dogged archival research. These revelations about Black medical contributions to the war will inspire historians and their students for years to come."

—**Margaret Humphreys**, author of *Intensely Human: The Health of the Black Soldier in the American Civil War*

"A monumental achievement, *Without Concealment, Without Compromise* is the first book on the Black physicians who served during the U.S. Civil War. Jill L. Newmark has meticulously researched city directories and census records, newspaper reports and pension applications, federal depositions and military documents to produce a breathtaking account of the Black doctors who wore Union blue. The portraits of these men are compelling. *Without Concealment, Without Compromise* is a must read for anyone interested in either the Civil War or the history of medicine."

—**Jim Downs**, author of *Maladies of Empire: How Colonialism, Slavery, and War Transformed Medicine*

"Newmark's book moves deftly among medical history, military history, social history, and religious history—in the process showing how some of those traditional boundaries vanish when examining an event like the Civil War. An important work for anyone interested in the African American experience during the conflict that ended slavery. The author resurrects the stories of dedicated medical professionals who broke through racial barriers and serve to inspire us still."

—**Zachery A. Fry**, author of *A Republic in the Ranks: Loyalty and Dissent in the Army of the Potomac*

ENGAGING
——*the*——
CIVIL WAR

Chris Mackowski and Brian Matthew Jordan, Series Editors

A Public-History Initiative of Emerging Civil War
and Southern Illinois University Press

WITHOUT CONCEALMENT, WITHOUT COMPROMISE

THE COURAGEOUS LIVES OF BLACK CIVIL WAR SURGEONS

Jill L. Newmark

Southern Illinois University Press
Carbondale

Southern Illinois University Press
www.siupress.com

*Publication of this book has been made possible in part through a generous contribution by
Russell Newmark.*

26 25 24 23   4 3 2 1

Cover illustration: From left to right: John H. Rapier Jr., c. 1863, *image courtesy Anne
Straith Jamieson Fonds, The J. J. Talman Regional Collection, Western University
Archives and Special Collections, London, Ont. (cropped)*; Anderson R. Abbott in
uniform, c. 1863, *image courtesy Anderson Ruffin Abbott Papers, Special Collections
and Rare Books, Toronto Public Library (cropped)*; William P. Powell Jr. in uniform,
c. 1863, *image courtesy National Archives and Records Administration, Washington,
D.C. (cropped)*; and Major Alexander T. Augusta in uniform, c. 1863, *image
courtesy Oblate Sisters of Providence, Baltimore, Md (cropped).*

Library of Congress Cataloging-in-Publication Data
Names: Newmark, Jill L., author.
Title: Without concealment, without compromise : the courageous lives of Black
    Civil War surgeons / Jill L. Newmark.
Identifiers: LCCN 2022044210 (print) | LCCN 2022044211 (ebook)
    | ISBN 9780809339044 (paperback) | ISBN 9780809339051 (ebook)
Subjects: LCSH: African American surgeons—Biography. | African American
    physicians—Biography. | United States—History—Civil War, 1861–1865—
    Medical care. | United States. Army—History—Civil War, 1861–1865—
    Biography. | Medicine, Military—United States—History—19th century. |
    United States—History—Civil War, 1861–1865—African Americans. | African
    American physicians—United States—History—19th century. | African
    American surgeons—United States—History—19th century. | Surgeons—
    United States—History—19th century. | Physicians—United States—History—
    19th century. | BISAC: HISTORY / United States / Civil War Period (1850-
    1877) | MEDICAL / History
Classification: LCC E621 .N55 2023 (print) | LCC E621 (ebook)
    | DDC 973.7750922—dc23/eng/20220921
LC record available at https://lccn.loc.gov/2022044210
LC ebook record available at https://lccn.loc.gov/2022044211

Printed on recycled paper ♻

SIU
Southern Illinois University System

This book is dedicated to my kind and loving mother, Marie DeVito Newmark, who instilled in me the belief that I could do or be anything I wanted, and to Margaret A. Hutto, who taught me that possibilities can become reality and gave me unconditional love and support throughout the creation of this book.

Contents

Illustrations

Preface

In 2007, I was in the midst of co-curating an exhibition on African American academic surgeons for the National Library of Medicine. The display was conceived as a way to provide a perspective on African Americans in medicine and help advance the diversity of exhibitions at the library. While conducting research for it, I stumbled across a pioneering Black physician named Alexander T. Augusta, who, in 1868, was the only Black professor among the first five professors in the newly formed medical department at Howard University in Washington, D.C. His accomplishment piqued my curiosity and led me to discover that Augusta had also been the first African American commissioned medical officer in the U.S. Army and had served as a surgeon during the American Civil War. I wondered what other African Americans had served as surgeons during that war. Augusta launched me on a journey of discovery that uncovered the hidden stories of thirteen other pioneering Black physicians who, like Augusta, had served as medical professionals during the Civil War. As I delved deeper into my research over the years leading up to the creation of this book, I found records, images, and letters that had languished in archives and repositories around the country. I was reminded how the contributions and accomplishments of African Americans are too often overlooked and undervalued, and I was committed to bringing these important and inspirational stories into the light.

As I began my research, the paucity of publications on the subject was not unexpected. Some of the materials that were available lacked accuracy and depth. A few authors focused on the story of a single physician, others only mentioned the physicians in passing, and some attempted to touch upon all known Black Civil War surgeons but were limited in their treatment of the subject. This book expands on the foundation established by those publications, often from a small reference or a name, and develops each man's story to include early life and influences, military service, and postwar experiences as much as the resources allowed. It is a collective biography illuminating the courageous stories of Black Civil War surgeons. Primary sources were the focus for information on the lives and service of the fourteen Black men who served as surgeons during the war, but in many cases, locating information was like finding a needle in a haystack. It required taking small amounts of information and piecing them together to tell the larger story. The available resources determined the lens through which each man's story could be told. And while this book focuses on these fourteen men, I must point out that one African American female physician, Rebecca Crumpler, served at the end of the Civil War, caring for formerly enslaved people, though she was not part of the U.S. Army. Crumpler's medical work was carried out under the umbrella of the Bureau of Refugees, Freedmen, and Abandoned Lands, through which she provided medical care to Black civilians.

One of the objectives of this book is to provide the most accurate and full accounting of the lives and service of all known Black physicians who served as surgeons during the Civil War. To that end, it is important to make reference to one physician, David O. McCord, who has repeatedly been represented in multiple publications as an African American commissioned military surgeon in the United States Colored Troops (USCT). This representation, however, was based on a misinterpretation by a researcher of an announcement in the *American Medical Times* of January 9, 1864, stating that "Surgeon D. O. Mc-Cord, 9th Louisiana Vols., of African descent, has been announced as Medical Director and Inspector of Freedmen in camps and on plantations within the Department of Tennessee and the State of Arkansas."[1] The words "of African descent" refer to the 9th Louisiana Volunteers and not to McCord. Based on my extensive research and review of the federal and nonfederal records, McCord was a white physician who enlisted in the Union army on May 9, 1862, and was appointed second assistant surgeon to the 66th Infantry.[2] He then served as surgeon with the 9th Louisiana Infantry Volunteers (African Descent), which later became the 63rd USCT.[3] In December 1863, by special order, McCord was appointed medical director and inspector of freedmen in Tennessee and Arkansas and, eventually, Mississippi.[4] If McCord had been identified as an African American man, it is unlikely he would have been appointed surgeon to an all-white regiment in 1862, prior to the start of the official recruitment of Black men that began in 1863. It is similarly doubtful that he would have been placed in such a position of authority as medical director of freedmen in 1863, as the U.S. Army was reluctant to accept a Black physician for a surgeon or assistant surgeon position. White surgeons would not serve alongside or be subordinate to a Black surgeon, as demonstrated by the fervent protest of white surgeons against the appointment and position of Alexander T. Augusta as senior ranking regimental surgeon of the 7th Infantry of the USCT.[5] In addition, the federal and nonfederal records for the fourteen known Black surgeons all make at least one reference to their color, identifying them as either "colored," "mulatto," or "negro." This reference does not appear in any of the federal or nonfederal records examined for McCord.

I spent a considerable amount of time during my research chasing down primary sources, often from the smallest clue. When researching a subject where scholarly publications are few and far between, it is necessary to think creatively when seeking primary sources. Sometimes it requires taking a less-traveled path or pursuing characters that may at first seem secondary to the story but in reality play a greater role than expected. Such was the case in my discovery of a single photograph of one surgeon featured in this book. On a spring day in 2009, I requested the pension records of contract surgeon William P. Powell Jr. at the National Archives in Washington, D.C. Pensions were not often given to contract surgeons who served during the war and less so to African Americans, but I had thought it was worth a try to see if a pension file existed for him and soon discovered one did. I was surprised when the staff member handed me two full folders. I carefully opened the top folder, and much to my surprise I found myself face-to-face with a man seated in a chair wearing a military uniform. I opened and closed that folder several times, each time glancing at the photograph in disbelief before I got up, walked to the window, and took several deep breaths. I realized at that moment that I had found a rare photograph of an African American Civil War surgeon and perhaps the only known photograph that existed of him. In the black and white image, Powell directs his gaze toward the viewer, projecting an air of confidence and pride. This photograph had likely remained hidden for over one hundred years, as did Powell's story, and it was time for that story to be told.

While doing research for the exhibition *Binding Wounds, Pushing Boundaries: African Americans in Civil War Medicine* at the National Library of Medicine, thinking outside the box was again crucial as I developed a story around Alexander T. Augusta, focusing on the significance of a Black man wearing a military officer's uniform in public. The story was compelling, but I needed an image of Augusta in his uniform to bring the story to life. My search for an image brought me to the Library and Archives Canada, where I located a line drawing of Augusta in his military cap and uniform. Although this was a good likeness of him, it did not have the impact that an actual photograph would have, so I decided to turn my attention to identifying someone who might have had a photograph of Augusta in uniform. The most likely candidate was his wife, Mary, as I remembered that all too often the stories of women are ignored or neglected.

I began researching Mary Augusta and learned that she and her devout Catholic family were from Baltimore. Two of Mary's sisters were nuns with the Oblate Sisters of Providence, the first religious order of women of color, established in 1829. As a result of her family's connection to the Oblate Sisters, Mary Augusta had become a benefactor of the convent, and after her husband's death in 1890, she moved back to Baltimore and lived the remainder of her life with the nuns at the convent. Mary outlived Alexander by eighteen years and upon her death left all her worldly belongings to the Oblate Sisters of Providence. This led me to contact the archivist at the convent about a possible photograph of Augusta in uniform that may have been among Mary Augusta's possessions. The archivist told me that she thought a photograph in their collections matched my description. I made an appointment to visit the archives, and when I arrived I again found myself face-to-face with history: staring back at me was a carte de visite of Alexander T. Augusta in his uniform that matched exactly the line drawing I had previously located at the Library and Archives Canada. These two anecdotes illustrate the challenges and rewards of my journey researching this book and underscore the complexities of taking on this subject matter. Though many hours of research often ended with little results, moments like these kept my eyes on the finish line and the momentum moving forward. It was a journey of enlightenment, illumination, and inspiration, one that empowered my commitment to bring these stories to light.

As I contemplated a title for the book, I wanted it to reflect in some way all of the surgeons who are featured. *Without Concealment, Without Compromise: The Courageous Lives of Black Civil War Surgeons* originates from the motto of the *National Anti-Slavery Standard*, a nineteenth-century abolitionist newspaper. It is a fitting title for this book that explores the experiences and accomplishments of fourteen Black physicians who were uncompromising in their fight for equality and freedom and did not conceal their voices or their actions in that fight despite the often violent opposition they faced. Their previously hidden stories are revealed in this book and become part of the Civil War narrative.

It is important to make some remarks about the format and structure of the book. In most chapters, I refer to the featured surgeon by his last name. When a father and son have the same first and last names, I have used the Jr. and Sr. suffixes, as in the case of William P. Powell Jr., John H. Rapier Jr., and Benjamin A. Boseman Jr., to avoid confusion. This designation was not always a part of their legal names or used by them but helps to distinguish between father and son.

The use of language throughout the book reflects nineteenth-, twentieth-, and twenty-first-century usage. Common terminology used in the nineteenth century to identify persons of color included "negro," Black, "colored," "mulatto," and "quadroon," often a reflection of the person's complexion or perceived quantity of "Black" blood. These were created by a white society and within the constructs of a predominantly racist as well as slave-owning country and not necessarily by the population of persons of color. References to regiments of Black soldiers are often to the United States Colored Troops and the designation "of African descent," which was used for some early all-Black regiments formed prior to the establishment of the USCT. When referring to the hospital in Washington, D.C., where half of the fourteen Black surgeons served during the war, it is important to note that the hospital when first established was called Contraband Hospital or Contraband Camp Hospital and later Freedmen's Hospital. The name change occurred when control of the hospital was transferred from the U.S. Army to the Bureau of Refugees, Freedmen, and Abandoned Lands. References made to the hospital in pension records and other government documents use "Contraband" and "Freedmen's" interchangeably, and this is reflected throughout the book.

Acknowledgments

Over the fifteen years in which I researched and wrote this book, an extensive group of extraordinary people assisted me along the way. The journey began at the National Library of Medicine, where the idea for this project was inspired by an exhibition I curated in 2009 on African American medical personnel who served during the American Civil War. As a result of this exhibition, my interest in the subject blossomed, and in 2014 I organized a panel for the Society of Civil War Historians conference on the impact of African American practitioners on the health and well-being of Black soldiers during the Civil War. Prior to the conference, I was approached by Sylvia Frank Rodrigue of Southern Illinois University Press, inquiring about a possible book project. I had considered writing a book on the subject and now was happily being pushed in that direction. I am grateful to Sylvia for reaching out to me and for her continued interest, advice, and support throughout my first book writing adventure.

I will be forever grateful to the late chief of the History of Medicine Division at the National Library of Medicine, Elizabeth Fee, PhD, who encouraged me in the process, provided invaluable editing suggestions, and was always enthusiastic in her belief that I could tackle book writing. Her successor, Jeffrey Reznick, PhD, was a great help in guiding me through the book proposal process and generous in sharing his own book proposals, which helped me in crafting my own.

With any book research there comes a need for an excellent interlibrary loan department. I was fortunate to work in the world's largest medical library, which made it easy to obtain a myriad of materials through our own interlibrary loan program with the help of Ruth Hill, Mary Wassum, and Liliya Gusakova. A special thanks goes to Erika Mills for her assistance in obtaining photographs of materials from the Anderson Ruffin Abbott Papers at the Toronto Public Library.

My friends and colleagues were generous in giving their time to read, review, and discuss chapters with me. It was essential to receive feedback from a diversity of people who could provide their own perspectives and interpretations of the book's content. I am beyond grateful for their time and effort, including that of Mary Beth Corrigan, Elizabeth Fee, Pamela Leconte, Manon Parry, and Mariola Rosser. Their invaluable comments and suggestions helped bring clarity to the content and ensure that I focused on what was truly essential.

The story of Black Civil War surgeons depends heavily on primary sources often found in the deepest recesses of archives and repositories around the country and abroad. My success in obtaining these primary source materials was made easier with the generous assistance from several librarians and archivists, including Joellen Elbashir at Moorland-Spingarn Research Center, Howard University; Sharon Knecht at the Oblate Sisters of Providence Archives in Baltimore; Cheney J. Schopieray at the William L. Clements Library, University of Michigan, Ann Arbor; and Tania Henley at the Special Collections Centre, Toronto Public Library. A special thanks is due Kalina Newmark, who while a student at Dartmouth College obtained invaluable primary sources from the Rauner Special Collections Library.

Primary resources were not limited to the United States, and I am grateful for the assistance and information I received from historians and archivists abroad, including Mary O'Doherty at the Mercer Library, Royal College of Surgeons, Dublin, Ireland; Maureen M. Watry, PhD, at the Special Collections and Archives, Sydney Jones Library, University of Liverpool, England; and Jeffrey Green, Liverpool.

It is a wonderful experience to share and discuss research with fellow historians. Several were generous with me, including Jim Downs, PhD, at Gettysburg College; Margaret Humphreys, MD, PhD, at Duke University; Carla L. Peterson, PhD, at the University of Maryland; Forrester "Woody" Lee, MD, at Yale University; William Forstchen at Montreat College; Loren Schweninger at the University of North Carolina, Greensboro; Richard M. Reid at the University of Guelph; and Jonathan W. White, PhD, at Christopher Newport University. A special thanks goes to Greg Harris, great-grandson of J. D. Harris, for contributing his research, and to Catherine Slaney, who generously shared her research, documents, and thoughts on the experience of her great-grandfather Anderson R. Abbott. She made an important donation of Abbott materials to the National Library of Medicine that expanded the library's collection.

Photographs were critical to telling the story of these Black surgeons, but finding them was no small task. I am grateful to the following individuals for their help in locating important images: Elaine Grublin and Rakashi Chand at the Massachusetts Historical Society in Boston; Wilma Moore at the Indiana Historical Society in Indianapolis; Stephanie Stodden at the Eureka Springs

Historical Museum in Arkansas; and Theresa Regnier at Western University Archives and Special Collections in London, Ontario.

This book would not have been possible without the support of my family. They were enthusiastic, encouraging, and loving. I am truly grateful to Russell Newmark, Mahalia Newmark, Kalina Newmark, and Laura McShane, who followed me on this journey from the beginning and generously gave of their time to read chapters and provide constructive comments. My deepest thanks goes to Margaret A. Hutto, whose invitation to co-curate an exhibition on African American academic surgeons first introduced me to the history of African Americans in medicine. Over the past fifteen years, she listened to the myriad of ideas and stories that became the chapters of this book. From the beginning of this writing adventure, she offered encouragement, enthusiasm, and invaluable editorial and intellectual content suggestions that were instrumental in bringing clarity to the subject matter. She was always there as a patient sounding board for issues and questions throughout the process, keeping me on the right track toward the finish line. This book would not have been possible without her.

I will forever be indebted to my wonderful mother, Marie DeVito Newmark, who instilled in me the values, confidence, kindness, and love that enabled me to write this book. She was my biggest champion, my greatest supporter, and my greatest friend. I will be forever grateful to her for the guidance, encouragement, and unconditional love she gave me throughout my life.

Finally, there would be no book without the extraordinary group of fourteen courageous, determined, and dedicated Black Civil War surgeons whose stories are told here. They defied convention, social mores, racist attitudes, and oppressive laws to reach beyond society's expectations and achieve success. Their commitment to freedom, justice, and equality helped change the course of American history.

Without Concealment, Without Compromise

ENGAGING
—the—
CIVIL WAR

For additional content that will let you engage this material further, scan the QR code on this page. It will take you to exclusive online material and related blog posts at www.emergingcivilwar.com.

Point your smartphone's camera at the QR code or use a QR scanner, which is readily available for download through the app store on your digital device.

Introduction

On a rainy morning in February 1864, Major Alexander T. Augusta, former surgeon-in-charge of Contraband Hospital in Washington, D.C., left his lodgings to head to a court-martial hearing downtown where he was called to testify. As he stepped outside, he hailed the approaching streetcar. He attempted to enter the car but was stopped by the conductor, who told him that he would have to ride up front with the driver because no Black passengers were permitted inside the car. Augusta refused and moved forward to take a seat when the conductor physically ejected him from the car, forcing him to walk to the hearing in the rain and delaying his arrival. Outraged, Massachusetts senator Charles Sumner introduced legislation to desegregate streetcars in Washington, which became law the following year.

Augusta's position and status as a military officer and surgeon enabled him to be a catalyst for change through his public activism. His streetcar incident and Sumner's response illustrate the challenges he and others faced in the fight for equality as well as the ability of an individual to be a force for social and political change. Historian Wilbert L. Jenkins noted that during the Civil War, Black people were "central actors in their own lives and not . . . passive objects of a white-dominated society."[1] This is certainly true of Augusta and the thirteen other Black men who became physicians and took positions as medical officers in the U.S. Army. They were not complacent or satisfied with only achieving their goal to become physicians but were committed to using their positions to advance the cause for freedom and equality.

The lives and accomplishments of these fourteen Black men who served as surgeons during the American Civil War are explored in this book through the themes of justice and freedom, patriotism and pride, and the individual as a force for change. The accounts of these men go beyond the obvious merits of their military service to explore the people and influences that shaped their early lives and the impact they made on their communities, their race, and their country. Their ambitions were not deterred by society's prejudicial dictates, and their dignified acts of resistance and pioneering new pathways challenged the status quo. They became symbols of an emancipated future.

In 1860, the enslaved population in the United States was nearly 4 million, and the country would soon be entrenched in a civil war fighting to unite the country and end slavery.[2] After the attack on Fort Sumter in April 1861 that launched the Civil War, many were anxious to fight for the United States, including Black men, both enslaved and free, who were ready to take up arms. They believed joining the U.S. Army would demonstrate their right to citizenship and their patriotism. The fourteen men featured in this book were among those who were dedicated to the fight for freedom. They were committed to using their medical skills in support of emancipation and in service to thousands of Black soldiers and civilians during the war. Many of these men had been activists and advocates for social and political change prior to the war. Some had participated in the antislavery movement and actively promoted education and advancement for African Americans. When they became military surgeons, they moved their activism into a larger theater where they could use their newly acquired positions as military officers to advocate for change and support fellow Black soldiers and formerly enslaved people.

The idea that Black men in the U.S. Army uniform used their positions and profession to make "claim to equality in the public sphere" and demand "a wider definition of freedom" for themselves and for all African Americans has been advanced by historian Gretchen Long.[3] Enlisted Black soldiers demonstrated this when they publicly paraded with their regiments, taking space on the city streets as free men. When Augusta, in full military uniform, refused to stand in an area for Black riders on a streetcar, he laid claim to equality in the public sphere. His act of defiance was a public protest against an unjust and discriminatory law. It was a demand for equality and an act of patriotism. As E. A. Bucchianeri writes, "It's not unpatriotic to denounce an injustice committed on our behalf, perhaps it's the most patriotic thing we can do."[4] Even the simple act of wearing a military uniform in public was patriotic. Black soldiers in uniform demonstrated their desire to unite the country and join in the fight for freedom despite the fact that they were not recognized as full citizens with all the rights of citizenship. Though their presence would not usher in a resistance-free movement toward freedom and equality for African Americans, it would serve as a stepping stone toward emancipation and citizenship.

Black soldiers were met with both acceptance and resistance when wearing the U.S. Army uniform. African Americans were proud to see Black men in the Union blue and cheered them when their regiments marched down city streets. When a battalion of Black soldiers in Little Rock, Arkansas, paraded in the city, they were described as "a sight to send a thrill through the heart of every lover of freedom."[5] But Black soldiers did not always face such a jubilant reception. While wearing the uniform in view of white civilians and soldiers, they were often met with resistance and violence. Augusta was attacked on a train in Baltimore by a group of white men while in his uniform.[6] When he mustered in with his regiment, he faced opposition to his position as the ranking medical officer by fellow white officers. The white medical officers were not shy to voice their objections to his presence as their superior and did so in a letter to President Abraham Lincoln.[7] Rank-and-file Black soldiers were often jeered and ridiculed by angry white soldiers and civilians, even suffering the indignities of having their insignia and stripes ripped from their uniforms.[8]

Resistance to the participation of Black soldiers in the war was not unusual. It was expressed by people at all levels of society. President Lincoln did not publicly support the recruitment of Black men before January 1863, when he signed the Emancipation Proclamation, as his primary concern was the preservation of the Union.[9] In the summer of 1862, when a visiting delegation of men from the West met with Lincoln, offering him two regiments of Black men from Indiana, he responded that "he would employ all colored men offered as laborers, but would not promise to make soldiers of them." The delegation left with the understanding that "unless some new and more pressing emergency arises," Black men would not be enlisted in the U.S. Army.[10] But as the war lingered on and army resources became strained and depleted, it became evident that the recruitment of Black men was a necessity for the United States to be victorious.

Recruitment of Black men began in earnest after the formation of the United States Colored Troops in May 1863 with only white officers appointed to lead Black soldiers. Resistance against the full participation of Black men in the army was deeply rooted in racism. It was fueled by the stereotypes and mythologies about Black people created by a dominant white society in a largely slave-holding country where white people believed that Black people were lazy, unintelligent, and irresponsible, had no ambition, and were best suited to menial labor. Although Lincoln eventually supported the recruitment of Black men, many white officers and soldiers clung tightly to their prejudices. Historian Joseph T. Glatthaar, in his study of the relationship between white officers and Black soldiers, makes note that Northern white officers of the USCT came to the war with preconceived notions about Black people primarily founded on the ideas and beliefs promoted by their Southern enemy.[11] Though some white officers proclaimed their support of emancipation and the advancement of Black people, many harbored biases against them. They were resistant to the advancement of Black soldiers and their full participation on the battlefield. These prejudices and the negative assumptions about Black people held by white officers and soldiers undoubtedly influenced their attitude toward Black soldiers, fueling the fires of discrimination and mistreatment.

Despite this resistance and the prejudice they faced, many African American soldiers took pride in wearing the U.S. Army uniform. A formerly enslaved man who donned the Union blue said, "This was the biggest thing that ever happened in my life. I felt like a man with a uniform and a gun in my hand." Another declared, "I felt freedom in my bones."[12] Their patriotism and pride palpable. Some memorialized this important moment of their lives in photographs while wearing their uniform. Historian Deborah Willis notes that photos of Black soldiers frame them in patriotism and manhood, allowing us to "imagine in an instant the sense of bravery and pride that accompanied the very act of pinning and wearing the emblematic eagle and brass button." Her understanding that these portraits of Black soldiers "are connected to the concept of democracy and citizenship" touches upon the significance of their presence and participation in the war and their sense of patriotism.[13]

A Black man in an officer's uniform had even greater significance, representing position and authority not previously available to Black people. When surgeon John H. Rapier Jr. took a position at Freedmen's Hospital in Washington, D.C., it became clear to him that wearing an officer's uniform sometimes garnered unprecedented respect for a Black man. In a letter to his uncle, he described how he had first decided not to wear his uniform, but after observing the respect that other Black officers in uniform received, he changed his mind and would now dress in full Union blues, pointed hat and all.[14] Rapier's recognition of how appearance affects the way one is perceived while instilling a sense of pride in oneself speaks to the knowledge of self-representation and the politics of appearance. What one wears can indicate rank, position, status, and authority and can influence how one is treated and respected. A white officer recognized the transition of the Black man when wearing the U.S. Army uniform when he said, "He completely metamorphosed, not only in appearance and dress, but in character and relations too. . . . Yesterday a slave, to-day a freeman . . . he is nothing of what he ever before was; he never was aught of what he now is."[15] African American soldiers, surgeons, and officers in uniform changed not only how Black men were viewed but also how Black people envisioned themselves and redefined the conventional notions of authority and the role of African Americans in society.

Wearing a uniform and receiving a rank also changed the relationship of Black people with "the state and white society."[16] Historian Kate Masur suggests that Black soldiers in uniform were bolstered by their new positions to challenge the "vestiges of slavery."[17] This seems evident by the newfound respect garnered by some Black soldiers in uniform, especially Black officers, and by the way their status and position broke through social barriers. The newly acquired positions of surgeons like Augusta and Rapier provided entrée into social and political circles, giving them unprecedented access to the influential elite. In Washington, D.C., their presence at public events did not go unnoticed, and their attendance was often as shocking to many as it was celebrated. When Augusta and fellow Black surgeon Anderson R. Abbott attended a reception at the White House, it represented a new level of social interaction and opportunity not previously afforded to African Americans at any level of society. Though their presence was met with mixed responses from those in attendance, its significance cannot be denied. Two Black officers in uniform, for the first time, walked among the white political elite with equal access to the president and First Lady. As U.S. Army officers, Augusta and Abbott held positions that helped open the door for Black people and change their relationship with white society.

Though their new standing as authority figures in the U.S. Army was met with resistance at almost every turn, their positions as officers allowed them to advocate on behalf of soldiers and civilians in ways not previously available. As the first African American to head a hospital in the United States, Augusta was able to hire additional Black surgeons, assist the newly arriving formerly enslaved people by providing medical care and employing them in paying hospital jobs, and advocate for improvements in facilities and care. While directing the Contraband Hospital in Washington, D.C., he attempted to improve the water supply by noting the deficiencies of the facility and their effects on the health of the residents of the Contraband Camp where the hospital was located. Later in the war, while serving as surgeon-in-charge at Freedmen's Hospital in Georgia, Augusta often confronted white city politicians regarding unfair and discriminatory policies affecting the health and well-being of his staff and patients. His rank and status placed him in a position where he could advocate for changes that would improve the lives of African Americans under his care and living in his community. As a symbol of emancipation and an agent of change, Augusta was not alone. Each of the fourteen Black surgeons who served during the Civil War possessed the educational credentials, self-respect, and awareness of the extent to which his influence could effect change. Collectively they helped shape a new view of African Americans and pave the way for greater opportunities for advancement and acceptance of Black people in American society.

Without Concealment, Without Compromise is a collective biography of these fourteen Black Civil War surgeons and the experiences that shaped their lives and influenced change. It adds to the existing and growing historiography on the subject by providing a more comprehensive examination of them. Several scholars have touched upon some of the stories of Black Civil War surgeons. For example, Margaret Humphreys's *Intensely Human* includes a chapter on Black medical personnel as related to the health of the Black Civil War soldier. In it, she explores the idea that Black soldiers received second-class medical care at the hands of white surgeons; perhaps a greater number of Black surgeons would have improved the health of Black soldiers. Jim Downs's *Sick from Freedom* incorporates the service of Alexander T. Augusta as it related to the health conditions of the formerly enslaved people at a hospital in Georgia. Downs explores how Augusta advocated on behalf of his patients and the local Black community.[18] Though Humphreys and Downs offer useful glimpses into the service of these men and the influences they had on health care during the war, their focuses are not on the life journeys that brought these men to positions of power that enabled them to influence the health and well-being of those under their care. My aim is to offer a more holistic approach that encompasses all aspects of the Black surgeons' lives and work.

Each chapter in this book is focused on a single surgeon or on a group of surgeons who share a common element. The organization was predicated on the available resources and information for each surgeon. As with any biography, the extent of the storytelling can often be limited by obtainable resources and previously published research. For several of the surgeons, published research is minimal and few primary sources were accessible; in those cases, surgeons were grouped around a common element or theme. Those with greater representation among primary and secondary sources warranted an entire chapter.

The paths these men traveled to become military surgeons in a nineteenth-century segregated army can be appreciated only by having an understanding of the era's medical education. This background is explored in chapter 1. The stories of individual surgeons are examined in chapters 2 through 10.

Alexander T. Augusta, William P. Powell Jr., and Anderson R. Abbott were the first African Americans to hold positions of authority at a hospital in the United States, and their stories are highlighted in chapters 2 through 4. Chapter 5 and 6 discuss the lives of John Van Surly DeGrasse, the first African American member of the Massachusetts Medical Society, and John H. Rapier Jr., a dentist, physician, and prolific writer. The life of the only known Black naval officer, Richard H. Greene, is explored in chapter 7, and chapter 8 reveals the story of Willis R. Revels, the only African American preacher-physician to serve as a surgeon during the war. Chapter 9 discusses the life of Benjamin A. Boseman Jr. and his rise from military surgeon to politician. Family tradition can influence activism, and this theme is explored in the story of Charles B. Purvis in chapter 10. The stories of Cortlandt Van Rensselaer Creed and William B. Ellis are told in chapter 11, framed around their medical education at two Ivy League schools, while the phenomenon of four Black medical students—John H. Rapier Jr., Alpheus W. Tucker, J. D. Harris, and Charles H. Taylor—attending a single medical school in Iowa is explored in chapter 12.

* * *

My hope is that by lifting the veil on these often-hidden stories, my book will reveal the dedication, commitment, courage, and patriotism these Black Civil War surgeons demonstrated as they served their country at a critical moment in American history. Their presence and accomplishments contributed to the U.S. Army's success, influenced change, and forged new pathways for African Americans in society.

1. ❧ Breaking the Color Barrier: The Medical Education and Military Service of Black Physicians in the Nineteenth Century

> The University has been thrown into convulsions during the last ten days because an "American of African descent" dared to present himself as a candidate for admission to the medical class. . . . The faculty . . . invited Mr. Tucker to leave the university. . . . So you see Col'd Men are not admitted here.
>
> —John H. Rapier Jr.

In 1863, a young Black man named Alpheus W. Tucker attended his first class at the University of Michigan medical school after being accepted to matriculate by the university. His appearance in class that day caused an uproar among his fellow students, who were not hesitant to communicate their displeasure to school authorities. Succumbing to the prejudicial protests of white students, the school's administrators requested that Mr. Tucker withdraw from class and leave the university.[1]

Similar scenarios played out at medical schools across the United States in the mid-nineteenth century. Medical schools had consistently excluded people based on race and sex, reflecting societal attitudes of the time, but a small number of African Americans and women began to gain admission to some medical colleges.[2] Admission did not mean acceptance and graduation was not assured, but enrolling Black students at medical schools was the first step in breaking the color barrier that would allow fourteen Black physicians to become surgeons in the U.S. military.

Black people who pursued a medical education faced obstacles and discrimination along the way. Even after gaining admission, many were forced to leave after pressure from fellow white students and school administrators, much like Tucker at the University of Michigan. Rejection by most mainstream educational institutions in the United States led some to seek out a

8

medical education in Europe and Canada, while others found acceptance at a few schools in the northeast and midwest United States, such as Dartmouth Medical College in New Hampshire, the Medical Institution of Yale College in Connecticut, and Keokuk Medical College in Iowa.

Before the Civil War, education for Black people was not encouraged and in most instances was banned, with states enacting laws that prohibited the education of both enslaved and free Black people. Historian Heather Andrea Williams notes that white people understood the revolutionary potential of Black literacy, and the timing of these laws "exposed the close association in white minds between black literacy and black resistance."[3] In North Carolina, a law was enacted to punish the education of enslaved Black people in part because legislators believed "teaching slaves to read and write, tends to excite dissatisfaction in their minds, and to produce insurrection and rebellion."[4] Education has power, and for white people, an educated enslaved or free Black person was a threat to the power and control that white people maintained. Elias B. Caldwell, acting secretary of the American Colonization Society, an organization that supported the emigration of Black people to countries outside the United States, believed that both "enslaved and free blacks would be best kept 'in the lowest state of degradation and ignorance' to avoid their unfruitful aspirations of wanting 'privileges which they can never attain,'" namely freedom.[5] This belief was pervasive throughout the country and made obtaining a formal education nearly impossible for Black people.

Any education was difficult to acquire at best and often banned at worst. The only options were to learn in secret or at Black-run schools that Black communities established to educate their own children. Without basic instruction in reading, writing, and arithmetic, medical school was not achievable.

Medical education in the United States during the eighteenth and early nineteenth centuries was chaotic and unregulated. Physicians could be self-taught, trained by a practicing physician, or educated at a medical school in the United States or abroad. There was no formal structure to medical education and no formalized requirements or regulations to practice medicine. Some physicians began their careers as apothecaries or surgeon-barbers, compounding medicines and performing treatments such as cupping and leech therapy. This often served as an entrée into the medical world, inspiring them to seek training to become physicians. An apprenticeship was the most common way to become a physician. Those established in the profession would serve as preceptors, taking on students as apprentices and providing them with theoretical and practical medical experience. Many physicians at the time believed that hands-on training at the bedside was the best method for teaching medicine.[6] With no regulations or legal restrictions to practice medicine, those desiring to become a physician could choose whatever method of training worked best for them. Apprenticeships often began with one student and one physician but over time became more systemized and standardized. Preceptors often formulated training courses for more than one student utilizing contemporary medical literature, illustrations, and other teaching aids in their instruction. By the mid-nineteenth century, the standard in medical education became a mix of apprenticeship and attendance at medical school lectures in subjects like anatomy, materia medica, chemistry, surgery, and obstetrics.[7]

Though Black medical practitioners existed before 1837, they were often self-taught or gained medical knowledge through study with another physician willing to take on a Black student. Prior to 1846, when David Jones Peck was admitted to Rush Medical College in Chicago, a formal medical education for Black people in the United States was nearly impossible. The first formally educated African American physician, James McCune Smith, had no choice but to leave the country for Scotland, where he received his medical degree from the University of Glasgow in 1837, after being rejected on account of color from medical programs at Columbia University and Geneva Medical College in New York.[8] After receiving his medical degree, Smith returned to the United States and established a medical practice in the Black community of New York City and a successful business with the first Black-owned pharmacy in the country. Smith's education, leadership, and community activism served as an example to other young aspiring African American men who would go on to seek medical degrees, including fellow New Yorkers William P. Powell Jr. and John Van Surly DeGrasse. A few African American women also gained admission to medical school, but only at those established for the sole purpose of providing a medical education to women.[9] Rebecca Crumpler and Rebecca Cole obtained medical degrees from the New England Female Medical College in 1864 and the Woman's Medical College of Pennsylvania in 1867, respectively. After receiving her medical degree, Crumpler traveled to Richmond, Virginia, in 1865, where, working as part of the Bureau of Refugees, Freedmen, and Abandoned Lands, she provided medical care to formerly enslaved people.

To gain admission to medical school, an applicant was required to present recommendations attesting to their good moral character and academic prowess and proof of an established educational relationship with a reputable physician. It was also generally assumed that an applicant was white.

Some students of color were more easily accepted if they were considered non-Americans. John H. Rapier Jr., who was born in Alabama but spent time living in Haiti and Jamaica before applying to medical school, had an easier time than other Black students because he identified himself as a man from Jamaica. He sarcastically remarked to his cousin Sarah, "What a blessed thing for me, that I was born in Jamaica, it enables me to enter any college without questions of lineage."[10]

African Americans seeking a career as a physician knew a formal medical education was required to be accepted into the profession. Although many qualified African Americans who applied to U.S. medical schools were rejected based on their color, some were able to overcome this barrier and gain admission through sponsorship of a prominent white physician or politician. Cortlandt Van Rensselaer Creed had connections to wealthy white alumni at Yale College through his father, who worked at the school. Benjamin A. Boseman Jr. provided letters of recommendation from prominent citizens of his hometown, including two respected physicians and a local U.S. congressman. Others, like Willis R. Revels, were admitted through a program established by the American Colonization Society where a Black man's medical education was paid by the society in exchange for his emigration to Liberia, where he would provide medical services to the local population. Harvard Medical School and the Medical School of Maine were among those schools that participated. It was an appealing offer that some chose to accept, but others refused to emigrate after receiving degrees and remained in the United States.

In 1850, Martin R. Delaney, a Black man from Virginia, was accepted to Harvard Medical School after meeting with Oliver Wendell Holmes, the medical school dean. The Massachusetts Colonization Society had already sponsored two Black students, Daniel Laing Jr. and Isaac H. Snowden, prior to Delaney's arrival.[11] The admission of a third Black student became too much for the white students to accept, and they adamantly protested the presence of all three students at the medical school. White students claimed that the "admission of blacks to the medical lectures [is] highly detrimental to the interests, and welfare of the institution" and that it would "lower the reputation in this and other parts of the country." They went on to say, "We cannot consent to be identified as fellow students with blacks whose company we would not keep in the streets, and whose Society as associates we would not tolerate in our houses," though they "had no objection to the education and elevation of blacks."[12] It is interesting to note that similar reasoning was used by white assistant surgeons who protested the presence of Alexander T.

Augusta as the ranking medical officer at the mustering of four regiments of the USCT in 1864. The white officers claimed "to be behind no one, in a desire for the elevation and improvement of the colored race in this Country," but they could not and would not accept or tolerate the humiliation of being subordinate to a Black man. Though the Harvard Medical School faculty at first objected to the protests of the white students, Delaney and his fellow Black students were eventually asked to leave the university under the pretext that it was in the best interest of everyone. Dean Holmes explained that the university's decision was based on the fact that "the intermixing of the white and Black races in their lecture rooms is distasteful to a large portion of the class [white students] and injurious to the interests of the school."[13] Despite the policy Harvard had established in 1848 to accept Black students on the merit of their qualifying examinations, the school capitulated to the pressure from white students and expelled the Black students it had previously accepted based on their academic excellence.[14]

Despite such restrictions and obstacles, fourteen Black men shared a desire to move beyond the boundaries of color created by a dominant white society to pursue a medical education and serve their country. They were committed to a better life for themselves, their families, and their communities. John H. Rapier Jr. focused on how he could best provide for his family when deciding to pursue a medical education. Alexander T. Augusta applied his medical education to serving the Black community in Canada, but when the United States began recruiting Black soldiers during the Civil War, he decided he would serve as a surgeon where he could "be of use to his race."[15]

Their first challenge to becoming physicians was acquiring a formal medical education. Each man knew the difficulties he would face in gaining admission to a respected medical school, but these fourteen were not dissuaded. Cortlandt Van Rensselaer Creed was accepted at the Medical Institution of Yale College but wondered whether he would be allowed to attend.[16] When Alpheus W. Tucker was asked to leave the University of Michigan, Rapier described the incident, noting that the faculty had caved in to the demands of white students to remove Tucker, proving "Col'd Men are not admitted here."[17] Tucker, in a letter to the editor of the *Detroit Advertiser and Tribune*, wrote that despite the abhorrent treatment he received from the students and the school, it "will not prevent my continuance of my medical education elsewhere."[18]

These future Black surgeons faced the same obstacles of prejudice and racism as all persons of color, but they possessed certain advantages from being born free—a certain amount of wealth, education, and community support. Historian Richard M. Reid notes that "social and professional advancement entailed geographical mobility."[19] Most of these men had the financial means to travel, giving them the opportunity to gain life experience, to obtain an education, and to seek employment. All came from families and communities that advocated for education and believed that education was the key to advancement, and they understood that it was only through "the cultivation of the mind" that they could become truly emancipated and free.[20] They hailed from communities committed to Black progress and were encouraged in their abilities despite white society's limited notions about what Black people could achieve.

The earliest medical graduate among these fourteen men was John Van Surly DeGrasse, who graduated from the Medical School of Maine at Bowdoin College in 1849. Alexander T. Augusta, although the same age as De-Grasse, completed his medical exams in 1855 at Trinity College of Medicine in Toronto, Canada, but did not receive his formal medical degree until 1860. DeGrasse's father was a wealthy landowner in New York City and the son of a French navy admiral. He had the financial means to provide a formal education for his son, including studies in Paris. He was raised among a community of Black elite, including professionals, educators, entrepreneurs, and community leaders. In contrast, Augusta came from a family of lesser means and was raised among a community of skilled craftsmen, barbers, and semi-skilled laborers in Virginia. In order to pursue a medical education, he had to secure a well-paying job to finance his education. He trained and worked as a barber for several years before attending medical school.

William P. Powell Jr. acquired his medical education outside the United States after finding American medical schools inaccessible to him on account of color. Like DeGrasse, he lived among the Black elite in New York City, and his father ran a successful boardinghouse for Black sailors. His family had the means to travel from New York to England to escape the repercussions of the 1850 Fugitive Slave Act, which permitted any white person to claim ownership of any Black person, free or presumed a fugitive slave, based solely on the white person's claim of ownership. Capture of a presumed fugitive slave was made without due process of law and without allowing or considering the captured individual's testimony in his or her own defense. Powell Jr. was able to receive his medical education at the University of Liverpool beginning in 1852 at no cost after his father appealed to the school's admission committee on behalf of his son.[21]

Others found success in medical colleges in the northeast and midwest United States. Cortlandt Van Rensselaer Creed became the first Black graduate from the Medical Institution of Yale College in 1857, while Richard H. Greene, who received an undergraduate degree from Yale College that same year, received his medical degree from Dartmouth Medical College in 1863. Both men received financial and personal support from their families. Benjamin A. Boseman Jr. also came from a family of means and received his medical degree at DeGrasse's alma mater, the Medical School of Maine, in 1864. Charles B. Purvis similarly hailed from a wealthy family in Philadelphia and attended Worcester Medical College, receiving his medical degree in 1865.

* * *

At the outbreak of the Civil War, African Americans from all walks of life sought ways in which they could participate in the cause. Whether free or formerly enslaved, rich or poor, female or male, formally educated or not, many individuals desired to be part of the fight for freedom. Their desire to serve demonstrated their commitment to emancipation and their patriotism. Patriotism is fighting for change that can move your country forward, not just blindly supporting your country or waving a flag. For many Blacks during the Civil War, patriotism was directly connected to emancipation—they wanted to end slavery and gain citizenship. Some Black soldiers wrote about this connection. In a letter published in the *Christian Recorder* in 1864, a soldier in the 55th Massachusetts Volunteers wrote that Blacks enrolled themselves "under the broad banner of freedom" to "strike a decisive blow for God and the Union . . . to lay down our lives and shed our best blood beneath the Stars and Stripes."[22] A year before, the newspaper's editor wrote that "never had men stronger inducements to enlist than those which now press upon our colored fellow-citizens. Their country, their race, their own welfare for all time, appeal to them; and sure we are that the appeal will be responded to in a spirit worthy of men who appreciate their rights and the cause for universal liberty."[23] Similarly, when publicizing the recruitment of Black soldiers in Indiana, the broadside advertisement appealed to Black men to answer the call of their country and "let your moral sensibility and patriotism respond."[24]

Like other men who wanted to serve, Black physicians were quick to answer the call. With medical degrees in hand, they were now able to seek appointments as military surgeons with the U.S. Army. Alexander T. Augusta, the first to receive a position as surgeon, expressed his desire to serve in a letter to

President Abraham Lincoln, writing, "[I] would like to be in a position where I can be of use to my race."[25] This desire was shared by all Black physicians who applied for positions. After learning that the United States planned to raise Black troops during the war, Anderson R. Abbott sent a letter to Secretary of War Edwin M. Stanton, saying, "Being one of that class of persons, I beg to make application for a commission as Assistant Surgeon."[26] In his application, John H. Rapier Jr. stated, "I am desirous of entering the Medical of the Gov. . . . and would beg of you the knowledge of the proper method of making application."[27]

A formal medical degree was essential for a Black physician to acquire a position as a military surgeon, but having a diploma did not guarantee that the application process would be easy for either the U.S. Army or the Black applicants. The Army Medical Board expressed opposition, hesitation, and confusion toward the Black physicians who applied, but board members were met by confident, intelligent, and well-educated Black men. Still, when Augusta applied, he faced numerous delays, including an attempt to prevent him from taking the board's examination. It was only the intervention of Secretary Stanton that allowed Augusta to finally be assigned a date to appear before the board. After passing the examination, he was given a commission as a full surgeon with the rank of major. Only one other Black physician, John Van Surly DeGrasse, was commissioned as an army medical officer, and he was the only Black surgeon to serve in the field with his regiment.[28]

All Black physicians who applied for positions with the army faced the same Army Medical Board. Anderson R. Abbott followed in the footsteps of his mentor and friend, Alexander T. Augusta, when he applied for a position as a surgeon, even though he was a Canadian citizen. He was offered a position as a contract surgeon with the rank of captain. Despite his appointment, he was dissatisfied with his inability to secure a commission and believed it was based on racial discrimination.

After white assistant surgeons voiced their objections to Augusta's top ranking position and white surgeons in the field protested DeGrasse's presence, the government followed an unwritten policy of offering only contracts—not commissions—to other Black physicians applying to serve. By appointing Black physicians as contract surgeons, the government could more easily dismiss them or end their contracts if protests by white surgeons developed. The remaining twelve Black physicians received only contracts to serve as acting assistant surgeons and were assigned duty at Black-only hospitals or recruiting stations where new recruits for the USCT were examined.[29]

As military surgeons, African Americans could affect change in the care and treatment of Black patients and could challenge the discriminatory attitudes and actions facing Black soldiers and civilians. Organized health care for Black people in America started as an economic invention of white enslavers to keep the enslaved healthy enough to work and thus create wealth and prosperity for themselves. White doctors evaluated Black bodies based on keeping the "machine" working and not on what was best for the patient. This attitude carried over to many white doctors who treated Black patients during the Civil War. Some dismissed and disregarded the complaints of Black patients, and others refused to even touch the body of a Black person during a physical examination. When visiting Black troops in Arkansas and Missouri, surgeon Benjamin Woodward found some white surgeons unwilling to physically examine Black soldiers. "Med officers of the 11th would not and did not examine the men," he wrote, "and cases of Pneumonia were undetected because he *would not put his ear to chest of Negro*! Men left sick without care until ready to die, and then *wonder why they died*!"[30]

The care that white doctors provided to Black patients was more often than not substandard, neglectful, and lacking in compassion. This carried over to the treatment of Black soldiers by white surgeons. In military hospitals where Black surgeons treated Black soldiers and civilians, however, treatment and care were sometimes improved. Black patients who had been fearful of white physicians based on a history of distrust and mistreatment were now more open to examination and care when provided by Black physicians. There was an unspoken commonality that existed between Black physicians and Black patients, regardless of social status or life experience. Early twentieth-century research has shown that patient-physician concordance by race can influence the health and well-being of patients. This was likely true in the nineteenth century as well. In a study conducted at George Washington University in 2001, researchers examined the patient-provider and patient-staff racial concordance and its relationship to perceptions of mistreatment in a health care setting. They concluded that "racial concordance between minority patients and staff (as compared to nonconcordance) was found to be associated with lower rates of negative perceptions among Hispanics and blacks." They also suggested that "having a staff with a similar race background to that of the patient may play an important role in reducing patient perceptions of disrespect and unfair treatment."[31] Physician and author Damon Tweedy points out, "As a general rule, black patients are more likely to feel comfortable with black doctors . . . and seek them out for treatment."[32] How one self-identifies often affects attitude and can influence perspective and the understanding of others. As historian Manon Parry notes, "Who we are affects which issues we prioritize . . . [and] our ability to comprehend the circumstances of others."[33] The changes in attitude and approach to health care for African Americans introduced by these early Black Civil War surgeons set an important precedent for improvements in health care for Black people in America.

African American doctors who served as hospital administrators attempted to initiate changes in hospital environments, resources, and patient care. In 1863, Alexander T. Augusta, while acting as the surgeon-in-charge at Contraband Hospital in Washington, D.C., made attempts to improve the camp's poor water supply, which was affecting the health of the residents and patients. While practicing at Freedmen's Hospital in Savannah, Georgia, he similarly tried to provide a healthy environment for his patients by appealing to the local government and the Freedmen's Bureau administration for resources, personnel, and procedures that would improve patient care. William P. Powell Jr., in 1864, had perimeter fencing installed around Contraband Camp and Hospital to protect the residents and the camp's resources.

Despite the efforts by Black surgeons to improve the physical and medical conditions for Black soldiers, those soldiers serving in regiments of the USCT were subjected to poor medical treatment, subpar living conditions, and mistreatment at the hands of white surgeons. Historian Margaret Humphreys explains that "even by standards of the time, African American regiments received decidedly second-class medical care." She points out that Black soldiers endured conditions that were unhealthy and caused significant illness among them. "Although it is difficult to quantify the impact of inadequate medical care on the high rates of disease among black regiments," she wrote, "the evidence indicates that poor care was an important factor in these outcomes."[34] It is possible that Black soldiers would have been provided with a higher level of care and attention if more Black surgeons had served with regiments in the field.

Poor care of Black soldiers was in part due to the fact that white surgeons assigned to Black regiments were often less competent than those surgeons assigned to white regiments. "The mediocre physician ascribed high mortality rates to differences inherent in the black body and spirit," Humphreys points out, "and drank the medicinal whiskey stores while minimally serving his Black patients. At his worst, the surgeon was cruel, capricious, and dismissive of the needs of the men under his supposed care." White physicians seemingly made medical decisions not based on science and examination but on stereotypes and myths about Black people and their health.

Some saw the need for qualified medical staff among Black troops. Major General Nathaniel P. Banks, commander of the Department of the Gulf, was aware of the medical mistreatment of Black soldiers and remarked that "well grounded objections were made from every quarter against the inhumanity of subjecting colored soldiers to medical treatment and surgical operations by such men." He noted that "hospital stewards had been appointed as surgeons because they were the only medical men available." Hospital stewards maintained and dispensed medicines, but most were far from qualified to serve as surgeons. Banks felt that inadequate medical care for USCT soldiers was a serious matter and one that brought "discredit to the Army and the Government." He appealed to Washington in 1864 for a remedy to the lack of adequate medical staff for Black troops to no avail.[35]

Although the U.S. Army easily promoted white hospital stewards to assistant surgeon positions, it would not promote a qualified Black medical doctor who was serving as a hospital steward because of his color. Theodore Becker was a trained physician when he came to the United States from Suriname in 1857. Despite this fact, he was unable to secure a position in the U.S. Army as a surgeon and was appointed a hospital steward with the 54th Massachusetts Volunteer Infantry Regiment. When a white captain in the regiment fell ill and no surgeon was available to treat him, Becker was called upon to attend to him. The captain recovered from his illness and several white officers expressed their gratitude by recommending that Becker be promoted to assistant surgeon with the regiment. But their recommendation was rejected by the commanding officer because Becker was a Black man, and he remained a hospital steward.[36]

Black surgeons represented more than a profession to Black soldiers. They were an example of what a Black man could achieve if given an opportunity. Black soldiers saw in Black officers men of ranking military positions who could understand them and could advocate on their behalf. Perhaps if more Black surgeons were engaged as military surgeons during the war, the care that Black soldiers received would have been improved in more substantial and significant ways.

As military surgeons, Black physicians served as officers with the uniform and status their rank and position afforded. With this elevated status, they gained entry into elite social circles and access to influential politicians and policy makers to whom they could advocate for fairness, equal treatment, and civil rights on behalf of all Black people. Their presence among society's movers and shakers was, in and of itself, a political statement marking an advent of change for Black people in America.

Fourteen Black men shared a desire to move beyond the boundaries of color created by a dominant white society to become medical doctors and surgeons and achieve a better life for themselves and their communities. They were raised among well-educated free African Americans who were committed to freedom, equality, and advancement. Influenced and inspired by the accomplishments and success of those around them, they navigated the world with a strong sense of identity and a belief in their ability to move beyond society's expectations. Their work as medical professionals during the Civil War challenged the prescribed notions of race and pushed the boundaries of the role of Black people in America. They played a crucial role in the evolving definition of freedom, citizenship, and patriotism.[37]

2. ✤ Catalyst for Change: Alexander Thomas Augusta (1825–1890)

> ... splendid among the shabby field hands ... the sight of his uniform
> stirred the faintest heart in faith in the new destiny of the race, for
> Dr. Augusta wore the oak leaves of a major on his shoulders.
> —Anderson R. Abbott

On the eve of the one-year anniversary celebration of the 1862 signing of the D.C. Emancipation Act that freed all enslaved persons in the city, the crowd that gathered at the Fifteenth Street Presbyterian Church in the nation's capital could not help but notice the presence of a distinguished Black soldier wearing a military officer's uniform. The oak leaves on the epaulettes of Alexander T. Augusta's uniform were newly received; he had been given an appointment as surgeon in the U.S. Army earlier in the month. His appearance at the gathering was cause for great celebration, as he was the first Black man to achieve such a position.

Augusta came from humble beginnings in Norfolk, Virginia, where he was born free in March 1825. The only known evidence of Augusta's ties to the city is found in a "List of Free Negroes Residing in the Borough of Norfolk on the First day of February 1836." Alexander Augusta, age eleven, appears as a "free black" along with five siblings, John, Jane, Taliaferro, "Ceaser," and Mary, but no parents are identified.[1]

Little is known about his parents or his early childhood, but some insights about his early life can be gained from an understanding of the Black community of Norfolk. Augusta would have been part of a community of both enslaved and free persons that included skilled craftsmen, barbers, and semi-skilled laborers. Although Virginia had the largest number of enslaved African Americans in the United States, it also had one of the highest percentages of free Black people during the pre–Civil War years.[2] Free Black people gained a level of respect even from some in the white community that enabled them to bring lawsuits against white clients for unpaid debts, testify against white people in court, and invest in land.[3] As the social and political atmosphere

20

changed in the mid-1800s, however, the white population of Norfolk became fearful of the increasing numbers of literate free Black people who became more politically aware and active. White citizens found ways to hinder the advancement of Black people by limiting their opportunities for education and employment, leading to an exodus of many Black people from the city. Education was a key to escaping the confines of Norfolk, and although there were "no laws against teaching [free] African Americans to read in the early 1820s," a law had been passed in 1805 that exempted enslavers from teaching their Black apprentices to read and write.[4] The infringement on educational opportunities for Black people continued with the passage of an 1831 law that outlawed all meetings organized for the purpose of teaching Black women and men to read and write.

Augusta found a way to overcome the restrictions and move beyond them to seek out better prospects for advancement, first by securing an education and then by leaving Norfolk and moving north. His early education was likely obtained in secret or perhaps from a school for Black children that had been established in Norfolk in 1824. An education would have been impossible to obtain without the support, involvement, and encouragement of his parents and his community.

When he was old enough, Augusta left Norfolk and made his way to Baltimore, where he joined his older brother, John, by 1847. Both were employed as barbers in the city, Augusta likely as a barber-surgeon. He probably learned his trade through an apprenticeship with a local barber or through training with his brother.[5] Barber-surgeons not only cut hair but performed surgical procedures like blood-letting and teeth extractions. Although popular from medieval times through the eighteenth century, fewer barber-surgeons were active in the nineteenth century, and the job eventually transitioned to only cutting and styling hair. For Black men in nineteenth-century America, barbering was considered a respectable trade and provided a good income. Through the business, Black barbers gained economic independence and became upstanding members of their communities. Many Black barbers in Baltimore owned real estate in the city, the value of which equaled or surpassed the value of real estate owned by white barbers.[6]

While living and working in Baltimore, Augusta met native Baltimorean Mary O. Burgoin, whom he married on January 12, 1847, at St. Mary's Catholic Church in the city. Mary was the daughter of Augustine and Cecelia Burgoin, who owned a confectionery in the city. Devout Catholics, the Burgoin family would send two of their daughters to the Oblate Sisters of Providence convent, where they would become nuns and serve the Black community of Baltimore.[7] The ties that were established by the Burgoin family with the Oblate Sisters would remain steadfast throughout Mary's life, and she and Alexander would become benefactors of this religious order.

Over the next several years, Augusta continued working as a barber, but he had higher aspirations. He and Mary moved from Baltimore to Camden, New Jersey, outside Philadelphia, in 1850, where he intended to begin a profession as a physician. They followed Augusta's brother John, who had moved to Norristown, Pennsylvania, about twenty-five miles from Camden. Norristown had become a stop on the Underground Railroad in the early 1800s, and by the 1850s, John Augusta had become a well-known Underground Railroad agent.[8] For Alexander, the move to the Philadelphia area allowed him to begin his medical education. He planned to attend the University of Pennsylvania but was rejected by the medical school because he was Black. Undeterred, he began studying under the private tutelage of Dr. William Gibson, a professor of surgery at the university. A native of Baltimore, Gibson had taken a special interest in Augusta. Augusta's income as a barber provided enough funds to pay for a private tutor.

Although he gained a knowledge of medicine through private instruction, Augusta was determined to acquire a formal medical education. His ambition motivated him to make a cross-country trip to California, presumably to take advantage of the gold rush, where he hoped to earn tuition money for medical school. The 1852 census for California's El Dorado County listed Alexander Augusta as a twenty-seven-year-old Black man, born in Virginia and employed as a barber in Pennsylvania. One other Black person was listed—C. N. Augusta, identified as a twenty-five-year-old Black man born in Virginia who was also employed as a barber. It is possible that this was Alexander's younger brother Caesar, who might have accompanied Alexander on his travels west. Of the forty-five individuals listed on this page of the census, only two were identified as Black and one as "mulatto." More than two thousand African Americans had traveled to California by 1852, lured by the prospects of egalitarianism as well as gold. But the reports of both proved to be untrue, and after the California state legislature passed a strict fugitive slave law in 1852, many Black people left the state as it was no longer safe to stay.[9]

By 1853, Augusta had returned to Philadelphia and, with his wife, Mary, made his way to Toronto, Canada, to begin his formal medical education. His rejection from medical school in the United States compelled him to pursue this course of study across the border. Canada was an appealing place for people of color, and many formerly enslaved people had arrived safely from the United States by way of the Underground Railroad after escaping their enslavers. Canada had banned slavery in 1834, and there was no legal means for white enslavers to repossess formerly enslaved people once they crossed the international border. Black newspaper editor William C. Nell wrote, "Canada is destined to support an immense population of hardy and happy freemen, and . . . the sentiment of the more numerous and better portion of the inhabitants is that 'the preservation of her good name demands that Canada should continue to be a land of genuine freedom, and the City of Refuge to the oppressed man of color, where he can fearlessly breathe the air of freedom.'"[10] Alexander and Mary found Toronto especially attractive because Mary's sister Josephine Burgoin Bird lived there with her husband, Peter, and daughter, Marie Cecile. The city offered the Augustas greater freedom, a chance to live near family, and, for Alexander, a long-desired opportunity to pursue a formal medical education.[11]

After arriving in Toronto, Alexander established a drugstore on Yonge Street and Mary opened a dressmaking shop on York Street. Together they grew successful businesses and advertised regularly in the *Provincial Freeman*, a Black-owned local weekly newspaper. Augusta promoted his barber-surgeon services of cupping, bleeding, and teeth extractions along with applying leeches and filling prescriptions, noting that "the Proprietor, or a competent assistant, always in attendance."[12]

The Augustas' thriving businesses no doubt provided the necessary income for Alexander's medical studies at Trinity College of Medicine, now part of the University of Toronto. He was enrolled and attended lectures in 1854 and 1855 and successfully completed the medical exams, but he was not awarded a degree at that time because he failed the classical examination. The requirements for a bachelor of medicine degree included professional studies for four years, studying in college during one year, and passing an examination in divinity, classics, and mathematics.[13] By early summer of 1860, Augusta, who was already a licentiate of the Medical Board of Upper Canada, passed his examination in the classics and received a bachelor of medicine degree at the convocation held in June.[14] Later, Dr. John McCaul, president of the University of Toronto, would praise Augusta in his testimony before the American Freedmen's Inquiry Commission, saying Augusta had done "very well in medicine" as a student.[15] After graduating, Augusta continued his drugstore operations and worked as a physician and surgeon.[16]

Life in Toronto for Augusta included an active role in civic and political functions. He took part in improving the condition and education of the Black community and in supporting the cause for freedom in the United States. An antislavery society had existed in Canada since 1851, and there was a great deal of organized activity intended to assist Black people who came across the border, including events sponsored by the Association for the Education and Elevation of the Coloured People of Canada, incorporated in 1857. Augusta was a founding trustee of the organization, which focused on the education and training of Black youth in Ontario. The association's mandate was clear—to send the students it assisted to "schools, academies and colleges that are not set apart as separate for colored persons."[17] He was also an active member of several civic groups, including the Colored Citizens of Toronto, which promoted the welfare of Black people in Canada and "the elevation of their condition."[18] As chair of this organization, Augusta publicly denounced the mistreatment of Black people and responded to disparaging remarks made by a member of Parliament, stating that Black people would "resist by every means in our power, any invasion of our rights as citizens; and will hold up to public scorn and contempt all such panderers to American prejudice against color."[19] Augusta held strong and steadfast views on equality and was not afraid to share them publicly. This public demonstration for equal rights and justice continued throughout his life.

Although Augusta and his wife had settled in Toronto, the changing tide of the American Civil War would soon weigh heavily on him and strengthen his desire to be of service to his homeland. By January 1863, both the U.S. and Confederate forces were feeling the effects of fierce battles and great loss of life. The number of dead and wounded soldiers increased and fewer white men were available to serve, making the recruitment of Black men inevitable. Black men had been excluded from joining the military since the federal Militia Act of 1792, which provided for the organization of state militias. The prohibition against their service ended with the passage of the Militia Act of 1862, which authorized the enlistment of "persons of African descent."[20] After the signing of the Emancipation Proclamation by President Lincoln in January 1863, recruitment of Black soldiers began in earnest. News of the recruitment spread throughout the United States and Canada, and Augusta took notice. On January 7, he wrote to Lincoln and Secretary of War Edwin M. Stanton to request a position:

Having seen that it is intended to garrison the U.S. forts with colored troops, I beg leave to apply to you for an appointment as surgeon to some of the coloured regiments, or as physician to some of the depots of "freedmen." I was compelled to leave my native country, and come to this on account of prejudice against colour, for the purpose of obtaining a knowledge of my profession, and having accomplished that object, at one of the principle educational institutions of this province, I am now prepared to practice it, and would like to be in a position where I can be of use to my race.[21]

Two weeks later, Augusta received a response from Assistant Secretary of War P. H. Watson: "A Medical Board for the examination of persons desiring to be appointed Assistant Surgeons of Volunteers, is now in session in this city. Your application has been referred to it, and you are hereby notified to report in writing to the Surgeon General, who will name a date for your

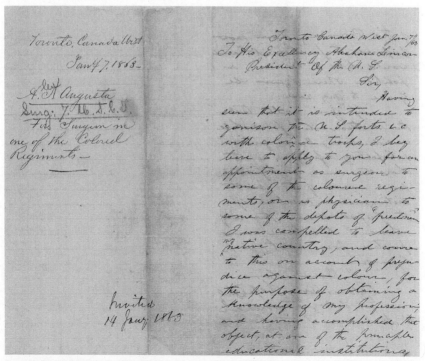

Letter from Alexander T. Augusta to President Abraham Lincoln, January 7, 1863, requesting a position as surgeon with the U.S. Army. *Courtesy National Archives and Records Administration, Washington, D.C.*

examination."[22] Augusta responded as instructed, and a date of March 23 was set for his examination before the board, to be held in Washington, D.C.

As the first African American to pursue a position as a medical officer in the U.S. Army, Augusta found that his application was met with confusion and resistance. Those in authority on the Army Medical Board did not know how to act on his application and were disinclined to accept such a request from a Black physician. Several delays occurred as a result of this uncertainty and confusion.

When Augusta arrived in Washington, he had to first obtain a permit for the examination, which was to be endorsed by Joseph R. Smith in the surgeon general's office. Smith assumed Augusta was the applying doctor's servant. But after Augusta informed Smith that he was indeed the applying physician, he received the endorsement and then personally presented his papers to Meredith Clymer, the president of the Army Medical Board. Clymer, though, refused to examine Augusta because of his color. Unsure how to proceed, Clymer forwarded Augusta's application to U.S. Army surgeon Brigadier General William A. Hammond. Clymer wrote Hammond that he believed an error had been made in accepting Augusta's application because Augusta was of "African descent," and he requested direction on how the board should proceed with the examination. "As no members of the Volunteer Medical Staff are of his descent or color," Clymer wrote, "and as he is an alien, and British subject . . . I respectfully ask that the Board may be directed as to the action they are to pursue in the case."[23] Hammond referred the matter to Secretary of War Stanton with a recommendation that the "invitation be recalled."[24] The unique situation of the medical board was noteworthy, prompting the *New York Times* to report on the reaction from the board and Meredith Clymer, noting that "opinion is divided here as to the action which Mr. Stanton will take in this novel but inevitable case."[25]

Three days later, Secretary Stanton made his decision. He directed the medical board to examine Augusta for the position of surgeon with the "Negro Regiments now being raised."[26] Meanwhile, understanding the confusion over his application, Augusta attempted to clarify his position in a letter to the medical board, stating that his case may not have been fully understood. He made it clear that he was Black and "expected to be employed in some colored regiments." Augusta noted that he traveled a long distance and at great personal expense "hoping to be of use to my country, and my race at this eventful period," and he wanted the board to look favorably upon his case.[27]

The board, following Stanton's instructions, questioned Augusta intensely for three days, officially announcing to General Hammond on April 1 that "the Board has examined Dr. A. T. Augusta, colored, and found him qualified for the position of surgeon in the Negro Regiment now being raised."[28] On April 4, 1863, Augusta became the first African American commissioned medical officer in the U.S. Army. His appointment as a full surgeon with a rank of major provided him with a salary of $2,230 a year. Acknowledging receipt of his commission in a letter to Secretary Stanton on April 7, 1863, Augusta formally accepted the appointment and enclosed his signed oath of allegiance.

Augusta shared his experience in a letter to the *Anglo-African* newspaper, making note that despite having faced a hostile medical board, the members treated him "with all the courtesy I could ask." He hoped that reading his words in the newspaper might encourage other Black surgeons to "send in their names," as he believed the government would support the appointment of Black surgeons, provided they were qualified and could pass the examination. Augusta explained that the week prior to his examination only one out of four white candidates had passed the written exam and that he had received an oral examination, which was more difficult.[29]

After earning his commission, Augusta made the rounds of the city's general hospitals. He told the *Anglo-African* readers that "the medical staff have treated me with every respect."[30] At Armory Square Hospital, Augusta encountered poet Walt Whitman, who served as a nurse there during the war. Whitman noted that he had spent the evening with "Dr. Augusta black surgeon, with the rank of major (the straps whereof I have seen Dr. A. wear)."[31] It was highly unusual to see a Black man in a military officer's uniform, and Whitman was impressed enough by the encounter to record his observations.

In one of Augusta's first public appearances in uniform, his presence was again singled out. On April 16, 1863, a celebration of the 1862 emancipation of enslaved people in the District of Columbia was held at the Fifteenth Street Presbyterian Church. The event was reported by several newspapers including Washington's *Evening Star*, which declared that "the appearance of a colored man in the room wearing the gold leaf epaulettes of a Major, was also the occasion of much applause and gratulation with the assembly. The individual thus distinguished was Dr. A. T. Augusta."[32] The *Liberator* also noted the special recognition of Augusta's presence made that evening: "The speaker then congratulated the audience on the fact that, for the first time in history of this country, epaulettes were seen on the shoulders of a black man."[33]

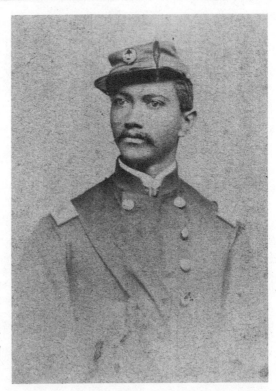

Major Alexander T. Augusta
in uniform, c. 1863. *Courtesy
Oblate Sisters of Providence,
Baltimore, Md.*

The appearance of a Black military officer in uniform continued to be worthy of recognition in the local newspapers. The *Daily National Republican* reported on Augusta's presence at the mustering of the first two companies of Black troops in Washington, D.C., on May 19, 1863: "Dr. Thaddeus Seeley, a surgeon at Armory Square Hospital, was detailed to make the examination of the men, as assisted by Dr. Augusta, the newly commissioned colored surgeon."[34] On that same day, Augusta's friend and fellow Black surgeon Anderson R. Abbott observed Augusta and described the impact of his public presence: "splendid among the shabby field hands . . . the sight of his uniform stirred the faintest heart in faith in the new destiny of the race, for Dr. Augusta wore the oak leaves of a major on his shoulders."[35]

Seeing a Black man in a military uniform stirred deep emotions. In some white people it provoked anger, including among those white soldiers who adamantly opposed the advancement of Black men. Some white soldiers expressed their anger through verbal and physical abuse of uniformed Black soldiers. When the 5th U.S. Colored Cavalry was detached to join white troops in western Virginia, the men were subjected to insults and physical assaults.

Colonel James S. Brisbin, the superintendent of the organization of Kentucky Black troops, noted that the Black soldiers were "made the subject of much ridicule and many insulting remarks . . . and in some instances petty outrages such as the pulling off the caps of the colored soldiers, stealing their horses, etc. was practiced by the white soldiers."[36] Many formerly enslaved and free Black people, though, had the opposite reaction and feelings. When a group of Black soldiers visited a Black church in Washington, D.C., they received a jubilant reception from church members. The *Christian Recorder* reported that "the excitement of the colored ladies knew no bounds, each trying to get a peep at the true Americans."[37]

The U.S. Army uniform was both a symbol of patriotism and pride for Black people during the Civil War and an instrument for change. Uniformed Black soldiers began to use "their elevated status to undermine some of the vestiges of slavery." They identified the city's streets and streetcars as places where they were entitled to equal access and respectful treatment.[38] Augusta certainly used his position as an army major to challenge the status quo and push for change. In a major's uniform, he was in a position of authority and prestige. He walked proudly through the streets of Washington and rode the streetcars demanding nothing less than equal access and respectful treatment, even though he was keenly aware of the hostility and violence he would face. Still, he never shied away from the controversy and anger that his appearance elicited. As Anderson R. Abbott observed, "He had a bulldog tenacity of temperament which cannot be deterred by fear."[39]

One particular incident demonstrated Augusta's strong belief in equal access and treatment and his determination to act on his beliefs. Soon after receiving his commission, he was approved for a fifteen-day leave of absence beginning April 25. Now a resident of Baltimore, he planned to head north by train, presumably to settle his outstanding obligations before settling into his duty in Washington, D.C. From his home in the city on April 30, he made his way to the President and Pratt Street railway station to secure a ticket to Philadelphia. He purchased his ticket and boarded the train, taking a seat in one of the cars. A few minutes had passed when a white teenage boy came up from behind him and, while swearing at him, caught hold of his right shoulder strap and pulled it off. Augusta confronted the boy and his companion, but the teenager continued to threaten him with a club and eventually grabbed hold of his other shoulder strap, tearing it from his uniform. Augusta turned toward the door but was soon surrounded by several other rough-looking men. A policeman entered the car and Augusta cried out, "If you are a policeman,

I claim your protection as a United States officer, who has been assaulted without cause." At the same time, the provost guards entered the car and Augusta applied to them for protection as an officer of the U.S. Army. After he proved his position as an army officer, they offered their protection. At that moment, Augusta could have continued traveling on the train, but he decided to pursue the incident in hopes that his efforts could be beneficial to others who might face the same predicament. He was "determined to stop back, so as to have the parties punished, knowing full well that the same thing might occur again, unless a stop was put to it at once."[40]

Accompanied by one of the guards, Augusta went to the provost marshal's office, where he filed a report with the lieutenant in charge, and then made his way back to the train station, where he intended to identify the assailants, who he believed were employed by the railroad. Arriving at the station with the full protection of the provost guards, he pointed out the parties who had attacked him and returned a second time to the provost marshal's office under the protection of the guards and with his attackers in tow. By the time he made his way back to the railroad station to catch his train, a large crowd had gathered. As he approached the station, he was assaulted by a man who, as he described, "dealt me a severe blow on the face, which stunned me for a moment and caused the blood to flow from my nose very freely."[41] The assailant was immediately taken into custody. Not knowing if there were any officers left to protect him, Augusta attempted to seek refuge inside a building but was refused entry. He eventually made it to the station under the protection of an armed officer and boarded the train. A military officer on the train who happened to be on his way to Philadelphia that day offered Augusta his protection. With his revolver drawn, the military officer escorted Augusta to his seat, but once the train was in motion, Augusta declined any further protection. He later learned that some of his attackers had been charged with assault and sent to prison.

In response to the incident, Augusta wrote to the *Christian Recorder* describing his experience and giving his opinion on his right as an officer of the U.S. Army to safely travel in the city. He believed that even though Baltimore was "a place where it is considered a virtue to mob colored people," he had a "right to expect a safe transit" through the city, especially as he "had volunteered to bind up the wounds of those colored men who should volunteer, as well as those rebels and copperheads whom the fortune of war might throw into my hands." But he took "higher grounds" to justify his course, saying that "my position as an officer of the United States, entitles me to wear the insignia of my office, and if I am either afraid or ashamed to wear them anywhere, I am not fit to hold my commission, and should resign it at once."[42] Augusta demanded respect and equal treatment because of his position and rank as a military officer, which he had obtained through the same process and by meeting the same requirements as white applicants. He knew that his color was the impetus for the attack, but as a man with his rank and position, he deserved respect regardless of color.

Augusta was not the only Black soldier to suffer the indignity of such an assault. In June 1863, Corporal John Ross was attacked by several white men while walking down a street in Washington, D.C. Ross was then struck with a baton by one of the policemen who arrived at the scene, and in the tussle the chevrons on his uniform were torn off. The police officer was arrested and a military hearing held. The hearing officials concluded "that the Negro had been shamefully and inhumanely treated; that whatever might be the private opinion of any one, the Government having authorized it, they [Black men] should be treated as soldiers." This incident "demonstrated that U.S. military officials could be a powerful force in defense of Black soldiers' claims to dignity and respect."[43] This does not imply that Black soldiers had the complete support of the U.S. government but suggests that the government could be influential in maintaining dignified treatment of Black soldiers by defending their right to serve and their right to wear the uniform of their military positions.

Following Augusta's train incident, he returned to Washington, D.C., and on May 20 received a notice to report for duty to R. O. Abbott, the medical director of Washington. Abbott had been instructed by the secretary of war to assign Augusta to Contraband Hospital in Washington as its surgeon-in-charge. This appointment made Augusta the first African American to direct a hospital in the United States. Contraband Camp and Hospital had been established by the U.S. Army in 1862 to provide temporary food, housing, and medical care to thousands of formerly enslaved men, women, and children who escaped their enslavers and sought refuge in the nation's capital. It was not uncommon to see forty to fifty arrivals at the camp in one day. By the end of 1863, Contraband Camp had processed over fifteen thousand individuals.[44]

When the hospital was first established, most cooks, laundresses, and nurses were Black women and men, while those in positions of authority, such as surgeons and head nurses, were white. The appointment of Augusta as surgeon-in-charge began a shift in the racial makeup of hospital staff, with Black men taking over leadership positions from white men. With Major

Augusta at the helm, it became clear to the army medical department that all white assistant surgeons and head nurses at the hospital would have to be reassigned and replaced by African Americans. Augusta could not be permitted to supervise white hospital staff, and the white staff refused to serve under the direction of a Black man. Medical director R. O. Abbott explained to General Hammond that "as difficulty will arise in placing Surgeon Augusta over the Hospital Staff as at present organized, I am of opinion that the interest of the Government will be best served by procuring, if practicable, colored, in lieu of white assistants for Surgeon Augusta." He followed up telling Hammond that the services of two white surgeons, C. B. Webster and J. B. Pettyjohn, would no longer be needed and they would be reassigned.[45]

Upon his arrival, Augusta made his own staffing changes. He began with a request to hire fellow Black surgeons William P. Powell Jr. and Anderson R. Abbott on contract as his assistant surgeons.[46] He also hired camp residents as nurses, cooks, and laundresses. As surgeon-in-charge, Augusta was responsible for training staff and for all hospital administration, including ordering supplies and rations, controlling sanitary procedures, performing surgery, and treating patients.[47] But he went beyond the standard responsibilities of his position to demonstrate a commitment to bettering the conditions at the hospital, not only treating his patients' illnesses but working to improve their overall well-being. Most formerly enslaved who arrived at the camp were illiterate and penniless. They had no food and no source of income and possessed only the clothes they wore when they arrived. Augusta provided hospital work for as many people as he could and helped others secure employment outside the camp. In the pension application of Jane Isabella Saunders, a Black nurse who served at the hospital, Saunders's daughter, Susan Burrell, recalled how Dr. Augusta hired her mother: "For I remember how he pitied my mother with six children when she found my father was dead, and he took two of my brothers to work for him and got us a place with the lady next door to him."[48]

Augusta's position enabled him to push for improvements in the camp and hospital. Built on land formerly used for brickmaking, the damp and swampy conditions, combined with an inadequate supply of fresh water, created a breeding ground for illness and placed a strain on the camp's hospital workers and medical personnel. These conditions made residents and hospital staff susceptible to sicknesses like diarrhea and respiratory infections. Augusta recognized that the environment was a direct cause of illness among camp residents. He told medical director Abbott that "we are at present suffering very much at this hospital for the want of water. The water inside the camp appears to produce diarrhea and the wells . . . are drying up."[49] He recommended the introduction of a water pipe system that would draw water from the city's main water line into the camp to replace the camp's only water source, a well that was dry half the year. A proposal was drawn up but ultimately rejected based on cost and on the plans to transfer the residents of Contraband Camp in Washington, D.C., to a newly organized camp in Arlington, Virginia. The identification of the environment as a cause of illness was not a popular theory with many medical professionals who believed that a "poor moral and spirit condition" was the cause of sickness. It was not until the late nineteenth century that "poor social and environmental conditions" began to be recognized as contributing causes to the spread of disease.[50] Augusta's understanding that the environment played an important role in maintaining good health put him in the forefront of this emerging theory.

After several months serving as surgeon-in-charge at Contraband Hospital, Augusta found his position at the facility "inconsistent." Hoping for something more regular where he could make an impact, he applied for an assignment as surgeon to one of the Black regiments and received an appointment as regimental surgeon for the 7th Infantry of the USCT. He left Contraband Hospital and reported for duty at Camp Stanton in Benedict, Maryland, on October 17, 1863. Camp Stanton was established to recruit and train African American men for the U.S. Army. Named after Secretary of War Edwin M. Stanton, the camp trained soldiers in the 7th, 9th, 19th, and 30th regiments of the USCT. Augusta arrived at the camp wearing his military uniform and carrying a standard surgical field kit and pocket kit.[51] He was the ranking medical officer among all four regiments. The white medical officers objected to being placed in a position subordinate to a Black man. Seven of these officers representing each of the four regiments protested to President Abraham Lincoln:

> When we made application for position on the Colored Service, the understanding was universal that all commissioned officers were to be white men. Judge of our surprise when, upon joining our respective regiments, we found that the Senior Surgeon of the Command was a Negro.
>
> We claim to be behind no one, in a desire for the elevation and improvement of the colored race in this Country, and we are willing to sacrifice much in so grand a cause, as our present positions may testify. But we cannot in any cause, willingly compromise what we

consider a proper self-respect; nor do we deem that the interests of either the country or of the colored race, can demand this of us. Such degradation, we believe to be involved with our voluntarily continuing in the service, as subordinate to a colored officer. We therefore most respectfully, yet earnestly, request that this unexpected, unusual and most unpleasant relationship in which we have been placed may in some way be terminated.[52]

Augusta's qualifications were not under attack by these white surgeons. What they objected to was a Black man's position as the ranking medical officer. This was based solely on the concept of racial hierarchy in society, which they were now perpetuating in the medical profession.[53] Their opposition to his presence as their superior officer was quite clear—he was Black, and they would not be subordinate to a Black man regardless of his rank.

Although the white medical officers who signed the protest letter claimed to support emancipation, a deep-rooted and institutionalized racism was demonstrably visible in their attitude and actions. It is not clear whether their letter reached President Lincoln, but by the end of 1863, Acting Surgeon General Joseph K. Barnes ordered the reassignment of Augusta to Birney Barracks in Baltimore, a USCT recruiting station, where he would examine Black recruits. Barnes explained the decision for Augusta's reassignment, saying "he was accordingly assigned to the 7th U.S.C.T. as surgeon, but on the representation of Asst. Surgeon Morse, 7th U.S.C.T., and Surgeon Suckley, Acting Director at Baltimore and at the request of this office he was removed from his regiment and assigned to the duty of colored recruits at Baltimore, MD where he now is."[54] Evidently, the opinions and feelings of lower-ranked white medical officers took precedence over Augusta's rank, senior position, and skill. They cared little about his reputation as a good physician and viewed him only as a threat to their own positions.

Augusta propelled himself forward despite living in a world where racism, bigotry, and discrimination created obstacles and blockades. His actions broke barriers and moved the cause for equality forward. In early February 1864, he was involved in an incident that led to a change in the laws governing streetcars in the District of Columbia. On the morning of February 1, Augusta, wearing full military uniform, left his lodgings at 14th and I Streets to head downtown for a court-martial. He had been summoned to appear at the trial as a medical expert in the case of an army private accused in the death of a Black man the previous year. Augusta was in a rush that morning to reach his destination. Standing in the rain, he hailed the first approaching streetcar. When he stepped into the car, he was blocked by the conductor, who told him that Black riders were not permitted to ride in the covered seated area of streetcars and that he would have to stand up front with the driver. Augusta flatly refused and questioned the conductor on his action. The conductor repeated that it was "against the rules for colored persons to ride inside." Augusta made a second attempt to enter the car and was physically ejected. He found himself in the street "compelled to walk the distance in the mud and rain," arriving late to the hearing.[55]

His tardiness forced him to provide a written explanation in which he described the incident as an "outrage committed upon me by the Conductor of Car No. 32, of the City Railway Co." He noted that he was "trusting that something may speedily be done to remedy such evils as those we are now forced to submit to."[56] Augusta focused on how his ejection from the streetcar affected his ability to fulfill his obligations as a military officer. He made a connection between his life as a public citizen and his duties as a professional surgeon employed by the nation's military using his "military status to extend his claim in the realm of civil rights."[57]

News of the incident spread quickly, reaching the ears of Senator Charles Sumner of Massachusetts, a staunch supporter of abolition. On February 10, Sumner initiated legislation to remedy the situation, introducing a resolution that would provide "by law against the exclusion of colored persons from the equal enjoyment of all railroad privileges in the District of Columbia." In the ensuing discussion Sumner described Augusta's expulsion from a Washington streetcar as his motive for proposing the resolution, noting that Augusta was a commissioned officer of the U.S. Army and had been wearing an officer's uniform. It was an "outrage on humanity and upon the good name of our country," Sumner said, one that "is worse for our country at this moment than a defeat in battle."[58]

Several senators commented on the resolution during the debate. Sumner noted that "it was just as great an outrage to eject him [Augusta] from the car as it would be to eject . . . [a U.S.] Senator . . . [which] would not bring upon this capital half the shame that the ejection of this colored officer from the car necessarily brings upon the capital." Sumner was presented with an opportunity to push forward the cause for equality, inviting Augusta into the chambers of the U.S. Senate, which put him in a place of power, persuasion, and progress. After an exhaustive discussion, a vote was taken. The resolution was adopted 30 votes to 10.[59]

Augusta was physically present in the Senate chamber when the resolution was first introduced, an unusual and noteworthy event. Senator Waitman T. Willey of West Virginia had "deep anxiety relative to the possibility of granting commissions to colored soldiers" and resented the presence of Augusta in the Senate chamber dressed in his major's uniform. A reporter referred to Augusta as the "obnoxious colored Surgeon" but also described him as "a modest, gentlemanly appearing man . . . probably as well qualified as many of his fellow butchers."[60]

As a direct result of this resolution and Sumner's influence, the charter of the Metropolitan Railroad in Washington was amended to prohibit the exclusion of persons from any car on account of color. When an amendment to the act to incorporate the Metropolitan Railroad Company in the District of Columbia was introduced in July 1864 and approved on March 3, 1865, the prohibition against excluding persons of color was extended to every railroad in the District of Columbia.[61] Although this amendment legally desegregated Washington streetcars, Black people still faced difficulties riding public transportation. In September 1865, Sojourner Truth, a well-known abolitionist who had come to Washington to assist with the Freedman's Relief Association, attempted to board a streetcar in the city. While holding onto the railing as she tried to enter the car, she was dragged several yards after the conductor refused to stop the vehicle and she refused to exit. On a second occasion, Truth was on an errand for Freedmen's Hospital where she volunteered as a nurse. As she attempted to board the streetcar, she encountered a hostile conductor. Threatening to pull her off the car, he violently grabbed her arm, causing injury to her shoulder. According to Truth, the incident was reported to the railroad president and the conductor arrested for assault and battery.[62]

Even though Augusta was late to the court-martial trial because of his ejection from the streetcar, the military court placed great stock in his expert testimony regardless of his color. The defendant, a white army private, was accused of attacking and killing a Black man on the street. The white defense attorney had implied that the medical treatment the injured Black man had received accelerated his death, in part by the lesser skill level of the attending surgeons at Contraband Hospital, where the patient died. Directly responding to the defense attorney's allegation, the judge advocate who prosecuted the case pointed out, "The last witness produced on the part of the Prosecution was Dr. A. T. Augusta, a gentleman whose rank acquired by his undoubted proficiency should entitle him to the position of a reliable authority on the case at issue."[63] The court found the defendant guilty of manslaughter, in part due to Augusta's testimony.

Augusta's refusal to accept the inequities of traveling on a Washington streetcar moved forward the cause for equality by bringing his experience to the attention of the U.S. Senate, leading to legislation desegregating streetcars in the city. His position as an army officer and surgeon-in-charge of Contraband Hospital garnered him respect and attention that were not given to most Black people. At a time when the reliability, truthfulness, and intelligence of African Americans were questioned, doubted, and mistrusted, Augusta broke this stereotype of Black people with his intellect and competence.

The positions that Augusta and Anderson R. Abbott held as regimental surgeon and acting assistant surgeon at Contraband Hospital, respectively, provided entrée into new social and political circles with unprecedented access to the influential elite of the nation's capital. In late February 1864, Augusta and Abbott attended a reception at the White House wearing full dress uniforms. It was the first time Black military officers were present at a White House event. President Lincoln graciously welcomed them, and they walked freely through the rooms. Not surprisingly, their fellow guests had mixed reactions to their presence: some showed friendly interest and greeted them, while others disdained the two Black men who were among them.[64] The presence of prominent military surgeons would not have been unusual, but as Black military officers, their attendance brought lively attention to themselves and pushed them further into the public eye.

Augusta continued to insist on equal treatment and confronted government officials on the issue. While still serving in Baltimore, examining Black recruits for the USCT, he attempted to collect his monthly major's pay of $169 from the army paymaster but was told that he would receive only the standard Black soldier's pay of $7 per month. Augusta protested to Secretary of War Edwin Stanton and Senator Henry Wilson of Massachusetts, chairman of the Senate Committee on Military Affairs, in April 1864. Augusta made it clear that the paymaster at Baltimore had refused to issue him his full pay and inquired whether the proposed legislation for equal pay for Black soldiers that was being considered in Congress would include Black commissioned officers.[65] Stanton's instruction to Wilson was to acknowledge Augusta's letter and reply that "the subject was submitted from the Paymaster General's Office, April 12th and it was decided that Surgeon Augusta was entitled to pay according to his rank."[66] Wilson was in favor of equal and retroactive pay for Black soldiers and introduced a provision to the equal pay legislation to achieve that goal.

The refusal of the paymaster to pay Augusta according to his military rank was part and parcel of a regular practice to pay Black soldiers less than their white counterparts. This practice began with the recruitment and enlistment of Black soldiers in 1863, when Black soldiers were paid seven dollars a month, which included a three-dollar deduction for clothing, while white soldiers were paid thirteen dollars per month. As Black soldiers became aware of the discrepancy in pay, they began to protest the discriminatory practice. The men of the 1st South Carolina Volunteers, later the 33rd Infantry of the USCT, refused to serve until they received equal pay, while the 54th and 55th Massachusetts regiments refused to accept any pay until it was equal to those of white soldiers. In the fall of 1863, Corporal James Henry Gooding brought this pay discrepancy to the attention of President Lincoln. Gooding made a passionate case for equal pay, noting that "the patient Trusting Descendants of Africs [*sic*] Clime, have dyed the ground with blood, in defense of the Union, and Democracy. . . . We have done a soldier's duty."[67] For Gooding, equal pay would bring a new incentive for Black soldiers' patriotism and enthusiasm in fighting for their country.

Black soldiers received some support for equal pay from white officers. Colonel Thomas W. Higginson, the commanding officer of the 33rd Infantry of the USCT, appealed to a sense of fairness when noting that the government pledged equal pay and rations for Black soldiers upon enlistment but failed to live up to that pledge once their service began. The "government," he said, "is degraded by using for a year the services of the brave soldiers, and then repudiating the contract by which they were enlisted."[68] The issue of pay became the subject of much discussion in the nation. *Harper's Weekly* reported that "there is no more pressing political issue than the payment of the colored troops," and "the people of this country are fully prepared for that policy and heartily approve it."[69]

Protests and objections voiced by Black soldiers and the support received from senators fighting for equal pay within the system effected change. In June 1864, Congress passed legislation that required equal pay and made it retroactive for all Black soldiers. The *Liberator* noted that "Congress, in equalizing the pay and bounty of white and colored troops, has maintained the honor of the national uniform."[70] The *Burlington Free Press* reported that "Congress has at last seen the injustice of allowing any longer the sentiment, that a black man is not worth as much as a white man. . . . Justice, even if tardy, is better than persistent injustice."[71] Although many Black soldiers protested openly against discriminatory pay, Augusta's protest brought with it his rank and position and his relationship with influential and politically positioned white people. His actions once again became a catalyst for change

Even though Augusta had been assigned to examine recruits for the USCT in Baltimore, he remained the regimental surgeon for the 7th Infantry of the USCT. White assistant surgeon Joel Morse, who had been among the seven white surgeons who first objected to Augusta's position as senior surgeon at the mustering of the regiment in late 1863, objected to Augusta maintaining the position of regimental surgeon, even though Augusta was not serving directly with the regiment. Morse told Senator John Sherman of Ohio that he considered Augusta's position as the ranking medical officer to be "a wrong to which I with others have been subjected." His hope was that Sherman would intercede on his behalf to "right this wrong which to my mind is grave, unjust, and humiliating." Believing that the government had guaranteed that all officers in the USCT would be white, Morse saw the present situation as a betrayal of white officers who had joined the army with that understanding. "If Surgeon Augusta were to return to the regiment," he wrote, "I should resign immediately; not from any personal feeling against him, but from principle." He claimed to have no objection to Augusta holding the position of surgeon, but not within a regiment where Augusta would be the ranking medical officer with white officers subordinate to him. Morse complained that Augusta's removal from direct service with the regiment in late 1863 was a burden and, although necessary, was "a great injustice to the regiment" as it left the regiment without a surgeon. He also viewed it as a burden on himself, since he was required to perform the duties of both the regiment's assistant surgeon and surgeon without additional compensation. Morse requested that "as a matter . . . of justice to all parties . . . Augusta should be reinstated as Surgeon of Volunteers of colored recruits, or placed in charge of some General Hospital for Colored Troops, and a white be given the appointment of Surgeon to the 7th Regiment of the U.S.C.T. Troops."[72] Although Morse pointed out that Augusta's reassignment away from the regiment was a burden, he did not believe that Augusta should return to his post with the regiment but should be permanently removed and replaced with a white surgeon. Perhaps Morse's own aspiration for advancement was motivation enough for him to appeal for Augusta's removal as the regimental surgeon. As long as Augusta remained in the position, Morse's hope for advancement within the regiment would be blocked.

While in Baltimore, Augusta continued to speak out when he observed unequal treatment. After witnessing the treatment of Black riders on streetcars in the city, he told Major General Lewis Wallace, the commander of the Middle Department of the 8th Army Corps in Baltimore, that the streetcar company "exacts of colored passengers the same fare it does for whites, and then huddles them together in the front car with all sorts of person, where smoking pipes and cigars continue all the time, and where they are subject to insults."[73] Augusta continued his campaign to highlight the unequal treatment of Black people.

By early 1865, the recruitment of Black soldiers in Baltimore had ended. After having examined nearly five thousand Black recruits, Augusta's services were no longer needed.[74] The army was in a quandary about where he should be reassigned. Colonel S. M. Bowman, chief muster and recruiting officer for the USCT in Maryland, requested advice on reassigning Augusta. Bowman recommended that he be sent to Hilton Head, South Carolina, where the recruitment of Black soldiers continued, and noted that Augusta was "a first rate examining surgeon."[75] The surgeon general's office agreed on the reassignment if Augusta's services could be useful elsewhere. A few days later, Augusta was relieved of his duties in Baltimore and ordered to report for duty in Beaufort, South Carolina.

Before his departure from Baltimore, President Lincoln was assassinated at Ford's Theatre in Washington, D.C. As Lincoln's remains passed through the city on April 21, Augusta, in full uniform, led a procession of seventy-five thousand troops to honor the late president.[76] A few days later, he left Baltimore, leaving his wife behind, and headed to South Carolina, where he reported for duty on May 3. Among the U.S. Army troops present in the city were several regiments of the USCT, including the 33rd from South Carolina, the 26th from New York, and the 104th organized in the spring of 1865. Augusta was assigned to examine USCT recruits and treat sick and wounded soldiers from these regiments.

After only a few months in Beaufort, Augusta was transferred to Savannah, Georgia, where he would begin a more permanent position. Arriving in early July, he was assigned to treat the freedmen of the Ogeechee, a job he performed for two months. By September, he was serving as surgeon-in-charge of Lincoln General Hospital for Refugees and Freedmen. Lincoln Hospital had been transformed from the Savannah Poor House and Hospital into a facility for freedmen and was controlled by the Bureau of Refugees, Freedmen, and

Abandoned Lands, more commonly referred to as the Freedmen's Bureau. Established by the War Department in March 1865, the bureau provided relief and medical care to formerly enslaved persons. Under the direction of General O. O. Howard, the Freedmen's Bureau established more than forty hospitals and employed over one hundred physicians.[77] In Georgia, its medical department consisted of five hospitals with a surgeon-in-chief, three medical officers, and seven private physicians.[78] By 1868, only eleven of the Freedmen's Bureau hospitals remained, and by 1872, all had closed except the hospital in Washington, D.C.[79]

Lincoln Hospital cared for both freedmen and Black residents whom other doctors and facilities in Savannah ignored, refused, or failed to treat. In early 1865, the hospital treated an average of eighty-five patients per week with 63 occupied beds. After the war's end in April, the number of freedmen increased dramatically, averaging over two hundred patients being treated each week with more than 150 occupied beds.[80] Augusta established himself at the hospital and became a well-respected medical professional, attending to both administrative and clinical duties. A hospital volunteer noted that "Dr. Augustus [*sic*], a colored man, a surgeon in the U.S. army and an elegant intelligent man, is now in charge of the 'bureau' Hospital, having both Black and white patients, under his care."[81] An Ohio reporter at the *Cleveland Leader* recalled meeting Augusta and being impressed by his decorum and his "sense of modesty which is commendable."[82]

Augusta's administrative responsibilities at Lincoln Hospital were similar to those he had performed at Contraband Hospital in Washington, including hiring staff. When he took charge, his two assistant surgeons were white, but he was permitted to replace them with Black assistant surgeons T. L. Harris and Charles H. Taylor.[83] This was likely an effort on the part of the Freedmen's Bureau to engage Black physicians rather than white, to avoid the issue of white physicians being subordinate to a Black surgeon-in-charge.

Managing the hospital's daily operations, Augusta administered its finances and supervised the care of patients. He was able to initiate and sign contracts, hire personnel, request services and supplies, and implement policies and procedures, a rare position of authority for a Black man, especially in the South. As the hospital's chief administrator, Augusta could advocate for Black patients in ways previously impossible for persons of color. Approaching white city officials, including Savannah's mayor Edward C. Anderson, he presented his professional medical opinions on issues affecting the health and well-being of the city's Black residents and hospital patients. Augusta was a reminder to city authorities that sick and wounded Black residents were human beings, worthy of respect and proper treatment.

One of the largest projects Augusta directed during his tenure at Lincoln Hospital was moving the facility's entire operations to a new site in March 1866. Tasked with selecting a vacant plot of land on which to establish the new hospital, Augusta found a suitable site, and once it was approved by Colonel Daniel E. Sickles, commander of the Department of the South, the first delivery of lumber was made for construction. Subsequently, and without consultation with Augusta, the location for the new hospital was changed. Although he made it known that the change occurred without his knowledge, he arranged to visit and examine the new site. He determined that its proximity to a swamp would be problematic. Augusta's experience at Contraband Hospital in Washington, D.C., made him keenly aware that environmental conditions were key to a person's health and well-being and reported the potential problems with the new location directly to Sickles. Despite Augusta's report, Sickles was determined to keep to the new plan. Augusta's concerns were not assuaged, though, and a month later he approached Savannah's mayor, asking that a drainage ditch be cut through the swamp to help improve conditions. A land survey was completed and funding was obligated, but despite Augusta's efforts, a delay in securing final approval pushed the project start date too late in the season for such construction, and the drainage ditch was never built.

The failure to provide a drainage ditch left the area ripe for unhealthy conditions and likely led to the increased incidence of cholera at the hospital and among the freedmen living in the adjacent area. Augusta prepared for a possible cholera outbreak by alerting his superiors. He informed Surgeon J. W. Lawton, surgeon-in-chief of the District of Georgia, in July 1866 that he had called upon the post surgeon and the chairman of the board of health in Savannah to determine what action they would take in case of a cholera epidemic, recognizing that an outbreak in the city "would send all colored persons attacked to this hospital," which would "be a heavier burden than we are warranted in assuming."[84] It was clear to Augusta that the city would not take on responsibility for Black residents who fell ill, so he was proactive in preparing for a possible outbreak. His understanding of the impact of the environment on health was in direct opposition to that of other white Freedmen's Bureau physicians who merely believed that Black people were inherently inferior and susceptible to certain illnesses while being immune to others.[85]

Augusta was proven correct when in the winter of 1865 and the spring of 1866 the outbreak of illnesses, including cholera and smallpox, placed an undue strain on the hospital. The city of Savannah regularly sent all of its sick Black residents to the hospital for treatment, and despite an increase in the occurrence of smallpox, this policy did not change. Augusta was forced to manage the increasing population of sick patients with very limited resources. He vehemently protested to Caleb Hornor, chief medical officer of the Freedmen's Bureau, about the city's failure to take responsibility for its destitute freedmen, insinuating that the city authorities would rather have smallpox spread throughout the city than attend to the care of its Black citizens.[86]

Despite the increased burden placed on the hospital, he knew it was essential to continue the hospital's medical services to Black city residents until the civil authorities could "be induced to take charge of them and give them that protection which humanity dictates."[87] To help with the increasing numbers of smallpox patients from the city, Augusta asked for an additional assistant surgeon, but his request was denied. Lawton agreed with Augusta's contention that the city should bear some responsibility for its residents and instructed him to "refuse any more patients except a few undoubted cases whom we cannot ask the city to take care of." Lawton did not believe it was the hospital's "duty to assume the charge of the cases of smallpox that may occur in the city of Savannah. The city is fully able to provide its own sanitary institutions and support its own poor."[88] It seems that Lawton's determined stance, along with Augusta's support, eventually influenced the city's policy, and by August 1866 the city had taken over most of the smallpox cases.

Among the many challenges faced by all Freedmen's Hospital administrators, including Augusta, was a lack of sufficient funds to keep the facilities operating. To keep expenses as low as possible, hospitals hired local freedmen and paid them in rations. Although this helped, increases in monthly budgets were still necessary as the sick and wounded continued to be admitted to the facilities, and the cost of rations and supplies drained hospital budgets. To lower costs further, Freedmen's Bureau physicians began cultivating their own food for their hospitals.[89] Augusta established a three-acre vegetable garden at the hospital in March 1866. He had hopes that the garden would provide food for the facility's use, offer work for convalescing patients, and provide garden produce to the elderly. Unfortunately, circumstances over the next few months, including drought conditions and grazing cattle, thwarted those expectations, and the garden yielded far less than was hoped for.[90]

Although he was working under the Freedmen's Bureau, Augusta remained a commissioned officer in the U.S. Army and the regimental surgeon of the 7th Regiment of the USCT. Once his regiment mustered out in 1866, he became a private physician under contract with the Freedmen's Bureau. He resigned from his position on March 27, 1867, and returned to Washington, D.C., to be reunited with his wife, Mary. For his faithful and meritorious service, Augusta was brevetted a lieutenant colonel in July 1867 and became one of the two highest ranking African Americans to serve during the American Civil War. The other was Lieutenant Colonel William N. Reed, who served with the 1st North Carolina Colored Volunteers, later designated the 35th Regiment of the USCT, and was considered "mulatto." He was one of the few men of color who achieved an officer's rank who was not a surgeon or chaplain.

Augusta's return to civilian life afforded him the opportunity to travel, and he spent some time abroad before returning to the United States, where he took on a short-term position as a faculty member of the medical department at Wilberforce University in Ohio.[91] This appointment gave him the distinction of being the first African American faculty member of a medical school in the United States. He next returned to Washington, D.C., and established a private medical practice. Among his patients were the children and grandchildren of Frederick Douglass, famed African American orator and abolitionist.[92] He also accepted a teaching position in 1868 at the newly formed medical department of Howard University. The university was established in 1867 as an institution primarily for the education of Black youth in the liberal arts and sciences. A medical department was organized the following year with the first three faculty appointments made in May 1868, followed by two appointments in September, including Augusta's. Augusta was the only Black faculty member among the first five faculty appointed. He was given the position of "demonstrator" of anatomy rather than "professor," which was the title given to the other four white faculty members. Though his title was different, he received the same $1,000 annual salary as the four white professors. Assigning Augusta a lesser title likely avoided conflict with the white medical faculty who might not have considered a Black man their equal and therefore not deserving of the title "professor." But by the 1869–70 school year, his designation was changed from demonstrator of anatomy to professor of practical anatomy. It seems this adjustment may have resulted from a change in the annual salary for demonstrators from $1,000 annually in 1868 to $500 annually in 1869. Perhaps the board had decided that Augusta was a valuable faculty member and a change in his title to professor would allow him to maintain his salary of $1,000 a year.[93]

By 1873, a financial crisis in the country caused the university to no longer be able to pay the salaries of their instructors. Resignations were requested and accepted, after which the university's trustees reappointed the same instructors at the same salaries with the understanding that salaries would be paid only if funds could be raised. Instructors accepting the new appointments would have to work pro bono. Augusta and several other professors accepted this arrangement and worked several years with no pay.

During his time at Howard University, Augusta continued to support the cause for equality for Black people. In 1868, four years after his ejection from a Washington, D.C., streetcar, he once again found himself embroiled in a similar case, not as the victim but as the victim's physician. On February 8, Kate Brown, an African American woman who worked as a restroom attendant at the U.S. Senate, was violently removed from a streetcar in Alexandria, Virginia, for refusing to sit in the car reserved for Black people. Brown had purchased a round-trip ticket in Washington, D.C., for the "ladies' car" and traveled to Alexandria that morning without incident. As she boarded the same car of the train in Alexandria for her return trip, she was confronted by a police officer hired by the railroad who insisted that she ride in the car reserved for Black people. Her refusal led to her forcible removal from the railroad car by the police officer, who pounded her knuckles, twisted her arm, grabbed her collar, and dragged her onto the platform. When members of the Senate heard that a Senate employee had been ejected from a streetcar because she was a Black woman, they convened an investigation.[94]

Many prominent members of the Black community supported Brown and were determined to see justice in her case. When Augusta was called to testify at the Senate hearing, he did not hesitate. As the victim's physician, he was determined to provide support for Brown's claims and do what he could to secure compensation for her pain and suffering. Intent on providing an accurate accounting of her injuries, condition, and treatment, he read his prepared statement as part of his testimony. He described Brown's injuries as severe and may have experienced a sense of déjà vu when treating Brown and testifying before the Senate hearing committee as he remembered his own experience on a Washington streetcar only four years earlier. Augusta likely felt empathy for Brown and used his medical expertise to provide evidence of the severity of her injuries and the extent of her suffering. He was determined to show Brown as a human being who was justified in her claims. When the hearing concluded, the Senate committee issued a report in Brown's favor. She went on to file a lawsuit against the railroad company and was awarded a $1,500 settlement. The railroad company appealed the court's ruling, but the decision was upheld by the U.S. Supreme Court in 1873.

Augusta's continued protests against the inequalities that Black people faced everyday was fueled not only by the blatant discrimination he observed and experienced daily but by his fair-mindedness and integrity. It was clear to Augusta that race and color played a part in incidents like Kate Brown's, and he took the higher ground by addressing them as human rights issues. He was determined to show that people of color were human beings and citizens and had the right to equal and fair treatment.

For Augusta, the fight for equality was not limited to public transportation or the daily activities of life but extended to his own profession. Black and white physicians had a common interest in the advancement of their profession and the sharing of medical knowledge among colleagues. They were eager to join medical societies to promote and disseminate medical and surgical knowledge and develop regulations for medical practice and conduct. The Medical Society of the District of Columbia was the local medical organization that licensed physicians in Washington, D.C., and through membership enabled physicians to hold consultations with one another and participate in discourse on medical cases for the benefit of their profession.

In early 1869, Augusta and fellow Black surgeon Charles B. Purvis sought membership in the Medical Society of the District of Columbia. At the same time, leaders of the Medical Society initiated an investigation of medical practitioners in the city whom they believed had no diploma or license from the society to practice medicine. Among those named under this investigation were Augusta and Purvis; the society said they were not members and suggested they were practicing medicine illegally.[95] These accusations put into question the qualifications and medical practices of Augusta and Purvis. The Medical Society implied that the licenses issued to them by the society gave them "all the legal rights requisite to practice in the District of Columbia" and that their desire for membership was solely for social advancement.[96] Augusta and Purvis publicly responded to the society's claims in defense of their right to membership and full access to the medical profession in Washington, D.C.

Augusta made clear that he believed the intentions of the Medical Society in refusing membership to him was motivated by the desire of white physicians to drive both himself and Purvis out of the profession because of their color, and by doing so the white physicians could lay claim to their "practice of medicine among colored people."[97] Augusta described how a white physician, Dr. Garnett, had "taken two of my patients while I was attending them, and without notice to me, except that my next visit I was informed that Dr. Garnett was attending."[98] Augusta's motivation in seeking membership in the society was twofold: first, to repair the damage to his reputation caused by the public statements made by the Medical Society implying that he and Purvis were practicing medicine illegally; and second, to avail himself of "the privileges of professional intercourse . . . by attending meetings where medical and surgical subjects are discussed, and where peculiar and interesting cases with their appropriate treatment are communicated for the benefit of the profession at large." It was Augusta's belief that the failure of the society to admit him as a member was a detriment to his patients. "I consider my patients are entitled to the same consideration that any other doctor's are," he said, "and the spirit which would exclude me from the counsel of those whom I have at least a moral right to look to for assistance in battling with varied elements of disease is inhuman and in direct antagonism with the feeling that should guide those who are members of so noble a profession as ours."[99] As Augusta had done many times before when confronted with blatant discrimination, he looked beyond his own personal advantages in the matter to acknowledge how the act of rejecting a person based on color affected the larger part of humanity. The rejection of his membership in the society, he believed, was not only a rejection based on color but a repudiation of the physicians' professional responsibilities and ethics that extended beyond the artificial boundaries of color.

Despite the fact that Augusta and Purvis had applied for licenses and, after submitting their diplomas and other papers documenting their education and experience, were issued licenses by the Medical Society, they were still denied membership. According to Augusta, "The license would be of no service to me unless I became a member of the Society."[100] As the provisions of the society's charter outlined, "No member of this association shall consult with, or meet in a professional way, any resident practitioner of the District, who is not a member, thereof, after said practitioner shall have resided six months in the District."[101] When Augusta and Purvis had their names put forward for membership in the Medical Society, its members lobbied strongly against their admission and encouraged as many members as possible to vote against their membership. A third Black physician, Alpheus W. Tucker, applied for membership three months after Purvis and Augusta and was also rejected by the Medical Society.

To be denied membership in the Medical Society of the District of Columbia limited Black physicians' ability to consult with white physicians on medical cases and take advantage of professional development opportunities. Augusta and Purvis had planned on attending the American Medical Association meeting to be held the following year in Washington, D.C., and hoped that as members of the Medical Society of the District of Columbia they could serve as delegates to the meeting. After their membership to the society was denied, Augusta and Purvis, along with Tucker, appealed to the U.S. Congress for redress, and a congressional investigation was convened. Their claim was that the Medical Society was acting against its own charter by refusing admission to all physicians in the District, regardless of color. Although Senate investigators determined that Augusta, Purvis, and Tucker had been discriminated against by the society solely based on the color of their skin, they offered no immediate remedy.

Again coming to Augusta's defense, Senator Charles Sumner introduced legislation in February 1870 that would repeal the charter of the society "to secure for medical practitioners in the District equal rights and opportunities without distinction of color."[102] In his accompanying report, Sumner described the Medical Society and its charter, making clear "that any test of membership, on account of color, is without any sanction in the charter or constitution of the society, in neither of which is there any limitation of 'white' or 'Caucasian.' The application of such a test is in the nature of an abuse or tyranny, not forbidden in positive terms, but condemned by reason and humanity."[103] The bill was blocked, and although it was brought before the Senate three more times, the last on December 18, 1871, it failed to move forward. Sumner acknowledged that "good men, practitioners in Washington have been excluded on account of color" and the society had acted "as if slavery still ruled with its proscriptions, exclusions and tyrannies."[104]

The Senate committee's findings were a small victory for Augusta and his colleagues, but they were still excluded from membership in the Medical Society of the District of Columbia. Undeterred by this setback, the three Black physicians helped form the National Medical Society of the District of Columbia and declared it a racially integrated organization.[105] Augusta, Purvis, and Tucker, along with several white physicians, assembled a delegation from the National Medical Society and attended the 1870 American Medical Association meeting in Washington. Augusta and the other National Medical Society delegates sought recognition from the AMA, but the Medical Society of the District of Columbia actively protested, urging meeting attendees to vote against the admission of the integrated delegation. Although the AMA made no mention of race in its charter or code of ethics, Augusta, Purvis, and Tucker were denied both admission and recognition on account of color, with no consideration of their qualifications or experience.

* * *

Settling into life in Washington, D.C., was not difficult for Augusta. By 1868, he had established a private medical practice and was living comfortably with his wife, Mary, in the northwest section of the city. They were active in social circles, often appearing in local newspaper society columns as attendees at prominent events or celebrations, hosting a party in their own home, or returning from travel. A regular churchgoer, Augusta participated in activities at St. Andrew's Episcopal Church, including singing in the choir and serving as an elected member of the committee that administered the church's daily business affairs. He was also a member of the Grand Army of the Republic organized for Civil War veterans, the Prince Hall Masonic Lodge, and the Anthropological Society that met regularly at the Smithsonian Institution.[106]

Augusta's time was occupied with his medical practice, his teaching position, and work as an examining surgeon with the Bureau of Pensions . He was a member of the Civil Rights League and served on the Board of Trustees of Colored Schools of Washington and Georgetown, where he reported on sanitary conditions and advocated for access to education. For a time, he taught anatomy and physiology in a local preparatory school for Black students and advocated for their educational opportunities. His free time was spent vacationing with his wife at resorts in Atlantic City, New Jersey. Augusta had a keen interest in real estate and invested in property in Washington, D.C., and Baltimore. He and his wife purchased a home at 1319 L Street, Northwest, where he maintained his medical practice. By 1870, he had amassed real estate holdings worth $10,000 and a personal estate valued at $600.[107] Augusta's income supported and maintained a household that included several live-in domestics.

As a civilian, he continued to be at the center of social justice activities, always willing to address the issue of equality in a public forum. In 1872, hotels and restaurants were required to serve "any respectable, well-behaved person, without regard to race, color, or previous condition of servitude."[108] This law was tested when Augusta and R. W. Tompkins, a clerk at the Freedmen's Bank, entered a local ice cream parlor in the city. They attempted to purchase some ice cream at the usual price of fifteen cents but were asked to pay two dollars in advance. After they refused to pay the inflated price, the proprietor refused to serve them. The matter was brought before a D.C. court, where the presiding judge ruled in Augusta's favor. The defendants in the case denied refusing service on account of color and testified that service was refused to Augusta and Tompkins because the two men would not remove their hats and had used abusive language. This argument was dismissed by the judge; on appeal, the District of Columbia Supreme Court dismissed the case claiming that the "complaint had been improperly drawn up and that the nature of the offense did not come within the scope of the act."[109]

During Augusta's tenure on the medical department faculty at Howard University, he served as the Gerrit Smith Chair of Anatomy and a clinical lecturer on the diseases of the skin as well as a member of the medical staff of Freedmen's Hospital, which functioned as the university's teaching hospital. He was the attending surgeon and clinical lecturer for both dermatology and urino-genital diseases from 1870 to 1875 and ward physician from 1875 to 1877. In addition, he served as attending surgeon to the Smallpox Hospital and Washington Asylum. Augusta was awarded an honorary medical degree by Howard University in 1869 and an honorary master of arts degree in 1871.

In September 1876, Augusta once again faced an apparently racially motivated obstacle, this time at Howard University. The medical faculty and the board of trustees recommended a transfer of appointments for him from professor of anatomy to professor of materia medica, but Augusta declined the transfer. It is unclear why the transfer was being made except for the enigmatic statement by the board of trustees that the decision was "merely . . . to promote the interests of the department not a reflection on the ability of either professors."[110] There was speculation that his transfer was racially motivated. Some believed that the university was attempting to remove Augusta, "a competent colored professor in an institution for the education of colored youth . . . to give a place to a poor white medical professor."[111] Whether or not the proposed transfer was racially motivated is unclear, but by the end of the 1877–78 academic year, Augusta was no longer on the faculty. He made an appeal to be reinstated as professor of anatomy in May 1879, but the board of trustees rejected Augusta's request, saying it was "unwise after the lapse of two academic years to reopen the question." Describing him as "a learned and able physician and anatomist and a thorough and faithful instructor," board members reiterated that the transfer was "merely a change designed to increase the efficiency of the whole."[112] Augusta's affiliation with the university's medical department ended in 1878, but he remained in Washington, D.C., maintaining a successful private medical practice.

Augusta had left the staff of Howard University's medical department by 1878, but he continued his association with Freedmen's Hospital and vied for the position of surgeon-in-chief of the hospital in 1881. He had an interest in obtaining the position as early as 1878, when he was called to testify before a congressional committee investigating the hospital. When asked about conditions at the facility, he testified that he found some of the wards "very offensive and filthy" and placed blame for such conditions on the current surgeon-in-chief, Gideon S. Palmer, and Charles B. Purvis.[113] Augusta felt it necessary to make clear his reticence to testify as he was an applicant for the position of surgeon-in-chief and likely feared his testimony might jeopardize his chances of securing the job. Palmer resigned in 1881, and both Augusta and Purvis laid claim to the vacated position. Purvis, seventeen years younger than Augusta, received the appointment despite Augusta's experience and long history with the hospital.

When Augusta reached the age of fifty-two, he prepared a will, which revealed his concern for the welfare of his family and the causes and organizations he supported. He made provisions for his wife and made bequests to several family members. He left money to religious and charitable organizations, including St. Mary's Episcopal Church in Washington, where he provided for a stained glass window to memorialize Secretary of War Edwin M. Stanton "for kindness bestowed on me before and after I was appointed Surgeon U.S.A."[114]

Throughout Augusta's remaining years, he continued to be involved in social activities and political causes until December 1890, when he fell ill with pneumonia at the age of sixty-six. After only ten days, he succumbed to his illness and died at his home on December 21. His funeral service was held at St. John's Chapel in Washington, followed by a memorial service a month later at the Ebenezer AME Church attended by prominent citizens and Black soldiers.[115] Augusta was interred at Arlington National Cemetery in Virginia, the first Black military officer to be buried there.

After Augusta's death, his wife, Mary, returned to her hometown of Baltimore. She lived out the remainder of her life at the convent of the Oblate Sisters of Providence until her death on September 17, 1908. Honoring Augusta's request, Mary's will bequeathed $300 to St. Mary's in Washington, D.C., for a stained glass window in honor of Stanton. Today, it serves as a reminder of Augusta's extraordinary life, the pride he felt in his wartime service as a U.S. Army officer, and the patriotism he demonstrated for his country.

3. ❄ For Race and Country: William Peter Powell Jr. (1834–1916)

> I am amongst the first to answer my country's call for medical men.
>
> —William P. Powell Jr.

William Peter Powell Jr. was among the first African American men to serve as a surgeon in the American Civil War, but what sets him apart from the other known fourteen Black Civil War surgeons was his unwavering determination to secure a government pension for his service. His twenty-five-year quest for a pension required navigating through the bureaucratic red tape of the federal government and perseverance in the quest for equality. Records of his experience as a military surgeon and his contributions to the Contraband Hospital in Washington, D.C., where he served are few. By contrast, there is considerably more information about his father and his early years growing up in a household devoted to the abolition of slavery. Extensive records are also available about his later tenacious efforts to obtain a military pension that reveal aspects of his life after the war.

Born free in New Bedford, Massachusetts, in 1834 to a Native American mother and an African American father, William Peter Powell Jr. began his life in a family committed to abolition and civil rights. His father, William P. Powell Sr., was a well-known, outspoken abolitionist with a long history as an advocate and supporter of the cause for freedom and equality. Surrounded by many of the nation's most influential and well-educated people of color and having a family legacy of activism, Powell Jr. gained the confidence to pursue a career in medicine, serve his country as a military surgeon during the Civil War, and follow a protracted journey in an effort to secure a military pension.

At the time of Powell Jr.'s birth, his father had established himself in New Bedford, a thriving nineteenth-century whaling port. A self-described mariner, he had received a U.S. Seamen's Protection Certificate in 1827 at the age of twenty-one and embarked on his first sea voyage to the Antilles. Born in New York in 1805, Powell Sr. was the son of the enslaved Edward Powell and the grandson of the enslaved Elizabeth Barjona, who served as cook to the founding fathers of the Continental Congress.[1] According to New York state law, at the time of Powell Sr.'s birth he was considered free. The state had passed a gradual emancipation act that freed all enslaved children born after July 4, 1799, although they were not considered truly free until they reached the age of twenty-five for females and twenty-eight for males. From an early age, Powell Sr. received some schooling, but he spent much of his youth on sailing vessels and apprenticed as a ship smith in his teens before settling in Massachusetts.[2] After arriving in New Bedford, he met and married Mercy Oker Haskins, a Wampanoag Indian in December 1832. Mercy was from a well-established New Bedford family, the daughter of Amos H. Haskins and Basheba Aucooch and the sister of Amos Haskins, a whaling vessel captain and one of the few Native Americans to achieve the rank of master mariner.[3]

New Bedford's established Black community, active seaport, and antislavery activities attracted African Americans such as Powell Sr. and abolitionist Frederick Douglass, who had come to New Bedford in 1838 after escaping from his enslavers in Maryland. In his autobiography, Douglass described the town as "clean, new and beautiful." He noted that the residents, especially the formerly enslaved people, enjoyed a comfortable economic status, possessing "more of the comforts of life, than the average of slaveholders in Maryland."[4]

Powell Sr. worked as a blacksmith in New Bedford and became an organizer and participant in antislavery meetings. By 1836, he was the proprietor of a temperance boardinghouse for Black sailors. Powell's experience as a Black mariner gave him firsthand knowledge of the often poor treatment and conditions under which Black men served on sailing vessels. Through his boardinghouse, he provided Black sailors with much-needed support and services. The boardinghouse also provided a safe haven for those escaping enslavement on the Underground Railroad and became a gathering place for abolitionist meetings attended by local residents.

Powell Sr.'s commitment to the welfare of Black sailors and his abolitionist activities continued after the family moved to New York City in 1839. The city had become a haven for those escaping enslavement after slavery was abolished in the state in 1827 and was a place where free Black people could find new opportunities. This burgeoning community included professionals, educators, entrepreneurs, and civic leaders who opened their own businesses and their own schools where Black children could receive an academic education. New York City was a place where Powell Sr. could provide a comfortable lifestyle for his family, a better education for his children, and a temporary home for the large number of Black sailors who frequented the port of New York.

Arriving in New York City, Powell Sr. again established a temperance boardinghouse for Black seamen where he lived with his wife and their three children: five-year-old William, three-year-old Edward, and one-year-old Sylvester. The family would grow to include daughters Mercy and Sarah and sons Isaiah and Samuel. Powell Sr.'s Colored Seamen's Home was the largest boardinghouse for Black sailors in New York City.[5] He strived to offer a safe haven that would provide not only for the sailors' physical needs but also for their spiritual and educational needs.

The atmosphere at the boardinghouse was active and enlightening. Filled with a strict moral code of temperance and respect, there were ample opportunities to expand one's education and participate in lively discussions among residents and guests about current events. William C. Nell, editor of Frederick Douglass's *North Star*, described it as having an "excellent library," and "at meal times, and every occasion of interview, conversations are introduced on the various questions incidental to the elevation of man."[6] The Colored Seamen's Home was the center of much of the Powell family's life. The children not only had access to the extensive library there but were exposed to the constant infusion of intellectual discourse and antislavery activities.

Powell Sr.'s position and reputation as an antislavery activist gave him and his family entrée into a social circle with New York's Black elite, who included politically minded activists and influential community leaders. Historian Carla Peterson notes that the Black elite often chose "professions that would enable them to alleviate their community's suffering," such as medicine, pharmacy, printing, and education. They lived comfortably in racially mixed neighborhoods and shared middle-class values.[7] Education was a central tenet of the Black community in New York City, and they understood that "it [was] only by the cultivation of the mind, that they [could] become truly emancipated and free."[8] Based on this view, they established their own private school system to provide a formal education for their children. Powell Sr. and Mercy shared that same belief, and it is likely that their seven children, including Powell Jr., were educated in the schools established for Black children by their own community.

After moving his family to New York, Powell Sr. continued his abolitionist activities. He established the Manhattan Anti-Slavery Society and hosted meetings and benefits for the antislavery movement at his boardinghouse, often involving residents and family members. Similarly, Mercy played an active role as a member of the group's board of managers. As the oldest child, Powell Jr. likely assisted his father both in running the boardinghouse and in the abolitionist activities that took place inside and outside the home.

Abolitionist meetings were attended by members of New York's Black elite who no doubt influenced Powell Sr.'s children. Among this circle were physician James McCune Smith and pharmacist Philip A. White, who likely had the most influence on Powell Jr. Smith was the first African American to hold a university medical degree, which he received from the University of Glasgow in Scotland, and the first to run a pharmacy in the United States. White apprenticed in Smith's pharmacy before becoming the first African American graduate of the College of Pharmacy of the City of New York in 1844.[9] White eventually opened his own drugstore in New York City. Both men were formally educated, were community leaders, and owned and operated their own businesses. Powell Jr. had contact with both Smith and White and was perhaps encouraged by them to pursue a career in pharmacy or medicine. Powell Sr. favored a career as a pharmacist for his son. He attempted to obtain a position for him as an apothecary apprentice but was told by the business owners that if they hired his son, they would lose their customers, presumably because he was Black. By 1850, the sixteen-year-old Powell Jr. was identified as an apothecary in the U.S. Federal Census.[10] Perhaps by that time he had secured employment in White's pharmacy.

The enactment of the 1850 Fugitive Slave Act marked a turning point for the Powell family. Powell Sr. believed the act "declared war upon blacks, free and slave," and he considered his options for providing a safe place for his family to live. He decided to relocate to England, where, he said, "character and not color—capacity and not complexion, are the tests of merit."[11] His family would escape the new fugitive slave law, and his children could have greater opportunities for education and advancement. Although Powell Sr. had the financial capability to move his family to England, he nevertheless petitioned the New York state legislature for financial support in their move. Acting on political principle, he claimed that the service of his grandmother to the Continental Congress as cook and the service his father had given the state as an enslaved person contributed to the welfare of the nation, and therefore he was entitled to receive the benefits put forth in the Declaration of Independence but were denied him because of color.[12] His petition was denied consideration. In response, the *National Anti-Slavery Standard* editor commented, "Had Mr. Powell asked permission to sell his children at auction to the highest bidder, or have asked assistance to emigrate to Liberia, he would have gained a hearing."[13]

Powell Sr. made at least one trip to England prior to relocating his family. He wrote Sydney Howard Gay of the *National Anti-Slavery Standard*, "I am here at last. I feel for once in my life though under a foreign flag—a man, indeed! One thing I know, yea two, in my own country—according to the letter and spirit of the Fugitive Slave Bill I am a –THING, but here according to British magnanimity, I am a MAN."[14] He returned to the United States in early 1851 and prepared his wife and children for their departure. By the end of the year, they boarded the packet ship *DeWitt Clinton* and set sail for England. After the long journey, they arrived in the town of Liverpool, where they would remain for nearly ten years. Liverpool was an active seaport where Powell Sr. felt comfortable and could continue his connection to the maritime world, offer aid to Black sailors, and assist the formerly enslaved arriving from America. He secured a position in the customs house of Christopher Bushell and Co. and made good on his promise to improve the condition and opportunities for his children. The youngest children enrolled in local schools, and the oldest began training in their chosen professions. Mercy Powell wrote to a New Bedford acquaintance in America that "we have apprenticed two of them to learn engineering [Edward and Sylvester], and one will be studying to be a surgeon and physician [William Jr.]." Another son, Isaiah, became a cooper or barrel maker, and daughters Mercy and Sarah developed their skills in what was considered the "female arts" of needlework and sewing. She described their life as "living comfortable in the pleasant suburbs of Liverpool."[15]

Emigrating to Liverpool was a welcome change for Powell Jr. He could now pursue a medical education that would have been denied him in the United States because of his color. To further his son's desire to begin training in medicine, Powell Sr. appealed to the faculty of the Liverpool Royal Infirmary School of Medicine in May 1852 for admission to the medical school for his son as a "free student." In his appeal, he noted that his son was "prevented from being educated at the colleges of America on account of his colour" and that their move to England was primarily to secure a better education for his children. After a lengthy discussion, the faculty committee accepted his appeal by a vote of three to two, and Powell Jr. began his studies in medical and surgical practice at no cost.[16] The Liverpool Royal Infirmary provided him with an opportunity to have both a theoretical and practical medical experience. The infirmary had ample operating and lecture theaters, a museum of anatomy, and over two hundred patient hospital beds.[17]

After completing his basic medical studies, Powell Jr. moved to Dublin, Ireland, and began a one-year course of study in "practical midwifery" at the Coombe and Peter Street Auxiliary Lying-In Hospital. The hospital offered a comprehensive education and training in midwifery, diseases of women and children, and practical pharmacy. It treated nearly six hundred in-house patients each year as well as several hundred patients in their homes. The hospital's connection to the Dispensary for Diseases of Women and Children, which treated over thirteen thousand patients annually, offered students an opportunity to perform minor surgeries and gain a knowledge of pharmacy.[18] Powell Jr. graduated from the program in 1858 and was admitted as a member of the Royal College of Surgeons of London.[19] He returned to Liverpool and began practicing as the house surgeon at St. Anne's District hospital and as a temporary surgeon at the Liverpool South Hospital.[20]

The Powell family maintained their ties to the United States and kept abreast of the developing volatile political situation in America. With the prospect of civil war looming at home in 1861, Powell Sr. decided to move the family back to the United States. It is likely his motivation was to allow his sons and himself the opportunity to participate in the fight against slavery. Traveling on the ship *Wyoming* in April of that year, the Powells sailed from Liverpool to Philadelphia.[21] They returned for a time to New Bedford, Massachusetts, renewing their participation in antislavery activities. Powell Sr. and Powell Jr. took an active role in a "colored citizen's group" as president and secretary, respectively.[22] Powell Jr. established a medical practice in the city, advertising his services in the *National Anti-Slavery Standard*.[23] His brothers Sylvester and Isaiah joined the crews of whaling vessels sailing in the Atlantic and to the South Pacific.[24]

The family eventually moved back to New York City, where Powell Sr. reestablished a boardinghouse for Black sailors and formerly enslaved people. Powell Jr. set up a medical practice in the city and in April 1863 applied for a position as surgeon with the U.S. Army. He was offered a contract as a private physician in May and appointed acting assistant surgeon with duty at Contraband Camp Hospital in Washington, D.C. His orders directed him to report to surgeon-in-charge Major Alexander T. Augusta. The *Boston Herald* reported that "Dr. Wm. P. Powell Jr., of New Bedford, a colored man, who received his medical education in England, has been appointed Assistant Surgeon in our army, and is stationed at the contraband camp at Washington."[25]

When Powell Jr. arrived, he quickly settled into his routine of examining and tending to patients. After only five months, he was given temporary charge of the hospital when Augusta was ordered to muster in as surgeon with his regiment. Powell Jr. served as the chief hospital administrator for only one year, during which time he managed hospital administration, treated patients, and performed surgery, including a leg amputation on a Black soldier from

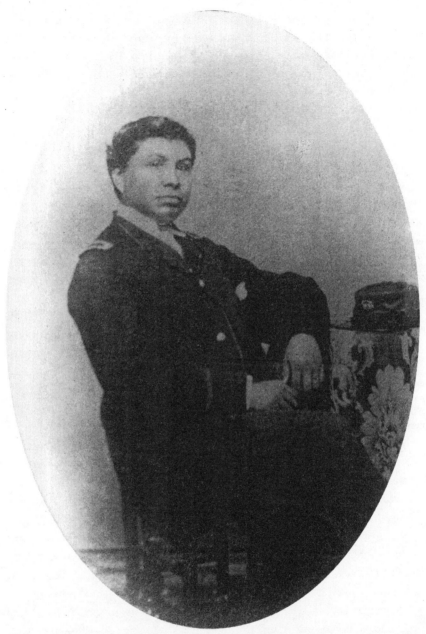

William P. Powell Jr. in uniform, c. 1863. *Courtesy National Archives and Records Administration, Washington, D.C.*

the 2nd Infantry of the USCT.[26] At the beginning of his tenure, he observed that the general health of the people was not good and reported many cases of smallpox, often five to six cases each day. During his first month in charge, he reported sixty-four new cases of smallpox resulting in thirty-three deaths with an overall number of sick at 143. Two to three deaths were reported on average per day across all ages and from all sicknesses.[27] Powell Jr. suffered from his own illness during his time at the camp, a common occurrence among hospital staff.

The hospital was the medical facility for the larger Contraband Camp, a refuge for the newly arriving formerly enslaved people where they received temporary food, shelter, and medical care. The combination of the camp's location on a damp, swampy parcel of land and the lack of an adequate supply of fresh water created a breeding ground for illness that affected the health and well-being of both the patient and hospital staff populations. It was a challenge to keep the staff sufficiently healthy to treat the sick and injured. Staff illnesses placed a strain on resources, resulting in other staff members being overworked and increasing numbers of patients. Sometime in 1864, Powell Jr. contracted a severe cold and catarrh that lasted several months and that, compounded by his inflamed rheumatism, made performing his duties very difficult.[28] He continued to direct hospital operations from his sickbed and often treated himself, as available medical personnel were limited.[29]

While Powell Jr. was in Washington, his father set up a comfortable life for himself and the family in New York. That life was soon shattered and its impact on Powell Jr. significant. In July 1863, over a four-day period, rioters protesting the new conscription laws ravaged the city and destroyed homes and businesses, especially those belonging to African Americans. The new laws required white men between the ages of twenty and forty-five to enlist in the army through a lottery process, while wealthy white men who could afford to pay the government $300 could avoid military service. Many working-class white men saw this as a move by the federal government to force their service in the army. Angered at the new draft law that many felt opened up opportunities for Black people to take their jobs while they served in the army, rioters targeted Black businesses and homes. Over three hundred people were injured and at least one hundred were killed during the four-day melee. Powell Sr. and his family lost everything as a result of what became known as the New York City Draft Riots. After barely escaping the mob's attack on their home, they sought refuge in the police department's 4th Precinct Station House along with over one hundred other African Americans from their neighborhood.

They spent twenty-four hours at the police station before they were escorted by the police to a boat bound for New Haven, Connecticut, and sailed back to New Bedford, where they spent time recovering from the assault.[30] As a result of the great loss suffered by his family, Powell Jr. became the family's sole supporter until his father was able to return to New York City and reopen their boardinghouse.[31]

Compulsory military service in the U.S. Army was instituted through the draft in March 1863, and that fall Powell Jr. received his draft notice. The official draft list identified him as a white physician living at 401 14th Street in Washington, D.C. Persons on the list were identified as either Black or white along with their occupations. Black people were generally listed as teamsters, cooks, laborers, and barbers, while white people were listed as bricklayers, carpenters, clerks, and physicians.[32] Perhaps Powell Jr.'s occupation as a physician prompted the recorder of the list to identify him as white, thinking that no Black man could be a medical doctor. When Powell received his notice, he expressed concern that if he was drafted, he would enter the army as a private rather than as a medical officer. He requested the intercession of R. O. Abbott, the medical director of the District of Columbia, stating his willingness to serve if he could do so as an acting assistant surgeon with a Black regiment. He pleaded his case by describing his position as the sole supporter of his parents since they had lost everything in the draft riots.[33] As a physician, Powell Jr. earned $100 per month, but as a private he would earn only $7 per month, which was not sufficient to support his family. However, he was never drafted and remained in his position as a contract surgeon at Contraband Hospital.

During his time as surgeon-in-charge, he was able to make some improvements to the camp and hospital and requested perimeter fencing around the entire facility to protect the camp and its residents. It was not uncommon for white people to attempt to search for and reclaim the formerly enslaved, and this perimeter fencing provided some security for the camp population. Powell Jr. also sought assistance from outside the camp for clothing and baby linens, which he felt would promote the health of residents and patients.[34] Although Powell Jr. had some successes, his leadership was not without controversy. He faced challenges both administrative and personal and was troubled by accusations of reckless drinking habits and questionable treatment of patients by some nurses and surgeons, both Black and white. Cornelia Hancock, a white Quaker from New Jersey and a volunteer nurse at the hospital, first described Powell Jr. in late 1863 as "part Indian—a good doctor." But her opinion changed by early 1864, when she described him as "neglectful" when treating patients and stated, "If I go to the Medical Director of this post and tell him what I know of Powell he certainly would have to leave his post."[35] In September 1864, Anderson R. Abbott, who also served at the hospital as an acting assistant surgeon, filed a complaint against Powell Jr., claiming that he was "in the habit of indulging too freely in spirituous liquors to a degree which renders him totally unfit to attend to his duties."[36] Powell Jr. made similar charges against Abbott and another Black surgeon, John H. Rapier Jr., who had joined the hospital staff in 1864, but these charges, as well as the charges against Powell Jr., were never substantiated. It is conceivable that personal conflicts between the surgeons led to these accusations in an effort to make a change in hospital leadership. Powell Jr. continued to serve as surgeon-in-charge despite the troubling allegations against him until he was relieved of his duties in November 1864. The reasons for his dismissal remain unclear.

Powell Jr. left Washington, D.C., and returned to New York City, where he reestablished a medical practice and rejoined his family in the boardinghouse, now called the Powell House. Although we find him in New York as late as 1870 along with his parents and siblings, the details of his life and activities between 1865 and 1891 are sketchy. Powell Sr. was now a notary public, the first Black person to receive such a commission, having been appointed in 1865 by the governor of New York, Reuben Fenton. Powell Jr.'s siblings were all gainfully employed, while his mother, Mercy, maintained the household. His sisters, Mercy and Sarah, were seamstresses and did needlework, while his brother Samuel was a druggist, Edward and Sylvester locomotive and marine engineers, respectively, and Isaiah, a cooper or barrel maker. Powell Jr. continued to help support his family.

By 1874, Powell Sr. had left the family in New York City and traveled west to San Francisco on his way to Hawaii. His trip was prompted by his development of an alleged cure for leprosy in the early 1870s, which he intended to demonstrate at the leper colony on the Hawaiian island of Molokai. His efforts were supported by the Hawaiian government, which provided him with $6,000 from the Kingdom of Hawaii's Board of Health through a legislative appropriation.[37] Powell Sr.'s son Samuel, who had been working as a druggist in New York City, joined his father there in August 1874. It is interesting to note that there is no evidence of the involvement of Powell Jr., the only medically trained professional in the family. After spending several months treating leprosy patients, Powell Sr.'s cure proved unsuccessful, as the patient he claimed to have cured was reconfirmed a leper and returned to the leper colony on Molokai. He was declared a "complete failure" by the Kingdom of Hawaii.[38] Powell Sr. and Samuel traveled back to San Francisco in October 1874. Samuel would eventually return to the East Coast and make a permanent home for himself in Cambridge, Massachusetts, where he would find employment as a janitor at Harvard University. Powell Sr. remained in California until his death in July 1879 at the age of seventy-three. After his father's departure from New York and subsequent death, Powell Jr. continued practicing medicine and remained the primary provider for his family.

Powell Jr. traveled to Liverpool sometime between 1870 and 1874, presumably to visit his brother Isaiah, who had taken up permanent residence there, but he returned to New York in October 1874.[39] Between the fall of 1891 and April 1892, he spent time in South America; the purpose of his trip and his activities there are unclear. By December, at the age of fifty-eight, he was serving as a ship's steward on a merchant vessel traveling from Europe. During the sailing he stuck himself with a fish bone in the middle finger of his right hand and developed blood poisoning that would affect his ability to work for the rest of his life. When he finally reached the United States, he settled in Baltimore. Powell's health began to decline in 1893; he was very ill with a badly swollen right arm and hand and an acute septic infection. His physician reported that Powell was "suffering with necrosis of bone of middle finger with sloughing of tendons of this finger and advancing cellulitis of arm."[40] The extent of his injuries led to the amputation of his middle finger, surgery on his right elbow, and a three-month stay in the University of Maryland hospital. He was left in diminished health with limited mobility of his right hand and arm and no family to care for him in his recovery.

* * *

From all indications, Powell never married and had no children. He lived a rather transient lifestyle after 1874, residing at times in Baltimore; Camden, New Jersey; and Philadelphia. By April 1902, at the age of sixty-seven, he had sailed to Liverpool to visit his ailing brother Isaiah. Although Isaiah had traveled back to the United States in 1897, he returned to England, where he died in June 1902, shortly after his brother's arrival. Powell remained in Liverpool after Isaiah's death. Alone and without a means of support, he sought out and secured employment as an assistant chemist with a local physician. After two and a half years, he fell ill with bronchitis and was admitted to the Workhouse Hospital for treatment. After recovering, he hoped to return to his job, but his former employer declined to hire him back because of his age, poor eyesight, and deafness. Once again, he was alone with no family to care for him, few friends, and no means of support.

Unable to live alone, Powell was moved from the Workhouse Hospital to the Kirkdale Home for the Aged, where he lived out the remainder of his years.[41] He described his life to Anderson R. Abbott in 1912:

I am an invalid at the Kirkdale Home. I have no one to look after me. All our family are dead. Out of a family of ten, I am the only one living of the Powell family.[42] I am suffering from Bronchial Catarrh and Rheumatism. Have had two operations performed on me. Have lost middle finger of right hand and an operation on the right elbow joint. My right elbow anchylosed for life. It renders me incapable of manual labor. Poor brother Samuel died January 1st, 1911 at Cambridge, Mass. He was a great help to me. Always sends me newspapers and magazines to read. . . . What troubles me the most at present is Bronchial Catarrh, Rheumatism at times, and also deafness. . . . Kindly let me hear from you. I have no one to correspond with since Sammy died. If it is not any trouble Doctor, please send me on a newspaper or a medical or surgical gazette. You must excuse my penmanship as my right hand is crippled for life. Accept my kind regards. Wishing you are in excellent health. Write soon. Yours faithfully. Wm. P. Powell.[43]

Much of the information about Powell's life between 1870 and 1915 comes directly from his application for a U.S. military pension. He initiated his Original Invalid military pension application in 1891 and continued to pursue a pension unsuccessfully for twenty-five years until his death in 1916. Applying for a pension began with the initial submission of an application by the claimant, followed by a review by the Pension Bureau. Applicants were required to provide proof of identity, military service, and pensionable disability. The bureau would then review the claimant's military and hospital records; obtain supportive depositions from medical personnel, fellow soldiers, family, and friends; and conduct medical examinations to determine the applicant's physical condition, ailments, and disabilities. The process could be long and drawn-out, complicated by legislative changes over time that expanded pensionable disabilities and modified claimants' eligibility requirements.

Initiated by Congress in 1861, the U.S. Army Pension system was as a means of compensation for veterans who served during the war and had sustained war-related disabilities. Instructions and guidelines were provided to pension examiners and examining surgeons who evaluated applications and an applicant's physical condition. The requirements for qualifying for a pension changed over the years. In addition to assessing illness and injury, examining surgeons were instructed by the 1870s to determine an applicant's "habits" and how those habits affected the origin and continuance of a disability.[44] A determination of "vicious habits," including excessive drinking, became a requirement in the Act of June 27, 1890, which stated that a soldier was required to have an honorable discharge, a minimum service of ninety days, and a permanent physical disability not due to vicious habits.[45] This act also removed the requirement that disabilities be a direct result of military service, making any disability pensionable. Benefit payments were no longer based on the specific disability but rather on a rating system that took into account an applicant's inability to perform manual labor.[46] With the Act of February 6, 1907, old age became pensionable.

Powell took advantage of the legislative changes and used them to advocate on his behalf that his disabilities were pensionable under the new laws. In October 1891, while living in Baltimore, he made his first Original Invalid pension application. He submitted three additional applications—in 1893 from Baltimore and in 1907 and 1912 from Liverpool— following on the heels of key legislative changes. In his original declaration of 1891, Powell claimed an inability to earn a living due to "rheumatism, resulting disease of heart, diarrhea, total deafness of left and partial of right ear."[47] In a subsequent declaration he submitted on March 22, 1912, Powell claimed his disability as "an attack of rheumatism and catarrh, owing to the hospital [Contraband Hospital in Washington, D.C.] being located on low and swampy ground . . . suffering from rheumatism, bronchial catarrh and deafness, the results from exposure in the time of duty." It is clear he described his disabilities as service-related and made a case for his inability to make a living from "manual labor" due to these disabilities following the legal definitions of a pensionable disability.[48]

During the course of his claim, his statement of disabilities remained essentially the same with only minor additions based on the current state of his physical condition at the time of each application. It is interesting to note that in 1864, while serving at Contraband Hospital, Powell revealed that he was "totally deaf in my left ear and have been since a child and also a sufferer of Rheumatism (chronic) and have been since I left Europe caused by exposure whilst practicing in that country."[49] This seems to indicate that some of the ailments he claimed were a result of serving as a surgeon during the war were actually preexisting conditions likely exacerbated by the poor conditions where he was working. Regardless of the origins of his ailments, the changing requirements to qualify for a pension should have been satisfied by Powell's age and disabilities that resulted in his inability to earn a living by manual labor.

Over the course of his claim, he was subjected to numerous medical examinations to determine the extent and origin of his disabilities—in May 1892 and November 1893 in Baltimore and in March 1899 in Philadelphia. In 1892, the examining surgeons described Powell as a fifty-eight-year-old male, five feet seven inches tall and 165 pounds. Although he claimed rheumatism, disease of the heart, and deafness, the surgeons found no evidence of the first two disabilities. Based on this examination, the Pension Bureau rejected Powell's claim on the grounds that he was "not disabled in pensionable degree under the Act of June 27, 1890." His examination in 1893 found that he possessed some disabilities, including limited motion in his right arm, a missing finger on his right hand, some deafness, scarring from blood poisoning, and an atrophy of muscles in the right arm but no evidence of heart disease or catarrh. The Pension Bureau during its review of his 1893 documents made note that Powell had signed his original pension application in October 1891 with a full signature, but his June 1893 application was signed with his "mark." Before considering approval of his application, they would need an explanation for the difference. Powell's response explained the injury and amputation of his finger in 1893 and the limited use of his right arm, which prevented him from signing his name. Although this seemed a reasonable explanation as well as a qualifying disability, a pension was again denied him. It seems the Pension Bureau was enforcing the letter of the law in evaluating Powell's applications and provided no leniency in their review. By May 15, 1894, Powell received formal notice from the pension commissioner that his claim was rejected on the grounds that his position as an acting assistant surgeon was not pensionable under the Act of June 27, 1890, and that he did not serve ninety days in the U.S. military service. This same reasoning was used to reject Powell's claim in 1907, when the examiners stated, "Rejection on the ground of no title to pension under Act of February 6, 1907 as claimant did not serve as an officer or enlisted man in the military or naval services of the U.S. during the Civil War."[50]

Powell's status as a contract surgeon was often questioned in relation to his pension eligibility. In May 1894, the Pension Bureau declared that he was not pensionable due to his rank as a contract acting assistant surgeon. In response, his attorney stated to the commission, "It seems clear that the decision of Assistant Secretary, April 30, 1891 in the case of Richard Mace, contract surgeon . . . distinctly declares: 'Contract surgeons having been made pensionable by the acts approved March 3, 1865 and March 3, 1878 are likewise pensionable under Section 2 of the Act of June 27th, 1890.'" The Pension Act of March 3, 1865, made it clear that "acting assistant or contract surgeons disabled by any wound received or disease contracted while actually performing the duties of assistant surgeons or acting assistant surgeons with any military forces in the field or in transit, shall be entitled to the benefits of the pension laws in the same manner as if they had actually been mustered into the service with the rank of 'assistant surgeon.'"[51] Despite this act, the Pension Bureau again rejected Powell's application in 1907, due to his status as a contract surgeon: "claimant did not serve as an officer or enlisted man in the military or naval service of the U.S. during the Civil War, his service as contract surgeon being that of a civilian employee."[52] It seems the Pension Bureau used the narrowest interpretation of the law regarding contract surgeons to deny Powell a pension.

In August 1898 and March 1899, Powell's claim for a pension was again rejected. His 1898 rejection was a result of his failure to show sufficient evidence that his disability from deafness was a result of his service and because his rheumatism, heart disease, and catarrh had not been seen since his previous examination. After his March 1899 examination, the Pension Bureau rejected his claim on the grounds that a pensionable degree of disability for his alleged ailments had not existed since July 14, 1893. Powell's last known physical examination and subsequent report by a physician took place in 1913, when his physician in Liverpool submitted a Physician's Affidavit describing Powell's present condition of chronic rheumatism and deafness and stated that it prevented him from regular employment. This examination, though corroborating his disability claim, still failed to secure a pension.[53]

Powell persisted in his quest for a pension, answering each rejection with a new application, medical examination, and letters of support. He even appealed to two sitting presidents. In 1900, he wrote to William McKinley, asking that the president "give my case favorable consideration." He also appealed to Theodore Roosevelt in 1908, soliciting the president's support to have his pension application reconsidered. He expressed concerns over the pension review process, saying, "I think there is considerable humbugging and favoritism in these pension cases before the Board of Pensions. Other contract surgeons got their claim without any trouble from information from one who has been connected with the Pension Bureau 27 years. I am amongst the first to answer my country's call for medical men in 1862. Gave up my practice in New York."[54] His letter to Roosevelt was certainly prompted by the president's 1904 Executive Order that declared old age a pensionable disability. The order was endorsed by Congress in 1907 through the enactment of the Service and Age Pension Act. It is unclear whether either McKinley or Roosevelt responded to Powell, but if either president did intercede on his behalf, that intercession failed to influence the decision of the Pension Bureau in Powell's favor.

Part of Powell's application included depositions and letters of support secured from former coworkers, surgeons, family, and friends. These were critical in substantiating his claims of disability and their origin. In 1893, depositions were taken from Charles Johnson, with whom Powell lived while in Baltimore; Johnson's granddaughter Elizabeth; and Powell's surgeon Dr. Frank Martin of the University of Maryland. Each of these depositions substantiated his claim of disability due to the loss of his finger and atrophy of his right elbow and arm leading to his inability to perform manual labor. Charles Johnson's deposition described Powell as being "in a bad condition" when he returned to Baltimore in May 1893. Johnson noted that the amputation of Powell's finger took place while he stayed at Johnson's home and testified that he required assistance for all of his daily activities, including "dressing and caring for himself."[55] Elizabeth Johnson also testified to Powell's "bad condition" and his confinement to the house. She described him as a "complete wreck unable to do work of any kind, totally dependent upon those not legally bound to support him."[56] However, the credibility of depositions offered by Black witnesses in support of a pension claim was often questioned and the testimonies considered unreliable, making it likely that the testimonies of Charles and Elizabeth Johnson were discounted. In his physician's affidavit, Dr. Frank Martin described Powell's medical condition and how he suffered from "an acute general septic infection" that led to the amputation of his middle finger.[57] But even with the testimony of Powell's white physician, he was still denied a pension.

Attempts were made by the Pension Bureau to obtain depositions from Powell's former fellow surgeons and hospital staff. Surgeon Charles B. Purvis submitted a statement corroborating Powell's claim that the hospital was located on "low ground and was without any drainage." He described how the patients and hospital staff were "subjected to severe exposure" and "among those afflicted was Dr. Powell who contracted a severe cold and rheumatism."[58] Hospital steward Samuel Powell (no relation to Powell) also submitted a deposition describing how Powell suffered from catarrh and acute rheumatism during his time in Washington and that these disabilities were "the result of exposure to the low condition and swamp in which the camp was surrounded. I use to see him daily during the whole time of his sickness. I should judge it lasted four or five months."[59] Despite these supporting statements from medical personnel familiar with Powell during the war, the pension commissioner claimed that "it is proper to add that the testimony of Charles B. Purvis and Samuel Powell is too indefinite to be accepted as satisfactory."[60] Could the racial identity of Purvis and Samuel Powell have influenced the pension reviewers' decision? Efforts were made by Powell and the Pension Bureau to contact other surgeons with whom he served, including Alexander T. Augusta and John H. Rapier Jr., but both surgeons had died before the requests were made. The only family member who supported his claim was his sister Mercy O. Powell Stowe. She wrote several letters to the Pension Bureau urging the examiners to review and approve her brother's application.

In June 1915, at the age of eighty-one, Powell made his last effort to prove his military service and sway the Pension Bureau in his favor. He sent the bureau a photograph of himself in uniform along with this sworn statement:

> I William Peter Powell take oath and say that I was born at 158 Purchase St., New Bedford, Mass. U.S.A. on June 15th, 1834 and on 19th May 1862 I joined as acting contract surgeon under Colonel R. O. Abbott Medical Director. I was stationed at Freedmans Bureau and Hospital for U.S. Colored Troops c/o 15th & T Street Washington, D.C. and on November 4th 1864, I retired on account of contracting catarrh, rheumatism and deafness in the service. Dr. A. Walters assistant Medical Director came to me during my illness. My diplomas and records were lost in the Earthquake at San Francisco. (I think in 1906 or 1907). I enclose my photograph taken in uniform August 1862. Signed Wm. P. Powell.[61]

This is the last known document that Powell provided to the Pension Bureau before his death on April 12, 1916, at the age of eighty-one.

Over the course of his twenty-five-years petitioning the U.S. government for a military pension, Powell faced an uphill battle. Met with numerous requests from the pension commissioner for more information, medical examinations, and depositions, his application was rejected at every turn. It is apparent that the system was neither lenient nor flexible with Powell's claim and that racism was a factor in his rejections and ultimate denial of a pension. Political scientist Sven Wilson writes that the statutes and regulations

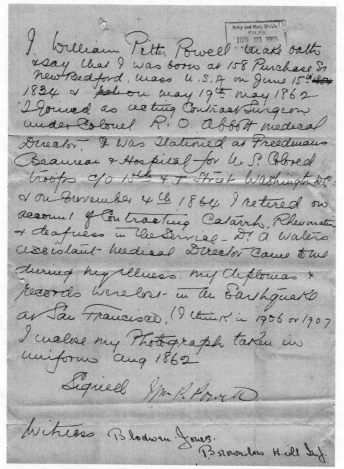

William P. Powell Jr.'s statement to the Pension Bureau that accompanied his photograph in uniform, 1915. *Courtesy National Archives and Records Administration, Washington, D.C.*

governing the pension system did not blatantly discriminate based on race, but long-held stereotypes that questioned a Black applicant's credibility and truthfulness and a legacy of discrimination against Black soldiers during the war influenced the special pension examiners' decisions to award pensions. Wilson points out that Black claimants who applied for a pension "were not extended the leniency and benefit of the doubt that whites often received."[62]

Historians Larry Logue and Peter Blanck expound on this discrimination, stating that "pension officials conducted no extensive discussion of race, but they did say enough to reveal solicitude mixed with suspicion of Black veterans and their survivors. A special examiner declared that 'those of that race who can be counted reliable and absolutely truthful, are a rarity indeed.'"[63] Although the statutes and regulations did not blatantly discriminate against Black applicants, the official instructions given to special examiners on how to deal with Black claimants were clearly biased. They cautioned examiners that "colored applicants, primarily widows, would falsify information in order to obtain a pension."[64] This directed pension examiners to doubt the credibility of Black claimants. It is interesting to note that during the period between 1890 and 1906, only 58 percent of Black applicants recommended for a pension by the examining surgeons were awarded one, compared to 80 percent of white applicants. Racism clearly played a part in the decisions of the Pension Bureau , and Powell undoubtedly suffered from this blatant discrimination.[65]

* * *

Powell's pursuit of a pension for his military service was unusually protracted, but his unwavering dedication and persistence in his quest was not surprising. His father's example of absolute commitment to the causes of antislavery and human rights clearly influenced Powell and empowered him in his pursuit of a medical career. His mother's strength, activism, and support were foundational to his self-confidence and his motivation to make a successful professional life for himself. Powell believed his Civil War service entitled him to a military pension, and he was willing to devote the remainder of his life fighting for that right. His efforts reflect his own personal journey for justice and equality. William P. Powell Jr. died having never received a military pension from his country for the service he gave as a surgeon during the Civil War.

4. ❈ Witness to History: Anderson Ruffin Abbott (1837–1913)

I am a Canadian, first and last and all the time, but that did not deter me from sympathizing with a nation struggling to wipe out a great iniquity.

—Anderson R. Abbott

On a winter evening in 1864, two U.S. Army officers appeared at the White House in their dress uniforms to attend a reception. The warm welcome from President Abraham Lincoln would not have been unusual for a White House guest, but the protests from Lincoln's son Robert about receiving these two visitors and allowing "this innovation" made it apparent that this was not a usual occurrence. That evening, two Black army officers, First Lieutenant Anderson R. Abbott and Major Alexander T. Augusta, made history by attending a levee at the White House. But breaking barriers was not unusual for either of these men.

Anderson Ruffin Abbott was born in Ontario, Canada, on April 7, 1837, the son of Ellen Toyer and Wilson Ruffin Abbott. Wilson had been born in Virginia to a white Scottish Irish father and a free Black mother in 1801. He was an ambitious man who began working as a carpenter at the age of fifteen before leaving Virginia to seek a better life. For a time, he worked in the hotel industry in exchange for room and board and then as a steward on a Mississippi riverboat. Ellen hailed from Baltimore and by all accounts was well educated. As a young woman, she was employed to accompany two girls from Boston on their travels. Wilson and Ellen met by chance during this time when she was asked to nurse him back to health after he suffered a serious neck injury while working at the dock where his riverboat was moored. Ellen and Wilson fell in love and eventually married in 1830, beginning their life together in Mobile, Alabama. It is unclear whether Ellen was free or enslaved at the time she met Wilson, but author Catherine Slaney, the great-great-granddaughter of Wilson and Ellen Abbott, suggests that Wilson bought Ellen's freedom soon after they met.[1]

With an enterprising nature, Wilson established a general store in Mobile. As greater restrictions were placed on free Black people in the South, he became concerned with the increasing animosity toward people of color. Tensions grew and his business and family were threatened by white people who resented his success. He decided to leave Alabama in 1835 and move his family north, eventually settling in Canada. Slavery had been abolished in Canada in 1834 with no legal means for white enslavers to repossess a formerly enslaved person once that individual crossed the Canadian border. It became a safe haven for many Black families from the United States who faced the same precarious conditions as the Abbotts. Wilson and his family settled in Toronto, where the Black population of over five hundred represented about 5 percent of the city's total population, and the Abbotts made a relatively smooth transition to life there.[2] Wilson and Ellen were involved in social and religious activities that included founding the British Methodist Church and supporting the Home Mission Society, which provided aid to the underserved. Through Wilson's astute business acumen, his wealth grew and he began investing in real estate. By the time of his death in 1875, he had acquired seventy-five properties, forty-two houses, five lots, and a warehouse.[3]

The Abbott family understood the importance of education. Ellen had taught Wilson to read and write, and both were committed to providing the best education possible for their five children, including Anderson. Wilson was part of a group of businessmen who managed the predominantly Black Elgin Settlement in Buxton, Ontario, where he moved his family for a short time and where his children attended the Buxton Mission School. Founded by William King, a white Presbyterian minister, the Elgin Settlement aimed to offer social and economic opportunities to Black people and provide a safe haven for the formerly enslaved people who had crossed the border into Canada from the United States. The town was primarily agrarian with a mill, a brickmaking facility, a school, and several churches. King and others in the community believed that "education and moral uplift were vital for citizenship" and that with the same educational opportunities, Black people could function successfully in society.[4] The Buxton Mission School was considered progressive and offered a classical academic curriculum. It had a reputation for providing a superior education such that it attracted both Black and white students and became one of the first racially integrated educational institutions in North America.[5]

Anderson Abbott attended school in Buxton, sharing a classroom with future Black Civil War surgeon John H. Rapier Jr. A proven scholar, Abbott remarked that he "was successful in carrying away either prizes or honors in all my classes."[6] While a student, he worked as a security guard at the local general store. Abbott's father, Wilson, was an advocate for greater educational opportunities for Black people and a member of the Association for the Education and Elevation of the Coloured People of Canada. His involvement with this organization and one of its founders, Alexander T. Augusta, likely provided an opportunity for Anderson to become acquainted with Augusta, who eventually became Abbott's mentor and friend. The two would serve together in Washington, D.C., as surgeons during the American Civil War.

Abbott completed his studies at the Buxton Mission School, becoming one of the school's first graduates, and went on to attend Toronto Academy as an honor student. He then began two years of study in the preparatory department at Oberlin College in Ohio in 1856. Oberlin had a reputation as a center for abolitionist activities, and many of the college's presidents embraced these efforts. The school attracted several other men who would go one to serve as surgeons during the Civil War, including Abbott's friend John H. Rapier Jr, Alpheus W. Tucker, and Charles B. Purvis. The preparatory department provided a course of study intended to ready students for "the classical or scientific course in the collegiate department." As a student, Abbott took general classes in English grammar, geography, history, mathematics, natural philosophy, and Latin. Those entering the department had to be at least sixteen years old and have testimonials of their good character. A fee of fifteen dollars per year was required for young men and twelve dollars per year for young women. Rooms with a stove were available for lodging on campus for a fee of four and a half to six dollars per year. To be "admitted to full membership" a student needed to "honorably" pass a probationary period of six months.[7]

As Abbott's interest in medicine grew, he pursued a course in chemistry at University College in Toronto after leaving Oberlin and then entered the Toronto School of Medicine at the University of Toronto. The school offered the standard course of study as well as provided access to anatomical and pathological models, a medical museum, a chemical lecture room and laboratory, and a cabinet of materia medica. Courses in obstetrics, midwifery, and diseases of women and children were offered through the Toronto Lying-In Hospital with fees of five dollars for six months or eight dollars for one year. The Toronto General Hospital gave students an opportunity to observe a variety of surgical and medical cases. Course lectures began on the first of October, and Abbott paid a fee of twelve dollars per course for those in anatomy, surgery, materia medica, practice of medicine, midwifery, and institutes of medicine. Lower fees were charged for courses in surgical anatomy, chemistry, botany, and medical jurisprudence. Candidates for the bachelor of medicine degree (MB) were required to pass one examination in law or art, to be at least twenty-one years of age, to have pursued medical studies for at least four years with regular attendance at lectures, and to have attended the "practice of some General Hospital" for one year as well as been present at clinical lectures on medicine and surgery for at least six months.[8] Abbott possessed a "perpetual ticket" for the Toronto General Hospital, indicating he practiced in the hospital from October 5, 1858, until April 1, 1861, covering the years he attended medical school.[9] In 1861, he became the first Black Canadian-born licentiate of the Medical Board of Upper Canada, giving him the credentials to practice medicine.[10] He would eventually receive his official bachelor of medicine degree in 1867 and be registered as a Member of the College of Physicians and Surgeons in Ontario in 1869.

With the outbreak of the Civil War in the United States in 1861, Black Canadians and American expatriates watched carefully as events unfolded, and many took an active part in abolitionist activities. Two years later, a local Toronto newspaper reported that the U.S. Army would begin the recruitment of Black men as soldiers, prompting Abbott's mentor, Alexander T. Augusta, to apply for a position as a surgeon. Following in Augusta's footsteps, the twenty-five-year-old Abbott appealed to Secretary of War Edwin M. Stanton "for a commission as assistant surgeon." He noted that he was "one of that class of persons" and desired to serve the cause.[11] Although Canadian by birth, Abbott's commitment to emancipation and justice was not confined by geographic borders. Later in his life, he wrote about his motivation to participate in the war, saying, "I am a Canadian, first and last and all the time, but that did not deter me from sympathizing with a nation struggling to wipe out a great iniquity." Abbott believed the war "was not a war for conquest or territorial aggrandizement nor for racial, social, or political supremacy. It was not a war for white men or Black men, red men or yellow men. It was a war for humanity, a conflict between beautiful right and ugly wrong, between civilization and barbarism, between freedom and slavery."[12]

Although he requested an army commission, Abbott was offered a position as a contract acting assistant surgeon with the U.S. Army, which he accepted on June 26, 1863. Still, he was unhappy about his inability to secure a military commission and believed it was based on racial discrimination. Abbott cited the commission of a white Canadian physician straight out of medical school to point out the difference in his own experience. When the

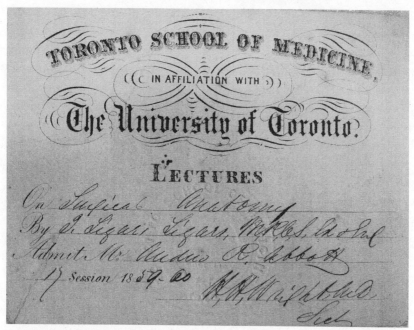

Anderson R. Abbott's surgical anatomy lecture ticket from the Toronto School of Medicine, 1859–60. *Courtesy Anderson Ruffin Abbott Papers, National Library of Medicine, Bethesda, Md.*

white physician applied for a surgeon's position, special arrangements were made for him to take the Army Medical Board examination. After passing it, the white physician was immediately given a commission and appointed to an army regiment.[13] Abbott was not afforded the same opportunity to serve with a full army commission and believed he was denied that opportunity because he was a Black man.

He traveled to Washington, D.C., in July 1863 to begin his contract at Contraband Hospital. Accompanied by Mary Augusta, wife of Alexander T. Augusta, they traveled through New York City, where they had a disturbing experience. While waiting in the train depot in New York, a man pretending to be drunk deliberately fell against Mrs. Augusta. In an effort to protect her, Abbott pushed the man away. The man turned toward Abbott with "a threatening attitude . . . and considerable violent language and profanity." He was then joined by a "big Irishman," and the two began threatening Abbott and Mrs. Augusta with physical violence. After seeing two soldiers enter the depot, Abbott and Mrs. Augusta saw their opportunity to escape. Making their way down a dark, deserted street, they eventually found safety on an avenue crowded with people. They walked back to the depot and waited for their train to depart. Abbott believed that he and Mrs. Augusta had experienced the early effects of the Draft Riots that took place in New York City that month.[14] White protesters attacked and destroyed many Black businesses in New York City in retaliation against the new draft laws, resulting in over three hundred injuries and one hundred deaths.[15]

After his harrowing experience in New York City, Abbott arrived safely in Washington and began working at Contraband Hospital alongside his mentor, Alexander T. Augusta, and William P. Powell Jr. Contraband Camp and Hospital had been established by the U.S. Army in 1862 as a place where formerly enslaved women, men, and children could find food, shelter, and medical care (see chapter 2). At the time of its formation, all persons in positions of authority, such as surgeons and head nurses, were white, while the majority of regular nurses were African American. After Augusta's appointment as surgeon-in-charge of the hospital in April 1863, all white assistant surgeons were replaced with Black assistant surgeons, since the white surgeons would not serve under the direction of a Black man.

As an acting assistant surgeon, Abbott treated patients and helped with hospital administrative duties. He settled into life in the city, but a month after his arrival he fell dangerously ill with miasmatic fever.[16] Abbott was confined to his bed for six weeks at the boardinghouse of Walter and Virginia Lewis. Miasmatic fever affected many Washingtonians at the time, including fellow Black surgeons John H. Rapier Jr. and William B. Ellis.[17] The residual effects of his illness would afflict him for the remainder of his life. Abbott was treated by Augusta, who traveled regularly to the Lewis home to administer care. Elizabeth Keckly, seamstress and confidante of First Lady Mary Lincoln, lived in the Lewis home and became friends with Abbott. She helped nurse him back to health and gained a great familiarity with Abbott and Augusta during his recovery.[18] The relationship between Abbott and Keckly would become an important and influential part of Abbott's life in Washington.

After his recovery, Abbott resumed his duties at the hospital, tending to the needs of Black civilians and wounded soldiers of the USCT. In late October 1863, Augusta was assigned to the 7th Regiment of the USCT and Powell assumed the duties of surgeon-in-charge. Abbott maintained his ties with Augusta, who was now stationed in Baltimore, often socializing with him and his wife. In early 1864, he and Augusta attended a reception at the White House hosted by President Abraham Lincoln and First Lady Mary

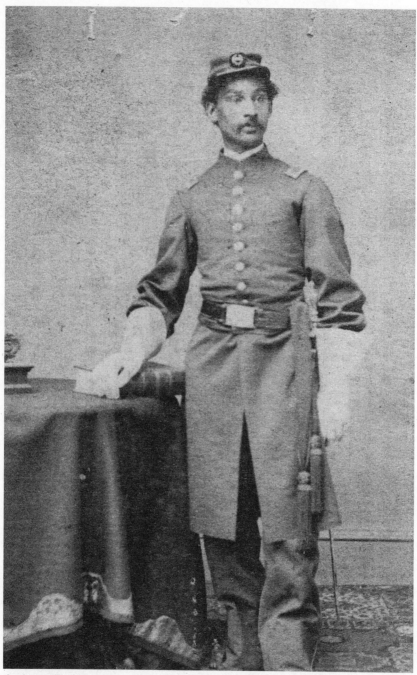

Anderson R. Abbott in uniform, c. 1863. *Courtesy Anderson Ruffin Abbott Papers, Special Collections and Rare Books, Toronto Public Library.*

Lincoln, as mentioned at the beginning of this chapter. In his memoirs penned later in his life, Abbott provided a description of his experience that evening. On a cold February night, he and Augusta had made their way to the White House. Wearing full dress uniforms, they entered the White House porch, where a cordon of soldiers guarded the entrance and where their coats were taken. The Executive Mansion was a "blaze of light" with "carriages containing handsomely dressed ladies, citizens and soldiers . . . depositing the elite of Washington at the entrance to the porch." They left the vestibule and were led along a hallway to a door where they were met by B. B. French, the commissioner of public buildings. French escorted them to the president, who was standing just inside the doorway. With an outstretched hand, Lincoln welcomed them cordially. Robert Lincoln, the eldest son of the president, was taken aback by his father's gesture. When he asked his father if he was going to "allow this innovation," the president responded, "Why not?"[19]

After greeting the president and First Lady, Abbott and Augusta made their way into the East Room, where they were the focus of everyone's attention. "We could not have been more surprised ourselves," Abbott said, "or created more surprise if we had been dropped down upon them through a sky-light. Colored men in the uniform of the U.S. Military officer of high rank had never been seen before. I felt as though I should have liked to crawl into a hole. But as we had decided to break the record we held ground."[20]

It was clear to Abbott that their presence at the White House was controversial and garnered mixed reactions from those in attendance. "Wherever we went a space was cleared for us and we became the center of a new circle of interest. Some stared at us merely from curiosity, others with an expression of friendly interest. While others again scowled at us in such a significant way that left no doubt as to what views they held on the Negro question."[21]

Augusta and Abbott's invitation to the reception was likely influenced by their prominence, but it was perhaps equally a result of their connection to Elizabeth Keckly. Keckly frequently visited the White House, which gave her extraordinary access to the First Lady and the president. She was involved with the Contraband Relief Fund, which raised money to help the formerly enslaved people in the city and specifically those at Contraband Camp and Hospital. Among the contributors to the fund was Mary Lincoln.[22] Keckly's association with the relief fund would have brought her in contact with both Augusta and Abbott. She was a close friend of Abbott's, having met him at the boardinghouse where they both resided and where Keckly helped nurse him back to health when he fell ill soon after his arrival in Washington. Perhaps the combination of their positions as Black surgeons, Keckly's friendship with Abbott, and her close ties to Mary Lincoln prompted the invitation that was extended to Augusta and Abbott.

Abbott was joined at the hospital in June 1864 by his school friend and fellow Black surgeon John H. Rapier Jr. They had become friends while attending the Buxton Mission School in Canada and were now working alongside each other at Contraband Hospital, known by this time as Freedmen's Hospital. When not on duty, they spent time socializing together outside of work.

When William P. Powell Jr. departed the hospital in November 1864, Abbott assumed the position of surgeon-in-charge and remained in the position until 1866. His duties included not only treating patients but also handling administrative responsibilities like ordering supplies and rations, controlling sanitary procedures, and hiring and training staff. One medical case in 1866, attributed to Abbott, involved the treatment of a thirteen-year-old "mulatto" boy who suffered from frostbite, from his feet to his knees, as well as jaundice and tuberculosis. The boy's condition was severe, and it was necessary for Abbott to amputate his left leg. Though the amputation was successful, the boy succumbed to his illnesses.[23]

Abbott again found himself at the White House in April 1865, but unlike the reception he had attended the prior year, this visit was on a more solemn occasion. On April 14, Washington, D.C. was in great celebration after the surrender of Confederate general Robert E. Lee five days earlier. "Washington was brilliantly illuminated and decorated," and the city was filled with an expression of "the intense joy which thrilled the heart of the nation." Abbott joined the throngs of people in the city's streets celebrating the U.S. victory. After enjoying supper with a friend, he watched a torchlight procession held in honor of Secretary of War Edwin M. Stanton that resembled "a fiery serpent winding its sinuous course through the streets and avenues of the city." After Stanton addressed the crowd, Abbott and his friend returned to their lodgings to continue the celebration.[24]

Their joyful evening was interrupted by a knock at the door bringing word that President Lincoln had been shot at Ford's Theatre that night. Abbott and his friends were overcome by the shocking news and anxious to learn of the president's condition. Deciding to venture out in hopes of finding some answers, the group headed toward the home of Secretary of State William H. Seward, who had been seriously wounded in a knife attack at his home that evening. "For the first time during my stay in Washington," Abbott remarked, "I was troubled with a feeling of uncertainty regarding my safety." As they reached Seward's house, a large and excited crowd gathered outside. Abbott kept himself and the women in his group a safe distance from the commotion while his friend went seeking information. When he returned, the crowd had grown even larger, and fearing for their safety, Abbott and his group headed home.[25]

He returned to his lodgings at the Lewis home and headed to bed, but his sleep was soon disturbed by a knock at the door. A messenger arrived at the house at two o'clock that morning "with a request from Mrs. Lincoln that Mrs. Elizabeth Keckley . . . should come to her." As a close friend of Keckly's, Abbott volunteered to accompany her as it would be improper for a woman to travel alone in the city at that hour. They entered the carriage and attempted to reach the White House, where they thought Lincoln had been taken, but it was cordoned off with troops, making it difficult to gain entry. After some persistence, they were able to present Keckly's calling card and learned that Lincoln was not at the Executive Mansion but had been taken to a house across the street from Ford's Theatre,[26] so the carriage turned back around and headed toward the theater. When they arrived at the Petersen House, they were again met by a line of soldiers, but once Keckly presented her calling card, they were permitted to enter the house. Abbott described the scene inside, where "in one room . . . was the dying president, while his companion was lying in an adjoining room prostrate with anguish." He stayed long enough to ensure that Keckly was safe before he returned home. Exhausted by the evening's events, Abbott retired to his room. Later that morning, he was "aroused by the first stroke of the bell, at twenty minutes past seven . . . which announced the painful intelligence that our beloved president was no more."[27]

Elizabeth Keckly wrote of the events surrounding Lincoln's assassination in her published memoir, but her recollection varies from Abbott's. In her story of what transpired, she never mentions Abbott. Her chronology has Walter and Virginia Lewis, owners of the home in which she and Abbott resided, accompanying her to the White House that evening after first passing by the large crowd that gathered at Secretary Seward's house. After being unable to gain entry to the White House, Keckly and the Lewises returned home. Abbott's chronology also refers to the crowd that gathered at Seward's house and his visit there with a group of friends who returned home after the crowd grew too large. Both Abbott and Keckly placed themselves at the scene near Seward's house that evening, but neither mentioned the other in their accounts. Keckly's recollection also differs from Abbott's regarding the carriage sent to take her to Mrs. Lincoln. According to Keckly, it was not until 11 o'clock on the morning of April 15 that a carriage arrived at her lodgings to take her to Mary Lincoln at the White House, accompanied by the Lewises. According to Abbott, it was much earlier, around 2:00 AM, when a carriage arrived, and it was Abbott, not the Lewises, who accompanied her to Mrs. Lincoln, first traveling to the White House and then to the Petersen House across from Ford's Theatre. It is interesting to note that in Keckly's account, when she finally reached Mrs. Lincoln at the White House the day after the assassination, the First Lady questioned her on why she did not come to her the night before, having sent a carriage for her that evening.[28] Perhaps this was the carriage that Abbott claims arrived for Keckly and in which he traveled with her to the Petersen House.

It is not clear why the recollections of Abbott and Keckly are so divergent. Both recalled being among the large crowd at Secretary Seward's house that evening, the cordon of soldiers surrounding the White House, and the difficulty in gaining entry there. The striking difference in their stories concerns their presence (or absence) at the Petersen House on the evening of the assassination. According to Abbott, both he and Keckly were there, but Keckly makes no reference to being at the Petersen House in her memoirs. Why would their stories not align? Abbott was considered a respectable and honorable man, and Keckly was a well-respected, upstanding citizen and close confidante of the First Lady.[29] Neither of them seem to have any discernible reason for being untruthful in their accounts. What does seem possible is that Abbott's recollection may have been affected by the passage of time. He put his memories to paper much later in his life than did Keckly, whose account was written and published in 1868, not long after the assassination. Could Abbott's memory have faltered after the passing years?

If Abbott's recollection is accurate, perhaps Keckly had other reasons for her version of the story, including two that seem plausible. She may have been hesitant to acknowledge Abbott's participation with her that evening to avoid any perception of impropriety due to the possibility that their relationship was more intimate than either of them publicly or privately acknowledged. In Keckly's 1896 deposition supporting Abbott's claim for a military pension, she referred to him as her "intimate" friend with a familiar knowledge of his life and his illnesses.[30] A second possibility may have been her desire to minimize her own involvement in the events that evening due to her relationships with Varina Davis, wife of Confederate president Jefferson Davis, and Mary Custis Lee, wife of General Robert E. Lee. Keckly had been the seamstress for both Mrs. Davis and Mrs. Lee before the war and was often privy to political conversations while working in their respective homes. She made note in her memoirs that "the prospects of war were freely discussed in my presence" by the Davises and other political leaders who frequented the Davis home.[31] Having access to the homes of Lee and Davis as well as to the Lincolns, Keckly would have been witness to discussions about the futures of both the Confederacy and the United States. Her "dual position straddling both worlds" must have been strange, if not uncomfortable.[32] She would have been careful to navigate both spheres with diplomacy and caution to avoid bringing attention to herself or soliciting concern for her presence in the homes of her clients. Dr. Francis Grimké, pastor of the Fifteenth Street Presbyterian Church in Washington, D.C., commented that Keckly's intimacy with influential U.S. and Confederate families "was a testament to her discretion, her business acumen, and not least the creative skills that placed her in such demand."[33] Though we may never know the real reasons that the recollections of Abbott and Keckly differ, the assassination of Lincoln was traumatic and profound for both of them. As close friends, they would have shared their experiences and perhaps been a comfort to one another as they struggled with the loss.

After Lincoln's death, Abbott went to the White House to pay his last respects to the president. Along the way, he noticed "the draping of public buildings, business houses, and residences" that were visible throughout the city and "the cabins of the freedmen" that displayed "emblems of mourning." He described the White House as "somber in the extreme" with "heavy mourning drapery, the deep gloom of the interior, the hushed voices and muffled footsteps." Abbott was escorted to the room where Lincoln's body was laid out. "As the writer looked upon the pale, cold face of the president as he lay in state in the guests' room," he remembered, "a great sorrow weighed heavily upon his heart, for he thought of the loss to the negro race in their nascent life of freedom, of the great guiding hand that now lay paralyzed by death."[34]

His description of the White House and the deceased president included only a small mention of the First Family: "It would be ungracious" to describe "the afflicted family, suffice it to say that the anguish of the widow in the privacy of her apartments, surrounded by her children, and with Mrs. Keckley as her sole companion, was pitiable in the extreme." Sometime after Lincoln's funeral, Abbott was presented a gift of a plaid shawl worn by the president, perhaps evidence of a more personal relationship with Lincoln or a result of his close friendship with Keckly.[35]

After the president's death, Abbott continued his work at Freedmen's Hospital. He often requested improvements in facilities and services including additional bathrooms, storage areas, and furniture.[36] Abbott was well-respected by his peers as well as by his white supervisors. R. O. Abbott, medical director of the District of Columbia, referred to Abbott as "efficient and zealous in the discharge of his duties."[37] A letter to Abbott from Major General G. B. Carse, assistant superintendent of the Freedmen's Bureau, expressed his "pleasure and satisfaction" in the "skillful manner in which you have discharged the duties of your position." He went on to say, "I consider you the most skilled of any Surgeon ever in charge of this post."[38]

Many years after leaving Washington, Abbott recorded some of his experiences during the war. In his article "Colored Female Corporal," he described an encounter with a young Black woman named Julia Ann Rogers who had escaped from her enslaver in Maryland on the way to church one Sunday. After reaching a friend's home, Rogers cut her hair and donned the uniform of a U.S. soldier as a disguise. She traveled on foot for two days to reach Fortress Monroe in Virginia, but while traveling across Confederate lines she was shot in the hip. After spending four months in the Fortress Monroe hospital she decided to enlist in Company K of the 28th Regiment of the USCT disguised as a man. Her skill as a soldier and "proficiency in drill" was evidenced by her promotion from private to corporal. She "took part in the battles before Petersburg . . . and afterwards was sent to City Point, Virginia," where she was discharged. She was admitted to Freedmen's Hospital "suffering from epileptic fits," and it was then that her sex was revealed. Abbott described her as a tall woman of about thirty-five years old with "a masculine countenance," and he was convinced that she could "carry out the deception very successfully."[39]

A second, more poignant recollection described the arrival of a young drummer boy at the hospital on Christmas Eve 1864 "who had been wounded in an ambush attack upon the flank of his line." Abbott finished his work for the day and was headed out of the hospital when he noticed an ambulance slowly approaching. "Being on duty at the time, as officer of the day," he recalled, "I followed the nurse, carrying a small boy in his arms." The ten-year-old was placed on a cot, where Abbott examined him. Abbott inquired about his name and age, but the boy remained silent except for "a tear trickling down" his cheek. When asked about his parents, the boy turned his face toward Abbott "with an intensity of anguish and a supplicating manner" and responded, "Secessh got 'em."[40] Abbott was deeply affected by his reaction and noted that "this one thought overshadowed all others and rendered him [the boy] insensible to all other impressions. Those endearing words, mother and father unloosed the lips that could give utterance to no other thought. They expressed most eloquently the pent-up emotion of that young life which was fast waning." He knew the boy had suffered a mortal wound and instructed the nurses to "care for him kindly." Abbott visited the boy throughout the night and "just as the Christmas bells were ringing in the dawn which heralds the advent of the child Jesus, this little child's spirit vanished into that better world where 'Secessh' can no longer rob him of all that is dearest to him on earth."[41]

The war ended in April 1865, but Abbott continued working at Freedmen's Hospital as well as at the Freedmen's Village Hospital in Arlington, Virginia, until the following April, when his contract expired. He returned to Toronto to continue his medical studies, earning a bachelor of medicine degree at the University of Toronto in 1867 and becoming a registered member of the College of Physicians and Surgeons in Ontario in 1869.[42] Abbott also took an active role in supporting the cause for equality, advancement, and opportunities for Black people. He was a prolific writer, penning lectures, essays, and letters in favor of equality, fairness, and justice. Favoring a united front among Black people in the fight for equality and justice, he said, "Numerically speaking we are in a minority in this country and if we become divided in sympathy and interest we render ourselves powerless in the hands of our enemies and incapable of accomplishing anything for the good of ourselves and our prosperity. Let us therefore be united in spirit and purpose."[43]

In 1871, Abbott married Mary Ann Casey, a well-educated young woman. They settled into life in Chatham, Ontario, and expanded their family to include three daughters and two sons.[44] He established a private medical practice in Chatham and accepted an appointment as coroner of Kent County, Ontario, in 1874, becoming the first Black man to hold such a position. Abbott's experience as a surgeon during the war, where he treated a variety of traumatic injuries and cared for dying and wounded soldiers, may have been a factor in his selection. His reputation as a skilled physician resulted in his election as chairman of the Kent County Medical Association four years later in 1878.

Abbott's commitment to educational advancement for Black people led him to join forces with Wilberforce Educational Institute in 1873 as its president, serving in that position for seven years. Wilberforce was established in Chatham to provide Black students with a well-rounded education, leading them to professions in teaching, art, law, medicine, and business.[45] Unlike his parents, who sought a private education for him and his siblings, Abbott and Mary Ann advocated for a public education for their daughters. He fought for the inclusion of Black people in the public school system and sought a seat on the school board to help achieve that goal.[46]

By 1881, Abbott retired from his position as coroner of Kent County and relocated his family to Dundas, where he reestablished a medical practice. When not attending to his medical responsibilities, he participated in civic organizations and supported educational institutions such as the Dundas Mechanics Institute, where he was director and managed the administrative responsibilities for the school. The institute was founded in 1841, with the goal of making education "accessible to the family of the working man," a concept that Abbott supported.[47] In addition to his civic engagement, he continued to write and took on an editorial position with a local newspaper. Never shy to express his opinion through his writing, he composed articles on a wide range of subjects, including civil rights and the achievements and ability of people of color.

The Abbotts moved several times before settling in Toronto by 1890. After only a year, they decided to leave their comfortable life in Canada and emigrate to the United States, where they found a welcoming and burgeoning Black community in Chicago with its own hospital and newspaper. Chicago was a destination for many African Americans who journeyed from the South. The Black population of four thousand in 1870 grew to fifteen thousand by 1890 and eventually reached forty thousand by 1910.[48] It is not clear why the Abbotts decided to leave Canada, but historian Catherine Slaney suggests it was "a regular practice of several family members to traverse the border and work in both Canada and the United States at various times over the years."[49] Life in Chicago provided new opportunities for Abbott and his family, where he and his wife joined social clubs and participated in local activities.

By the time the Abbotts arrived in the city, the new Provident Hospital and Training School began offering its services to Chicago's Black population. Founded by Daniel Hale Williams, MD, it was the first Black-owned and Black-operated hospital in the United States. In the late nineteenth century, few hospitals would treat Black patients, and Black doctors were excluded from practicing at most hospitals. With the opening of Provident Hospital, the African American community was provided with much-needed care, and Black physicians found a place to practice and acquire advanced medical training. The hospital also offered a program where Black nurses could be trained. Daniel Hale Williams had gained prominence after performing the first successful heart surgery in 1893, when he opened up the chest of a man and repaired an injury to the pericardium (the sac surrounding the heart). As a result of this groundbreaking surgery and his reputation as a hospital director and educator, Williams was offered and accepted the position as surgeon-in-chief at Freedmen's Hospital in Washington, D.C.

With Williams's departure in 1894, Abbott came out of retirement to take on the position of superintendent of Provident Hospital. His reputation as a respected hospital administrator and an accomplished surgeon made him an easy choice to replace Williams. His appointment was lauded by a local newspaper describing him as "well-known and universally recognized as one of the ablest colored surgeons in the country." The paper went on to say that "in him the public will have the most perfect confidence for he has proven himself worthy and capable in the highest degree."[50]

Abbott served at the hospital for three years, directing its operations, participating in fundraising activities, and making presentations as an invited speaker at various events in the city. As an able and captivating orator, he gave many public addresses, including one at the celebration of Queen Victoria's birthday in 1897. In his address, he spoke about the "days of slavery" and the activities of the Underground Railroad in guiding the enslaved people to freedom and aroused the audience's interest "to a state of excitement by his vivid pictures and anecdotes."[51] Abbott resigned his position at Provident Hospital in June 1897 but remained in Chicago with his family for a few years before returning to Toronto.[52]

For Abbott, the Civil War remained an important experience in his life. In 1890, he became a member of the Grand Army of the Republic, a fraternal organization established for veterans who shared the experience of military service during the Civil War. The purpose of the society was one of fraternity, charity, and loyalty. The GAR provided camaraderie among veterans and support for medical, burial, and housing expenses and honored deceased veterans with memorials, statues, and gravesite remembrances.[53] Abbott rose up through the ranks of his local post to be appointed its surgeon and aide-de-camp.[54]

Proud of his service as an army surgeon, Abbott believed he was deserving of an honorary or brevet rank in the U.S. military. In February 1891, he appealed to Secretary of War Redfield Proctor for an honorary rank. "I am one of those that left Canada during the late Civil War," he said, "to assist the government of the United States in suppressing the rebellion in the South." He described the particulars of his service and mentioned the shawl that was given to him after Lincoln's assassination as "evidence that I was held in some esteem during my Sojourn in Washington."[55] Though he served admirably during the war and received numerous letters of praise from his white supervisors, his request for an honorary rank was denied. Abbott was informed by the surgeon general's office that a brevet rank would require a "direct and specific enactment of Congress" and that "no general provision for such rank, applicable to Acting Assistant Surgeons, has ever become law."[56]

Following the rejection of his request, he applied for a military pension from the U.S. government. In June 1891, he submitted his Declaration for an Original Invalid Pension, basing his claim on liver disease, impoverished blood, chronic bronchitis, asthma, and rheumatism that were incidental to his military service and "in the line of professional military duties." Abbott claimed his chronic conditions led to heart disease and a poor physical condition, compelling him to abandon his professional calling as a physician and rendering him unable to support himself and his family.[57] He complied with the required physical examination to substantiate his claims of disability. The examining surgeon described Abbott as a man of five feet six inches in height and a weight of 128 pounds who was "well nourished" but "not a strong man." The surgeon noted that whatever disability he suffered from was likely due to "the repeated attacks which he alleges."[58]

To assist him in navigating through the pension claim application process, Abbott engaged the services of an attorney. Affidavits on his behalf were collected from several people and submitted with his application. Several affiants corroborated Abbott's claims. Isaac Mills, an electrician specialist, confirmed Abbott's claim of rheumatism and the electrical stimulation treatments he provided to Abbott for "muscular rheumatism and spinal irritation."[59] Other witnesses attested to the longevity of their relationship with Abbott and noted their familiarity with his health, describing him as in "physically sound health" throughout his childhood and until the time he entered the service of the U.S. Army in 1863, when his health was compromised by his service during the war and seriously diminished after the war. A Canadian pharmacist testified to the care Abbott received from a local Toronto physician and the myriad of prescriptions he provided to him, thus confirming Abbott's claim of various ailments.[60] A local Canadian physician said he knew Abbott as both a physician and a patient and testified that he treated him for "bronchitis, asthma, and hemorrhage of the lungs," which resulted in Abbott's inability to continue his own medical practice.[61] Abbott wrote to the Pension Bureau commissioner in his own defense, telling him that "I entered the service a robust and exceptionally healthy young man," and "I continued in this condition until the month of August 1863."[62]

Regular inquiries were made regarding the status of his claim by Abbott and his attorney, and additional affidavits were secured and submitted supporting his application, including one from Elizabeth Keckly. In her deposition, Keckly noted that she first became acquainted with Abbott while he visited friends at the home of Walter Lewis, where she resided and where they "became intimate friends." She corroborated his account of being "seriously ill" and confined to his bed at the Lewis home for six weeks during his illness. She remarked that he "was prostrate with the miasmatic fever that prostrated so many residents in Washington at the time" and that when he was recovering "he was very much emaciated . . . had a distressing cough . . . and was frequently lame and disabled by rheumatism."[63]

Abbott's application was rejected in 1897 on the grounds that he failed "to furnish competent evidence showing origin of the alleged disability and his physical condition for several years after his discharge."[64] He appealed the decision and submitted further affidavits, including from two Freedmen's Hospital nurses—Laura V. McCool and Mary Dorsey Glasgow. Both women corroborated Abbott's claim to poor health contracted during his service at the hospital and described frequent visits to Abbott, where they found him "seriously ill, suffering a fever." Their knowledge of his condition was based on their duty as nurses that kept them in continual contact with Abbott.[65]

Despite the depositions of Keckly and two nurses, Abbott's appeal was rejected. Reviewers based their reasoning on his service as a civilian on contract to the army medical department and their assessment that he had failed to furnish evidence from fellow officers. It is interesting to note that the review board commented that the evidence presented by the depositions of "two army nurses, both of who sign by mark, has been considered but is cumulative and is not regarded as materially affecting the status of the claim."[66] It seems that the review board disregarded the affidavits of the two Black nurses, judging their inability to write their names as a factor in establishing their credibility and determining the value of their depositions. A similar scenario played out in the pension application of William P. Powell Jr., where the depositions of several Black witnesses, including surgeons, were discounted and considered insufficient. It was common for the Pension Bureau to discount the credibility of Black witnesses. Historians Larry Logue and Peter Blanck note that though discussions of race were not generally conducted by pension officials, they did make statements revealing their distrust of Black witnesses and depositions.[67]

Abbott had been reticent to apply for a pension. He found it "repugnant to my sense of honor to ask any thing that savored of alms from the government, which I served for the cause of freedom and which had paid me for my services. It was not until I had been stripped of means of support by misfortune that I yielded to what I supposed was my right to, to make claim."[68] As late as 1907, he was still defending his right to a pension, but despite his continued efforts, he remained unsuccessful in convincing the Pension Bureau to change its decision in his favor.

Throughout the remainder of his retirement years, Abbott spent time writing and lecturing on a variety of subjects. Historian M. Dalyce Newby refers to him as a "latter day renaissance man" with his interests in poetry, music, and writing.[69] Among his many papers are poems, including "A Mother's Love." He lectured and wrote articles on subjects ranging from astronomy, science, and anatomy to literature, politics, and civil rights.[70] In his twilight years, Abbott was active and remained open to expressing his opinions on life, work, and history. On December 29, 1913, at the age of seventy-six, Anderson Ruffin Abbott died as a result of complications from surgery for appendicitis. He left a legacy of service to his community and to humanity in the name of freedom, justice, and equality.

5. ✤ Serving in the Regiment: John Van Surly DeGrasse (1825–1868)

From the hour I landed at New Berne [*sic*], N.C. to raise this Regiment to the present time, my zeal and interest in its welfare have been unabated.

—John Van Surly DeGrasse

John Van Surly DeGrasse was the second of only two African Americans to receive a commission as a medical officer in the U.S. Army during the Civil War and the only Black surgeon to serve in the field with his regiment. During the Civil War, Black surgeons were primarily assigned duty at recruiting stations or Black-only hospitals, as white surgeons would not work alongside them or be their subordinates. As the only Black surgeon in the field, DeGrasse was exposed to discrimination and mistreatment in an isolating environment, far from the support that other Black surgeons had working alongside each other in hospitals.

Born free in New York City in 1825, DeGrasse was one of five children of Maria Van Surly and George DeGrasse, a wealthy landowner. His grandfather Admiral Count François Joseph Paul DeGrasse had been a French naval commander whose fleet of ships assisted George Washington in the victory at Yorktown in 1781, resulting in the recognition of American independence from Great Britain.[1] Admiral DeGrasse had served in the French navy in India, and it was during this time that George was conceived. After George's birth in Calcutta around 1780, Admiral DeGrasse took some responsibility for the young boy and arranged for him to travel to America in 1799, where he settled in New York City, America's capital. During the American Revolution, Admiral DeGrasse had come to know Aaron Burr, later vice president, and it is likely through this relationship that George became employed as Burr's servant. Burr referred to George as "my man George (late Azor Le Guen now George d'Grasse)."[2] Burr was not only politically powerful but also a wealthy landowner and lawyer. In November 1802, he transferred a parcel of land to George, and this transaction ignited George's interest in landownership. The property, located in what is now lower Manhattan, was one of twenty-eight parcels of land George DeGrasse owned over the next fifty years.[3]

Eager to establish himself in America, George petitioned the Common Court of Pleas for citizenship in 1804. After proving, to the satisfaction of the court, that he had been a resident of the country for the required five-year period and of New York State for the required one-year period, along with demonstrating a good moral character, DeGrasse was granted citizenship without hesitation. It was unusual for a man of color to be granted citizenship in the nineteenth century, and it is likely his acquaintance with Aaron Burr and his father's assistance to George Washington at Yorktown influenced the court's decision.

DeGrasse integrated himself easily into the Black community of New York City. He met and married Maria Van Surly, a woman of Dutch and Moroccan ancestry, and they settled into life among the accomplished and successful Black elite who had established schools, churches, and organizations in their community. DeGrasse lived among his peers, free to pursue his political, social, and economic ambitions. The family grew to include five children, Isaiah, Serena, John, Maria, and Theodosia, named after the daughter of his former employer Aaron Burr. John, along with his siblings, was educated in the local private and public schools in New York City, including the African Free School established in 1787 to educate both girls and boys. Originally a one-room schoolhouse, it grew to include several schoolrooms that offered classes in reading, writing, and arithmetic, along with astronomy and geography for boys and sewing for girls.[4]

After receiving his early education in New York City, John DeGrasse entered the Oneida Institute in 1840 at the age of fifteen. Located in upstate New York, the institute was led by fervent abolitionist Beriah Green, who encouraged the acceptance of Black students to the school. It was among the first colleges to enroll Black and white students on an equal basis. The school provided a progressive education and was a leader in the fight for emancipation. It produced an abolitionist newspaper and was a stop on the Underground Railroad. Everyone was encouraged to participate in abolitionist activities, including students who founded New York State's first antislavery society dedicated to the immediate emancipation of all enslaved persons.[5] New York State had passed a gradual emancipation act in 1799, meaning all children born into slavery after July 4, 1799, were freed, but not until they reached the age of twenty-five for women and twenty-eight for men. In 1817, an additional law was passed that granted freedom to those born prior to 1799, but it delayed their emancipation for ten years.[6] Gradual emancipation was unacceptable to most, and the students protested this policy through their antislavery society.

DeGrasse attended the Oneida Institute for only one year before he transferred his studies to the Clinton Seminary, where his education was expanded to include Latin. The Oneida Institute did not offer Latin, and as DeGrasse's interest in pursuing a medical education developed, a working knowledge of the language would be essential. After studying at the Clinton Seminary for two years, he traveled to Paris around 1843 to begin studies at Aubuck College and gained a proficiency in the French language. He returned to the United States in late 1845 and continued his medical education by establishing an apprenticeship under the tutelage of New York physician Samuel Russell Childs, with whom he studied for more than three years.[7] While still an apprentice, DeGrasse was accepted at the Medical School of Maine at Bowdoin College in Brunswick, Maine, where he was among eighty-one medical students enrolled in 1847. Dr. Childs supported DeGrasse's pursuit of a formal medical education and in a letter to the school certifying his apprenticeship described DeGrasse as "diligent in his studies, exemplary in his conduct" and noted that he "sustains a good moral character."[8]

The Medical School of Maine offered a comprehensive course of study that included anatomy, physiology, surgery, chemistry, materia medica, pharmacy, obstetrics, and the theory and practice of physic. As a student, DeGrasse paid an admission fee of fifty dollars as well as a matriculation fee of three dollars and a graduation fee of eighteen dollars that included an engraved diploma on parchment. The medical courses began in February each year and ran for thirteen weeks. Examinations were conducted on a daily and weekly basis covering all lecture subjects. DeGrasse had access to the school's medical library with over 3,200 volumes as well as an anatomical cabinet with a variety of specimens and a collection of medical instruments and apparatuses. Students were able to observe surgical operations as a part of their regular course of study. DeGrasse fulfilled all the requirements for graduation, including three years of study under a regular practitioner of medicine, attendance at two full courses of medical lectures, and possession of a good moral character.[9] He completed and submitted his thesis on syphilis to the medical faculty and on May 19, 1849, passed his final examination and received his doctor of medicine degree. The *Salem Observer* made note of the graduation, referring to DeGrasse as one of "two colored medical students at Bowdoin Medical College."[10]

After graduating, he returned to France to study under famed French surgeon Alfred Armand Louis Marie Velpeau, known for his innovative surgical skill, his knowledge of surgical anatomy, and his prolific publications on medical subjects.[11] Many American physicians traveled to France to further their education and gain clinical experience that was not readily available in the United States, and even less so for Black physicians. It was observed that "the best seats in Velpeau's amphitheater have the name of American seats, as they are always filled by the Yankees, who have gone and occupied them long before the lecture commences."[12] Daniel Laing Jr., a Black medical student who had been accepted at Harvard Medical School in 1850 and then asked to leave the university because of his color, also studied with Velpeau in Paris in 1850 and 1851.[13] A Paris correspondent for the *Chicago Tribune* noted that "the attention of an American in Paris, is the equality and freedom that the colored man enjoys here. The great surgeon Velpeau," the writer reported, "had a Negro taking down his lectures." Some of Velpeau's students remarked that "the Negro has the inside track of all in the confidence and esteem of the world-renowned surgeon."[14]

DeGrasse remained in Paris for about a year before returning to the United States sometime between 1850 and 1851. He established a medical practice in Boston, where he treated patients in their homes and had consultations at his medical office. His practice included treating wounds, administering prescriptions for illnesses, providing vaccinations, delivering babies, and performing medical procedures, such as applying leeches and cupping. In one case, he resuscitated two people in their home who were suffering from asphyxia due to the inhalation of coal gas.[15]

In 1852, DeGrasse married Cordelia L. Howard, daughter of Peter and Margaret Howard, a prominent Black family in Boston. Cordelia was known for her musical talent and often performed with her sister for fundraisers supporting abolition and equality.[16] DeGrasse grew his medical practice and developed a reputation as a respectable physician. He was described as "skillful and faithful in his practice" and qualified "for administering to the various ills that human flesh is heir to."[17] His reputation and good standing as a physician gained him admittance to the Massachusetts Medical Society in 1854, its first African American member. *Frederick Douglass' Paper* lauded the accomplishment as "the first instance of such honor being conferred upon a colored man in this State, and probably in the country," and expressed its hopes that DeGrasse's admittance would encourage other young Black men to make "the most of their talents and opportunities" and "rise superior to circumstances, compel respect and confidence, and fill stations of honor and eminence much oftener than they have done, or perhaps have thought it possible to do."[18]

DeGrasse was committed to antislavery activities and began volunteering with the Massasoit Guards, a Black militia organized in Boston to protect the Black community from threats resulting from the passage of the 1850 Fugitive Slave Act. Many Northern states were no longer a safe haven for those who had escaped enslavement, and Black communities had to depend on themselves for protection. A number of them formed vigilante groups and independent militias to protect their residents from enslavers who used the Fugitive Slave Act to capture free and formerly enslaved Black people. DeGrasse was a member of the guards by 1855 and served as its surgeon.[19]

At the end of 1855, DeGrasse and his wife welcomed the birth of their daughter, Georgenia Cordelia. The family lived a comfortable life in Boston, and by 1860 DeGrasse had accumulated a personal estate worth $6,500.[20] He participated in social and political activities, contributed content to a monthly abolitionist publication, and was a member of the Prince Hall Grand Lodge of Masons fraternal organization. DeGrasse sometimes presented talks to its membership and was considered a learned and eloquent speaker.[21]

The outbreak of the Civil War in 1861 changed DeGrasse's life. In 1863, when the U.S. government began recruiting Black men for the war effort, DeGrasse applied for a position as a medical officer with the U.S. Army. After passing the Army Medical Board examination, he received a three-year commission as an assistant surgeon on April 28, 1863, a few weeks after Alexander T. Augusta. DeGrasse and Augusta were the only Black physicians to be commissioned as army medical officers. All other Black applicants were placed on contract with the army as acting assistant surgeons. This decision may have resulted from protests by white medical officers who refused to serve under the direction of any Black man.[22] With Black medical officers in ranking positions within regiments, white medical officers believed the possibility for their own advancement would be obstructed. By hiring Black physicians only as contract surgeons, the U.S. Army avoided any possible conflict. Black contract surgeons could easily be discharged or assigned to recruiting stations where white surgeons would not have to serve alongside them. White officers would no longer have cause to complain about their positions or feel their opportunities for advancement within regiments were restricted by ranking Black medical officers.

DeGrasse was eager to serve as an army medical officer, and in early May he received his assignment to join the 1st North Carolina Colored Volunteers (soon the 35th Regiment of the USCT). He was instructed to report to New York City on or before the morning of May 10 by the commander of the

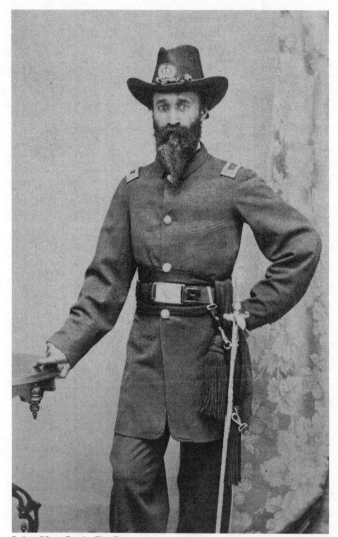

John Van Surly DeGrasse in uniform, c. 1863. *Courtesy Boston Athenaeum.*

regiment, Lieutenant Colonel James Beecher.[23] DeGrasse complied with the order, traveling to New York City where he boarded a vessel with several other regimental officers bound for New Bern, North Carolina. Upon their arrival, they began recruiting Black men for the new regiment. Many people opposed the recruitment and arming of Black soldiers, believing that Black men were best suited to fatigue duty like building trenches and latrines and setting up tents for white troops. The 1st North Carolina Colored Volunteers was unique as its commanding officers openly supported both the recruitment and the arming of Black soldiers. Formed in early 1863 through the efforts of Massachusetts governor John Andrew, the unit was part of a brigade commanded by Colonel Edward A. Wild and was referred to as Wild's Brigade. Wild was an experienced military officer recruited by Governor Andrew to organize and lead the newly formed units of Black soldiers in North Carolina. After his appointment, Wild set out to recruit officers for the regiment who were well experienced and committed to abolition. One such officer was Colonel Beecher, an experienced military man from a prominent abolitionist family that included his father, Lyman Beecher, a minister, and his sister, writer Harriet Beecher Stowe. As commander of the newly formed regiment, he championed the rights of his men and made efforts to improve their condition. Beecher and Wild continued to recruit officers, including Lieutenant Colonel William N. Reed as second officer, rumored to be "mulatto"; Reverend John N. Mars as the regiment's Black chaplain; and John V. DeGrasse as assistant surgeon.[24] Though these selections reflected the desire of Wild and Beecher to include men of color as officers, it was an invitation to controversy that would soon test their commitment to these officers and to their belief in the advancement of Black people.

Although he was part of the contingent of officers who had just arrived, DeGrasse's presence as a Black man in an officer's uniform was unusual and met with the disapproval of many white soldiers. Thomas Hale, of the 45th Massachusetts Regiment, wrote home about the arrival of Wild's Brigade and its Black surgeon. He mockingly described DeGrasse as wearing "the uniform of a major and is of course to be obeyed and respected accordingly. I wonder," he wrote, "how the nice young men of Boston, the ladies' pets, the gallant 44th will like the idea of presenting arms, the most respectful salute they can make, to a negro?"[25] Some enlisted white soldiers remarked that as their enlistment period was nearing an end, they would not reenlist if they were obliged to "salute a negro."[26]

DeGrasse's presence prompted some to act out their displeasure. It seems an order existed that forbade any Black soldiers from wearing shoulder straps or military buttons. While walking down the street, DeGrasse "was accosted . . . by one of the guards belonging to the 44th Massachusetts, notified of the order and compliance with its requirement demanded." It is not clear whether he complied, but it was said that he did "not appear at all concerned about the sentiment that prevails against him and his color as a soldier. He carries himself with considerable dignity and mingles with the officers composing Gen. Wild's staff as if he were morally and socially one of them."[27]

DeGrasse was tasked primarily with performing medical examinations of new recruits. One soldier, some years later, recalled that a fellow soldier was "stripped stark naked and carefully examined at New Berne [*sic*] by Dr. J. V. DeGrasse."[28] He also assisted the regiment as it established itself in the town. When a building occupied by the staff of the 5th Rhode Island Regiment was assigned to Wild and his staff, DeGrasse was among those who inspected the premises. A complaint was made against him for his supposed gruff behavior and for dislodging papers from the desk of the quartermaster. The quartermaster strong-armed DeGrasse and ejected him from the building. He assumed that DeGrasse was responsible for disturbing the documents, but it was later determined that a young boy of color who had accompanied DeGrasse had done so.[29] As a result, Wild ordered the quartermaster's arrest.

The regiment had reached its full contingent of soldiers by June and by the end of July left New Bern for Folly Island, South Carolina. DeGrasse went with the regiment, but the white assistant surgeon, Daniel Mann, remained behind, leaving DeGrasse the sole medical officer for the regiment for more than a month. During Mann's absence, a junior surgeon was temporarily detached to the regiment to relieve the burden on DeGrasse, who had fallen ill. Sickness within the regiment had increased after the troops' arrival at Folly Island, which added to the workload. This was due in part to the increased fatigue duty to which the soldiers were assigned coupled with a lack of decent water and supplies and the cold, wet climate of the coastal location.

When Mann eventually arrived, he took over responsibility for all sick officers and soldiers in camp while DeGrasse was kept in charge of the hospital. Mann objected, and tensions grew between DeGrasse and Mann. Mann felt that as the senior medical officer, he had sole authority to make duty assignments, including those related to the hospital, and vehemently complained to his superiors. His objections may have been boosted by a belief among many of the white officers that Lieutenant Colonel Reed, who was second in command, gave special treatment to DeGrasse. As a ranking officer, Reed was often placed in command of the regiment, and some, including Mann, felt he favored DeGrasse over white surgeons because he himself was "mulatto." The regiment had only an assistant surgeon on duty at the time, with no ranking regimental surgeon. This placed control of medical services in the hands of nonmedical officers. When Mann's complaint was received by the medical director, the commander of the Department of the South was notified of the difficulties of having a white surgeon and a "negro" working alongside each other.[30] Both Mann and the commander believed the favoritism and special treatment Reed showed toward DeGrasse put a Black surgeon at an advantage over a white surgeon, which was unacceptable. It was no secret that Reed was a staunch abolitionist and supported the rights of Black soldiers under his command, but the records of the regiment made no reference to his race that could substantiate the accusations made by the medical director and Mann that Reed's race influenced his treatment of DeGrasse.[31] A new regimental surgeon, Henry O. Marcy, was eventually appointed to the regiment in November 1863, but that did not alleviate the tension between DeGrasse and Mann.

By early February 1864, the regiment, now designated the 35th Regiment of the USCT, was ordered to join forces with several other regiments in Florida to block Confederate supply lines. Once there, the burden of care for sick and wounded soldiers fell on the shoulders of DeGrasse and Marcy, as assistant surgeon Mann remained behind. The regiment was now under the temporary command of Reed, who led the regiment in the Battle of Olustee on February 20, 1864. Reed suffered serious wounds in the battle, and a decision was made to transport him to the coast and move him to a hospital in South Carolina.[32] DeGrasse accompanied Reed to Jacksonville, Florida, and assisted in placing him on board a hospital ship headed to Beaufort, South Carolina, where Reed died.

After the Battle of Olustee, DeGrasse received some relief from the war when he was granted leave in March 1864 to attend to his sick daughter in Boston. He remained in Boston through April before rejoining his regiment in Florida. His time away may have given him respite from the horrors of war, but when he returned, he continued to be subjected to the same hostile environment he had left the month before. Marcy and Mann were relentless in their attacks on his reputation and his medical professionalism, making allegations against him of drunkenness and insubordination. Without the support of Reed, DeGrasse was left unprotected and vulnerable. In mid-September, as a result of the continued accusations made by his fellow white officers, DeGrasse was brought up on charges and would have to face a court-martial hearing in Jacksonville.

Throughout the army, drinking was a serious disciplinary problem. Officers accused of drunkenness were said to be neglectful of their duties and acting in an ungentlemanly way. Moral behavior and being "gentlemanly" were a requirement of officers, and those violating these requirements, especially through drunkenness, often faced disciplinary action and court-martial.[33] Accusations of drunkenness was an easy way for white officers to pursue the removal of a Black officer from the army.

DeGrasse's hearing was based on five counts of drunkenness, misappropriation of medicinal liquors, and conduct unbecoming an officer. These incidents were said to have occurred in February 1864 after the Battle of Olustee, in June 1864 while near Darby's Station, Florida, and in July 1864 while on board the steamer *Mary Benton* on the St. John's River in Florida. Seventeen witnesses were called, including eight for the prosecution (five white and three Black) and nine for the defense (five white and four Black), each giving testimony before a panel of eight white military officers, including Lieutenant Colonel Ulysses Doubleday of the 3rd USCT, president of the panel, and Captain Frank W. Webster of the 3rd USCT, judge advocate. DeGrasse represented himself during the proceedings and was permitted to present a written statement in his defense before the panel of judges made their final decision.[34]

Two charges were brought against DeGrasse with five specifications to those charges. The first charge was drunkenness on duty with three specifications: (1) when on duty with his regiment and ordered to assist in caring for the wounded, he failed to obey and in a state of intoxication retired to his quarters; (2) while on duty with his regiment he neglected his duty, deserted his post, and, when he arrived at camp, took to his bed in a state of intoxication; and (3) when he was sought to attend to a wounded soldier, he was found "entirely incapacitated to perform his duty caused by excessive drinking of alcoholic stimuli." The second charge was conduct unbecoming an officer and a gentleman with two specifications: (1) "while under the influence of liquor insult[ed] a colored woman name unknown using indecent and obscene language," and (2) "misapplied and appropriated to his own use liquor belonging to the Medical Department."

The court-martial proceedings began on September 17. Captain Webster, as judge advocate, represented the prosecution. On the first day of the trial, evidence was presented by prosecution witnesses addressing the first charge, drunkenness on duty. Both Webster and DeGrasse questioned each witness. Two white witnesses, hospital steward Delos Barber and surgeon Henry C. Marcy, and two Black witnesses, Private Benjamin Hawood, ward master, and Private Freeman Grice, testified for the prosecution. Barber and Marcy claimed that after the Battle of Olustee, DeGrasse arrived in camp intoxicated. Barber told the court that DeGrasse was "stupefied or under the influence of liquor" and his breath "was very strong smelling of liquor" while he slept in his quarters, which were shared by all medical officers. When asked by surgeon Marcy to arouse DeGrasse and order him to assist with the wounded, Barber said he could not wake him because of his intoxicated condition. Marcy corroborated Barber's statement, telling the court that DeGrasse's "breath smelled very strongly" while in his quarters and that it "caused the close quarters of the shelter to be effusive." He claimed DeGrasse had been drinking earlier in the day and was "suffering abnormal effects" as a result of drinking. Although a witness for the prosecution, Grice's testimony contradicted that of Barber and Marcy. Grice, who had been working on the stretcher corps that day, told the court that he helped DeGrasse "take off a couple of men" from the battlefield who were injured, and then they both made their way into camp. DeGrasse's condition "was all right," he told the court, and he had noticed nothing unusual. Hawood's testimony corroborated Grice's testimony; he stated he observed DeGrasse when the regiment arrived at camp and that DeGrasse was not drunk.

In his own defense, DeGrasse told the court in his written statement that if the charges were legitimate, Marcy or any other officer of the regiment would have reprimanded him for such behavior at the time the incident occurred. "Nearly seven months is allowed to elapse," he noted, "without a reprimand or without a single remark . . . that I had been guilty in the least of being under the influence of liquor." He admitted to having a small amount of whiskey that day but said he was not drunk. Describing the "long and tedious march" the regiment made going from the battlefield to the campsite, he contended that it was exhaustion that made it difficult to rouse him from his sleep that night. "During the battle," he says, "having sent my horse off the field, I devoted my entire time with the stretcher corps in bringing the wounded off the field. Later still in the afternoon till dark I was untiring in my efforts in caring for the wounded." Without his horse, DeGrasse walked nearly twenty miles to reach camp from the battlefield and, once he arrived, was "so physically exhausted, caused by the extraordinary work of the day," that he was "no more fit to comply with the order of Dr. Marcy than though I had been wounded." Marcy admitted to the fact that DeGrasse told him of his "excessive fatigue" and claimed he responded to DeGrasse by telling him "that all were excessively fatigued, but the care of the wounded was the first consideration."

More compelling evidence refuted the charges made by Marcy and Barber about DeGrasse's condition after the Battle of Olustee. During the battle that day, Lieutenant Colonel Reed, who was in command of the regiment, was mortally wounded. Marcy wrote a letter to Reed's widow, making note that he personally took charge of the wounded officer until he was called back to the regiment, at which time "Dr. DeGrasse went with him [Reed] to Jacksonville where he was placed on board the Hospital Steamer."[35] It is extremely doubtful that Marcy would have entrusted the care of the acting commander of the regiment to an intoxicated surgeon.

A second claim of drunkenness on June 2, 1864, charged DeGrasse with being intoxicated while riding his horse with the regiment as they traveled between Milton and Jacksonville. He was accused of misappropriating liquor that day from the medical department for his own personal use. Once again, Barber, the hospital steward, claimed to have seen DeGrasse "under the influence of liquor" while riding with the hospital cook outside Jacksonville. He was "settled in his saddle like a drunken man," Barber testified, and "was incoherent in his talk." Barber also claimed that DeGrasse had taken a bottle of liquor from the hospital dispensary for his own use. Marcy corroborated Barber's claims, telling the court that he himself had filled the canteen with liquor to be used for medicinal purposes and had observed DeGrasse drinking from it throughout the day. One other officer, Lieutenant Holland W. Batchelder, believed DeGrasse was drinking, making that determination based on the way DeGrasse "looked" as he passed Batchelder. White officer Lieutenant Henry L. Stone contradicted the testimonies of Barber, Marcy, and Batchelder when he told the court that he saw DeGrasse in the morning and then later in the ambulance and his condition was not altered on either occasion. Two Black soldiers, First Sergeant Jesse Smith and Private John Lee, corroborated the testimony of Stone, telling the court that they both observed DeGrasse that day and saw nothing wrong. Lee described how he carried the medical knapsack containing medicines and supplies as he traveled alongside DeGrasse during the march to Jacksonville. They both came into camp ahead of the regiment, and upon their arrival DeGrasse asked for a tub of water and took a bath. Lee observed DeGrasse as being "very well" and not in an altered state. Elizabeth Dernsey, the regiment's laundress, corroborated Lee's testimony when she told the court "he appeared to be a sober man" when she saw him that day. Lee admitted to seeing DeGrasse take a small drink in the morning but did not see him drink at any other time during that day. Another Black private, Freeman Grice, clearly stated that on the march that day to Jacksonville, DeGrasse was not under the influence of liquor. "No sir," he told the court, "at no time that I know of."

DeGrasse remembered that day to be "excessively warm," and when he reached the camp he was drenched with perspiration, dirty, and fatigued. He called for a tub of water, bathed, and changed his clothing before lying down to rest. He had performed all of his duties that day and tended to the many soldiers who "fell out of the ranks requiring medical care." DeGrasse claimed that if he had been intoxicated on his arrival into camp, he would not have bathed and changed clothes first but would have gone straight to bed. It seems likely that if DeGrasse was intoxicated, his superior officers would have mentioned it to him the next morning or reprimanded him, but "on the contrary," he told the court, "not a word has been spoken or intimated until these charges were preferred."

As to the charges that he misappropriated liquor from the medical department, DeGrasse denied the claim, telling the court that although he did use the liquor for his personal use, it was within appropriate parameters: "In admitting the personal use of the Hospital Whiskey, I will state . . . that I used it for myself under the same circumstances, and in the same proportions that I administered to others—both officers and men. I would not gentlemen hesitate one moment in using Hospital Quinine, Hospital Morphine, or Hospital Castor Oil if I felt that I needed it, and Dr. Marcy would never had thought of preferring charges against me for so doing." It is interesting to note that on a previous occasion when DeGrasse had been accused of misappropriating liquor from the hospital stores for his own personal use, Beecher, the regiment's commander, responded to the charges by saying that DeGrasse was within army regulations when "dispensing hospital liquor to nurses and stretcher corps when on extra duty."[36] It was common for a regimental surgeon to dispense whiskey for medicinal purposes along with other medicines. Dr. Nathan Mayer of the 11th Connecticut Volunteer Infantry, who was with his regiment in the South, described in his unpublished memoirs how he administered whiskey to soldiers on an extended daylong march, writing, "In one pocket I carried quinine, in the other morphine and whiskey in my canteen."[37] Whiskey was often mixed with quinine and given to soldiers as a stimulant for fatigue and exhaustion. DeGrasse admitted to using the whiskey for himself and that he gave it "as often to men who manifested signs of fatigue and exhaustion." DeGrasse noted that the two ounces of whiskey Barber claimed he drank was taken because he was ill. Surgeons often self-administered medicines to themselves if they determined there was a medical need to do so.

A presumed third incident occurred on June 24, 1864, when Lieutenant Batchelder observed DeGrasse to be "rather the worse for liquor." In this instance, contradictory testimony was offered by Marcy, who admitted that he knew of "no neglect of duty during said time," though he did not definitively state that DeGrasse was sober. The final incident of drunkenness occurred at Darby's Station on July 25, when DeGrasse was found asleep on a stretcher after the regiment's arrival at camp. Beecher and Hawood both testified that DeGrasse was "under the influence of intoxicating liquor." Hawood claims he observed DeGrasse drinking during the day and Beecher found him in an "unsettled position on horseback," presumably from being intoxicated. Later that evening, after their arrival in camp, Beecher claimed DeGrasse was asleep on a stretcher and could not be roused due to his excessive drinking. Several other witnesses, including Sergeant Major Austin L. Topliff and Sergeant Harlan Loomis, both white, testified that DeGrasse was not intoxicated. Topliff had been riding near DeGrasse while the regiment was heading to camp. When they stopped, he spoke to DeGrasse and told the court he noticed "nothing unusual." When asked about DeGrasse's general deportment within the regiment, Topliff described him as a "gentleman." Loomis testified that he saw DeGrasse that day and during the march to camp. DeGrasse was "attending to his duties," he said; "I should say he was not intoxicated."

Although several alleged charges of excessive drinking and drunkenness were made against DeGrasse, the harshest and most damaging charge was conduct unbecoming an officer. The alleged incident involved a Black woman who worked on board the steamer *Mary Benton*, a transport vessel moving soldiers north and south on the St. John's River. DeGrasse was accused of making lewd remarks and gestures to the woman while on board the vessel. Lieutenant Batchelder testified that on July 23, he observed DeGrasse "in close proximity to a colored woman . . . using words and making gestures insulting to a woman" and sexual in nature. He said he had no doubt that DeGrasse "had been drinking too much" because of his "language and general appearance" and characterized him as "quiet and gentlemanly" when sober but "argumentative" when drunk. Batchelder's account of DeGrasse's drunkenness was corroborated by Second Lieutenant Isaac R. Barbour, who also observed DeGrasse as "under the influence of liquor" while he talked with "a colored woman the laundress." When Barbour was pressed to explain how he could tell DeGrasse was intoxicated, he said, "From his general conduct," but couldn't specify except to say "silliness perhaps." The Black witnesses, including Grice, Lee, Smith, and Patty, the woman DeGrasse allegedly insulted, all testified to his sober state. Patty told the court that she was the only woman on board the steamer and that DeGrasse had "behaved to me very well he didn't behave to me bad." Two white officers, Captain Benjamin F. Pierce and Second Lieutenant Samuel C. Ambler, also testified that DeGrasse was not drunk and they saw no unusual behavior from him. When Pierce was asked to describe DeGrasse's general reputation and deportment, he said it was "that of a Gentleman." He admitted seeing DeGrasse intoxicated before but never to the extent that he was "not able to attend to his duties as surgeon." In his own defense, DeGrasse pointed out that Barbour's determination of his intoxication based on the observation of "silliness" was ridiculous and unreasonable. Of the eight witnesses testifying to DeGrasse's condition and behavior that day, six observed him to be sober and proper while two claimed he was drunk and behaved poorly. The preponderance of the evidence seems to suggest that he was sober and his behavior reasonable.

After all testimony had been given, DeGrasse submitted a written statement to the court in his own defense. He presented his evidence refuting each charge based on the testimony given in court and his own account of the events. DeGrasse believed there were other intentions behind the charges: "Motives, hidden motives . . . prompted the preferment of these charges." He told the court, "These motives I can feel, though I can bring no evidence before this court to prove malicious. The uncommon and untiring assiduity with which Surgeon Marcy has worked up this case. His pretrial and constant attendance here for the past five days, using every effort and all the means in his power to procure a conviction—manifesting inside and outside the court as much interest as though it was a personal matter or a suit where his money interest was at stake."

There is evidence that substantiates DeGrasse's claims that the charges brought against him were racially motivated and intended to permanently remove him from the regiment. Numerous complaints had been lodged against DeGrasse by white officers, including those made by assistant surgeon Daniel Mann, who questioned DeGrasse's authority and his position in the regiment primarily because he was Black. Mann complained to medical director Major Horace R. Wirtz that DeGrasse had been placed "in the superior or at the least the most important position" and was "disposed to dispute my right to rank him." Wirtz expressed his concern to Major General Quincy Gilmore of the Department of the South over the presence of a white man and a Black man working alongside one another. He said, "As might be expected from this unfortunate combination difficulties have arisen of a much serious nature," namely the elevation of "the Negro doctor over the white one."[38] These complaints were a catalyst to the formal charges brought against DeGrasse and the court-martial that followed.

Equally damning to DeGrasse was the testimony of hospital steward Delos Barber, who portrayed DeGrasse as a drunken thief who was unable to fulfill his responsibilities as a regimental assistant surgeon. Barber had made it quite clear a year prior to the trial that he had an aversion to Black people when in June 1863 he requested a transfer to the 1st North Carolina Colored Volunteers in order to secure a promotion to hospital steward, but after learning about the Black surgeon who had been appointed to the regiment, he retracted his request. "When I wrote that request," he said, "I understood . . . that all the non-commissioned staff of the Reg were white men. I find upon examination that this is not the case. I also find one of the surgeons of the regiment to be a mulatto (which I did not know before). Under these circumstances I protest against the transfer and most humbly hope that it be not made."[39] Barber clearly did not want to serve with or be subordinate to a Black man, and by testifying against DeGrasse with a claim that he was unfit for his position, Barber hoped to have DeGrasse removed from the regiment.

Barber was not alone in the desire to remove DeGrasse, as evidenced by the testimony given by several white officers, including commanding officer Lieutenant James Beecher. Though considered an abolitionist, Beecher sided with his white regimental officers in DeGrasse's court-martial, testifying that he had seen DeGrasse drunk on several occasions. His testimony contradicts a response he gave to assistant surgeon Mann before the commencement of the court-martial proceedings. Mann had accused DeGrasse of intoxication and misappropriating the medical department's liquor. On this occasion, Beecher responded to the charges by saying that "there was not one instance brought to my notice of an intoxicated officer . . . a thing which can probably be said of no other regiment." He believed DeGrasse was within army regulations when "dispensing hospital liquor to nurses and stretcher corps when on extra duty."[40] In this instance, Beecher's response seems to be a defense of DeGrasse, but in reality, it was likely elicited from a concern with his own reputation. Beecher was a religious man and a strong proponent of temperance. An accusation that the regiment he commanded abused liquor was unacceptable and a direct reflection of his command. Further, alcohol abuse was a deeply personal issue for Beecher as his wife had been committed to a sanitarium for her abuse of alcohol and drugs. Although Beecher defended his regiment when this accusation of alcohol abuse was made, he was unwilling to defend DeGrasse for the same offense. If he had done so, he would have gone against the testimony of his white officers. Although he supported the idea of appointing Black officers to the regiment, he was unable to extend that support to DeGrasse during the court-martial proceedings. When his abolitionist ideals were put to the test, Beecher unequivocally failed.

It seems the motivation behind the court-martial was racism. Those who testified against DeGrasse and the panel of judges who decided his case intended to rid the regiment and the army of this highly educated, intelligent, and successful Black surgeon whom white officers saw as a threat to their dignity and their authority. In his defense, DeGrasse emphasized to the court his patriotism and his service as surgeon: "From the hour I landed at New Berne [*sic*], N.C. to raise this Regiment to the present time," he told the court, "my zeal and interest in its welfare have been unabated. My character as a gentleman and my upright deportment have never been questioned by officer or men until these I think unfounded charges were preferred. I am of course gentlemen, peculiarly interested in them, as my honor and reputation are at stake, not alone here in the army, but at home and wherever I am known. Trusting implicitly in your judgment and impartiality, and feeling you will do me justice." He spoke his truth as a good soldier but left his fate in the hands of the judges, hoping they would administer a fair and impartial decision.

After all testimony had been given and DeGrasse's written statement admitted as evidence, the courtroom was cleared. The panel of judges conducted what they considered a "mature deliberation" before returning with a guilty verdict on all charges. DeGrasse was sentenced to be cashiered. It seems the judges were neither fair nor impartial in rendering their decision. On October 27, a final statement was added to the written transcripts of the proceedings: "The proceedings, findings, and sentence in the foregoing case, having been approved by the officer ordering the Court, and submitted to the Major General Commanding the Department for this action thereon, are hereby approved and confirmed. Assistant Surgeon John V. DeGrasse ceases to be an officer of the United States service from this date." And thus, DeGrasse's military service was abruptly terminated.

DeGrasse returned to Boston and resumed his medical practice. It is hard to imagine that he was not affected by his experience as a surgeon during the war. He had witnessed the horrors of war while treating wounded soldiers on the field and faced blatant discrimination and a court-martial with little support from his superior officers. Notwithstanding the circumstances of his departure from the army, DeGrasse's service was recognized by Massachusetts governor John Andrew when he presented him with a gold-hilt sword for meritorious service during the war. Perhaps Governor Andrew recognized the difficulty that a Black soldier would have in finding favor in a military court against a white accuser and decided to honor DeGrasse because of his dedicated service in the army and his good reputation as a medical doctor. In 1868, four years after leaving his army service, DeGrasse fell ill with tuberculosis and died on November 24 at his home in Boston. He was forty-three years old.

6. Adventure and Ambition: John H. Rapier Jr. (1835–1866)

> Coloured men in the U.S. Uniform are much respected here, and in visiting the various Departments if the class is that of an Officer, you receive the military salute from the ground as promptly as if your blood was a Howard or Plantagenet instead of a Pompey or Cuffee's.
>
> —John H. Rapier Jr.

On August 14, 1864, John H. Rapier Jr. received his first pay for service as an acting assistant surgeon with the U.S. Army while serving at Freedmen's Hospital in Washington, D.C. His pleasure at receiving his monthly salary of $100 and his desire for advancement were palpable as he told his uncle of the "most eventful event of my life. My draft was in favor of 'Acting Asst. Surgeon Rank 1st Lieut. U.S.A." He added, "In the Spring, I want my drafts payable to Maj. John H. Rapier, Surg., U.S.A."[1]

John H. Rapier Jr. had an appetite for knowledge, and his search for a meaningful existence was never stilled throughout his short life. An eloquent writer, Rapier spent many hours writing letters to his family and friends, documenting his daily life in a diary, and composing expressive poetry and prose about his life, loves, and innermost feelings. Through his writings, he revealed himself to be an intelligent and sensitive person with a sense of duty, compassion, and humor. He was a keen observer of the world with a passion for purposeful adventure and an ambition to be more than what was expected of a Black man in nineteenth-century America, and he filled his days with travel, politics, study, family, and service. His family roots and the examples set by his strong grandmother, loving father, and successful uncle influenced and encouraged him in his pursuits. Their strength, perseverance, hard work, and commitment to attaining a free and better life fostered the self-sufficiency and self-preservation that stayed with him as he navigated through the world.

John H. Rapier Jr. was born free to Susan and John H. Rapier Sr. on July 28, 1835, in Florence, Alabama, the second of four sons.[2] He was part of a family that included both free and enslaved family members—a free mother and father, an enslaved grandmother and stepmother, and free and enslaved siblings. He was raised primarily by his grandmother Sally Thomas in Nashville, Tennessee, after the death of his mother. His grandmother's example of strength and determination helped set him on a path to success.

Sally Thomas was born enslaved in 1787 and grew up on the plantation of enslaver Charles L. Thomas in Virginia. She had three sons, John Sr. and Henry, born in Virginia and likely fathered by a member of the Thomas family, and James, fathered by John Catron, a white Tennessee lawyer and U.S. Supreme Court justice.[3] Although Sally's three sons were born of white men of wealth and position, they were considered enslaved persons as dictated by law that declared all children of enslaved women were also enslaved. This did not deter Sally from finding a path to freedom for her children.

Sally and her two oldest boys lived on a plantation in Albemarle County, Virginia, in the early 1800s. When their enslaver died, they were shipped off to Nashville, Tennessee, to another member of the Thomas family. Nashville was a city that offered new opportunities for enterprising Black people. By the time of her arrival, the city's overall population numbered more than three thousand with a market-house, two banks, two printing offices, several factories, a courthouse, and a jail.[4] Enslaved Black people sometimes hired themselves out for work with their enslavers' permission, which enabled them to earn their own money while providing much-needed services to the white community. Sally could not read or write, but she was a smart, skilled, hard-working, and entrepreneurial-minded woman driven by her desire to secure freedom for her sons. Sally established her own laundry business within the city with the permission of her enslaver. She rented a small house where she washed and cleaned clothes for wealthy white Nashvillians and manufactured soap. Her children helped her run errands, assist in the shop, and gather wood for the stove. Sally's business allowed her to approach employers, arrange for work, and retain a portion of her earnings.[5] Working independently benefited her enslaver by relieving him of responsibility for her while still retaining a share of her earnings.

She grew her business, being careful not to appear arrogant, dispute a customer, or cause controversy that could threaten her business or her position. Sally navigated through the white world cautiously, remaining observant and learning the nuances of nineteenth-century race relations. Her mind was focused on securing freedom for her children. She used her business as a means to achieve that goal by saving as much money as she could and becoming familiar with her white customers who might be able to assist her.

As her business grew, so did her reputation for quality work. As a result, she had a long list of loyal customers and more work than she could handle.[6] Still, Sally knew it would be nearly impossible to save enough money to buy her sons' freedom, so she set out to find another path for them utilizing her good reputation and her connections with her white clients. For her sons to be free, she knew they would have to leave Nashville. She made arrangements for her oldest son, John Sr., to be hired as a "pole boy" and personal servant to barge captain Richard Rapier. John Sr. would help propel the barge through the water and provide for the needs of the captain. Captain Rapier was well known in Nashville with a good reputation, and he willingly took on the ten-year-old in his employ. When he moved his business from Nashville to Florence, Alabama, John Sr. went along and would eventually make Florence his permanent home.

Sally hoped that someday Rapier would free her son. She learned some years later that he had made a provision in his will that set aside money to purchase John Sr. from the Thomas estate in Virginia. After Captain Rapier's death in 1826, the executors of his estate carried out the barge master's wishes by purchasing John Sr. for $1,000, even though it took three more years to obtain permission from the Alabama General Assembly to finally make him a free man.[7] While working for Captain Rapier, John Sr. had learned to read and write, proving invaluable to him as he navigated the business world in Florence. He paid homage to his emancipator by permanently taking the name John H. Rapier. Now a free man, he was able to establish a business of his own in town and begin his new life in freedom.

Life in Florence was relatively good for John Sr. He built a thriving barbershop business and married Susan, a free "mulatto" woman from Baltimore with whom he had four sons, Richard, John H. Jr., Henry, and James Thomas. He was a hardworking man who was dedicated to providing a good life for his family. John Sr. believed in the importance of education and always encouraged his children in their studies. He impressed this upon John Jr., telling him, "I hope you will not omit any opportunity of emproving your self for knowledge is cappitle."[8] John Sr. kept up regular correspondence with his sons throughout his life. A loving and caring parent, his letters were filled with fatherly advice and guidance on farming, real estate, business, education, and daily living. He encouraged them to find suitable employment, settle down, and live an exemplary life. "I am tyard of seeing that rambling disposition in my children for it no pleasure to me my Son," he wrote to John Jr.[9] "You will do what is right and submit to nothing that is wrong. You know my son I have all ways advise you to do what is right to all men. Treat your self right is the next thing my son. In doing that you must keep clear of gambling and drinking, use industry and economy."[10] He knew as a parent that his sons might not always appreciate his advice and said, "It true, I may write things to you that may be unpleasant to your feeling at this time, you should remember that is from one who have the love of your welfare at his heart and feel it his duty to write plain to you."[11]

John Sr. and his young sons suffered a devastating loss in 1841 when Susan died in childbirth along with her twin boys, Jackson and Alexander.[12] It was a profound loss especially for six-year-old John Jr. Many years later, the death of his mother was still raw. "Death! Relentless Death! . . . ," he wrote; "I have nursed my irreparable loss to keep its voice ever before my eyes as it is ever in my heart. . . . The clods that pressed my mothers bosom, have weighed heavily on mine since that unhappy event, and time only makes my sorrow the deeper, my grief the more poignant."[13] After Susan's death, it was difficult for John Sr. to maintain his business and raise four young sons. His only option was to send two of his children, John Jr. and James, to live with his mother, Sally, in Nashville.[14] Sally provided a stable home life for her two grandsons along with her own youngest son, James, only eight years older than John Jr. She understood the importance of education and sent John Jr. and James to the same school that their uncle James had attended. John Jr. was a precocious child and showed great promise in his studies. His father was proud of him and told his oldest son, Richard, that John Jr. "wrote me two letters and he writes very plain for a boy of his age and practice, and has much taste for reading as any child I know and very good in arithmetic."[15] John Jr.'s precocious nature was reflected in his relationship with a local attorney. After a fire in the attorney's home, John Jr. was given several damaged books from the lawyer's library that he "eagerly devoured" in his thirst for knowledge.[16]

Though they were separated by over one hundred miles, John Sr. was an attentive father to his two sons. "I have not been to Nashville since last April," he wrote in a letter to his brother Henry in 1843. "I want to see them all very much. John and James are well pleased with their grandmother and don't want to come home."[17] The two boys had settled in with their grandmother and remained with her until her death in 1850, when they returned to Florence. John Jr. was eventually sent to live with his uncle Henry Thomas in Buffalo, New York, where he could further his education.[18]

Henry Thomas was an enterprising man who had been born enslaved in Virginia. As a young man and with his mother's encouragement, he escaped

and traveled north, settling in Buffalo, where he established a successful barbershop. Henry lived a relatively comfortable life with his wife and two children, but his concerns for the safety of his family weighed heavily on him
because of his status as a formerly enslaved man. The passage of the Fugitive
Slave Act in 1850 and news that an enslaver was in Buffalo to "retrieve one of
his runaway slaves" increased his concerns for the safety of himself and his
family. He decided to sell his business and move his family across the border
into Canada.[19]

Along with his wife, children, and nephew John Jr., Henry moved to the
newly established Elgin Settlement in Buxton, Ontario. Canada had become
a safe haven for Black people since slavery was abolished in the country. As
free persons violating no law, they were protected against extradition by an
enslaver. Buxton was the ideal location for John Jr. and his uncle Henry, who
both sought greater opportunities for education and advancement. Located
close to Lake Erie, Buxton was a predominantly Black community that offered social and economic opportunities to Black people. Residents could own
land and children could receive an academic education at the Buxton Mission
School.[20] The school was considered progressive and offered a classical academic curriculum.[21] Many residents of the community had settled in Buxton
specifically for the educational opportunities offered to their children. Among
those who attended the school were John Jr. and Canadian-born Anderson
R. Abbott, who would, like John Jr., serve as a surgeon during the American
Civil War.[22]

John Jr. returned to the United States in 1853, after spending eighteen
months attending school in Buxton and living with his uncle Henry. His
return to Alabama gave him an opportunity to spend time with his father,
stepmother, and younger siblings. He corresponded frequently with his uncle
James, with whom he had lived nearly ten years at his grandmother's home.
They had developed a close relationship that would last throughout his life.
"Those years I passed in your house and under your kind supervision," he
wrote his uncle, "are often secured to with all the respect that filial regard
gratitude and respect can inspire. No Father, I am fully aware, ever en-
vinced kinder interest and deep solicitude in his own childs welfare than you
for mine."[23]

James P. Thomas, the youngest son of Sally Thomas, was an example of
intelligence, adventure, curiosity, ambition, and success. As a child, he was
adventurous and inquisitive. He would "visit the slave quarters on nearby
plantations, attend Black religious gatherings, listen to speeches at political

gatherings, and venture into back alleys along the river front."[24] At age twelve, his mother arranged for him to work as an assistant to a prominent Nashville physician. From that experience, James transitioned to the barber trade, taking a position as an apprentice with a local barber in town. After a five-year apprenticeship, he opened his own barbershop at the age of nineteen, in the same house where his mother had her laundry business. As his business grew, he began to acquire real estate. He traveled widely, opening his eyes to the world and gaining a better understanding of the place and position of Black people in society outside of the South. John Jr. admired his uncle James and shared many of the same concerns over the increasing hostility toward Black people in the United States and the desire to seek out a place outside the country where conditions and opportunities for Black people would be improved. The concerns and desires they shared strengthened their relationship and motivated them to seek a freer, more prosperous life.

The Rapier-Thomas family had achieved great success for a southern Black family in the mid-nineteenth century. But despite their achievements, they still felt discontent living in a country where most Black people were enslaved and prejudice was a part of daily life. No one felt this discontent more than John Jr. His disenchantment with the United States was so deep that he made a solemn vow to his uncle James, saying, "Rest assured that never, so help me God if I can help it, will I ever again live in any country where I am a 'damn nigger' and nothing more."[25]

John Jr. kept up with world current affairs while in Florence and began following the news of William Walker, a white Nashville native who was intent on establishing English-speaking colonies in Mexico and Latin America. John Jr. was intrigued with this idea as a possible solution to finding a place where people of color could immigrate in order to gain freedom and prosperity. He had already expressed an interest in leaving the country. In late 1854 and early 1855, he spoke of his desire to join with the American Colonization Society and immigrate to Liberia. "I am serious in my idea of Emigrating," he said; "in this Country I can not live."[26] When he learned of Walker's plans, it reignited his interest in emigration. Walker was a well-educated, charismatic physician and lawyer as well as a sometime journalist. Easily bored with a routine life, Walker constantly sought out new challenges. A proponent of the idea of "manifest destiny," the belief that the United States was destined to expand its domain and gain control over North America, Walker decided to establish a colony outside the United States in 1853. He was among like-minded people in the mid-nineteenth century known as filibusters, who would form armed expeditions against outside nations in order to gain private rule over a country, eventually leading to complete control of North America by the United States.[27]

During a visit to his uncle James in Nashville in late 1855, John Jr. spoke enthusiastically about Walker's intentions in Central America to uplift the people and provide a safe haven for Black people emigrating from America. He showed his uncle a newspaper article describing Walker's invasion of Nicaragua and his plan to form a new government that would offer emigrants two hundred acres of free land and free passage to the country. James had known Walker when James was a boy in Nashville, so when his nephew announced his intention to go to Nicaragua and join forces with Walker, he agreed to join him, although he was at first reluctant.[28]

John Jr. and his uncle James boarded the steamer *Daniel Webster* on February 12, 1856, in New Orleans bound for Greytown, Nicaragua.[29] A few weeks after their arrival, they realized Walker's plans were far from what they expected. Walker intended to create a dictatorship that would reintroduce enslavement with no system to improve the condition of the country's inhabitants or emigrants from the United States. John Jr.'s hopes that this newly formed government would be a safe haven for people of color was not to be. Disheartened and disenchanted, John Jr. and his uncle made plans to return to the United States. In April, they sailed from Nicaragua to Panama, then on to Cuba, and finally to New Orleans. In Cuba, they were joined by Parker H. French, a white associate of Walker's who was also traveling back to the United States. During the voyage, French offered John Jr. a job as his personal secretary, which he accepted. He traveled on with him to New York City, eventually settling in Little Falls, Minnesota. When John Sr. learned of his son's employment with French, he said, "I believe your good sence will promp you to do what you know to be right and when you have done that I am shore that gentleman will do nothing but what is Honorable and may be the means of placing you in a way of doing better then you have been doing in the way of making a living for your self as he is a man of standing."[30] John Sr. always encouraged and advised his son on how to succeed in life and conduct himself in a honorable manner.

By the spring of 1856, John Jr. was settled into life in Little Falls. Centrally located in Minnesota, Little Falls sits along the northern Mississippi River, a major source of transportation and commerce that attracted white explorers and speculators to the area. A fort was established in 1848 by the federal government to maintain control of the area's resources and monitor several

Native American tribes that had settlements on the outskirts of the city. A dam and sawmill were built in 1849 and a town formally established in 1854.[31] John Jr. lived a relatively uneventful life in Little Falls but fell ill with a fever at the beginning of the new year. His illness resulted in the loss of his job and the refusal by French to pay him the wages he was owed. Incensed about the situation, he proclaimed that "while I was in this helpless condition, Col. P. H. French saw fit to discharge me."[32] Adamant about getting his back pay, he reluctantly accepted an offer from French to travel with him to California in exchange for his past wages once he recovered. Although he agreed to make the journey, John Jr. had no intention of going to California with French. His diary entry for February 5, 1857, made note that his agreement to accompany French was only "to get my pay from him for past services. I will go with him to St. Paul and there bid him a final adieu. The d——n scoundrel."[33] French had a reputation as an adventurer, entrepreneur, and swindler. He had executed several dubious plans in the past that conned people out of money, and when he served in Walker's government in Nicaragua, he had been dismissed as a result of legal problems. Whether John Sr. knew his son was working for a man with a sullied reputation is not clear, but he expressed concern for the company that John Jr. might keep. "My son," he said, "I hope you will take my advice I have often give you that is to mind your own business and keep out of bad company. I hope your sence will prompt to pursue that course."[34] In an effort to discredit John Jr., French vilified him in the Minnesota press, accusing him of quitting his job and stealing.[35] John Jr. made efforts to discount French's slanderous remarks by writing rebuttals to several newspapers. In his diary, he made note that he "replied through the same medium, but as yet am uninformed with what result."[36]

He finally parted ways with French and moved on to other opportunities to make a living. Little Falls and the surrounding area were still in their infancy when he had arrived, and he took advantage of new prospects in the growing area. He joined forces with an Englishman in early February to establish a hotel in a nearby town, but nothing came of the venture. He found employment for a time as a clerk and wrote articles for several newspapers, including the *Little Falls Northern Herald*, the *Minnesota Weekly Times*, and the *St. Paul Democrat*. His writing touched on a variety of topics, from politics and civil rights to snuff and the weather. He did not shy away from expressing his opinion on current events. In "Have Colored Children Rights?," he admonished the St. Paul Board of Education about its plan to place limits on the number of Black children who could attend school. He argued that all

Black citizens paid taxes the same as white citizens and were entitled to an education without restriction.[37]

In an effort to make ends meet while living in Minnesota, Rapier attempted to economize his lifestyle by cutting some of his "most expensive acquaintances" and giving up drinking, smoking, and gambling.[38] He was pleased when he was able to save money. "I have by dint of hard labour and economy," he wrote, "been enabled to place to my credit at Truman Smith's Bank the sum of $100. More money than I ever had before at one time of my earnings." He admitted at the end of 1858 that he had not economized as strictly as his "necessities and even wishes advised." Acquiring wealth was, for Rapier, a sign of achievement and stature. He believed it was "natural to desire the accumulation of wealth and the world believes it to be a laudable ambition to indulge this desire. . . . It is man's first duty to make money and his second, but no less imperative one is to save it." Earning and saving money was a strong motivation in all Rapier's endeavors. He believed having wealth elevated one's reputation. "The most reserved and select parlors are thrown open to you," he said, and "your faults are never seen through your Gold, your virtues are enhanced a hundred times."[39]

Though he had tightened his purse strings, he was able to maintain a moderate social life, occasionally attending concerts and the theater and going out with friends and female companions. John Jr. was affable, charming, and attractive, often professing his love for his female friends through prose and poetry. He spoke kindly and lovingly about them and was a thoughtful romantic who was unafraid to express his deepest feelings through his writing. He declared his undying love to them, and they, in turn, wrote back to him with "nothing but protestations of eternal attachment."[40]

Despite participating in social outings and cultural activities, life in Little Falls did not hold much excitement for him. When listing his expenses for 1857, he made note that "this year like the last has been ushered in on my part by idleness."[41] He aspired to more than his current situation afforded: "I feel often, very often that fate decreed me for a more bustling, busy life than the quiet and monotonous me that I lead. I feel that I am destined to rise to a point above my present."[42]

Though he found nothing of real interest in Little Falls, he was captivated by the Minnesota winter. It made such an impression on this Southern-born man that he wrote about the season in several diary entries and newspaper articles. The inclement winter weather kept him inside much of the time, and he often contemplated the conditions outside his window. It was "stormy and disagreeable," he wrote, with temperatures forty degrees below zero. While his observation of how winter "strips the magnificent trees of their lovely foliage" seems almost as harsh as the season, he also welcomed winter as a time to "gather in social circles about the broad and blazing hearthstones and forget the cares and sorrows of life." Despite the winter's invitation to socialize with friends in front of a warm fire, he did not fail to recognize those in need, reminding his readers not to "forget the poor and homeless wanderer who hath not where to lay his head . . . if he falls in your way, relieve his wants." He revealed a level of awareness and sensitivity to those less fortunate than himself. When winter finally ended, he couldn't be happier: "It scarcely seems a day since the cold breath of winter chilled all upon whom it chanced to fall," he wrote, " . . . but now instead of freezing breath of 'Father Grey Beard' we have the genial atmosphere of Summers."[43]

Much of what we learn of John Jr. during the late 1850s is revealed through his diary entries between 1857 and 1859. He made notes on his moods, his reflections on life, and his observations of the weather and other eventful experiences. In addition to his intellectual streams of thought and his beautifully crafted poetic words, he recorded the mundane aspects of his life, including letters received and written, names of correspondents, and monthly expenses. Money was spent on room and board along with purchases of clothing and supplies like pants, socks, undershirts, and blank books for writing. He also logged expenditures for washing, medicine, and the occasional theater ticket. In one notation, he casually referenced money "given away to a beggar." These few years of his recorded thoughts and impressions are invaluable in gaining insight and understanding of the daily life of a free, educated Black man in America.

John Jr.'s twenty-second birthday brought these reflective words about his own existence and death:

> Curse the day that first witnessed my advent into this mundane sphere and home of woe. Had I but fallen still born from my mother's womb, what a world of humble would I have been saved. . . . But all mariners on the Sea of Life is doomed to sail through the breakers of death ere they reach the Harbour of rest. Tis only in the grave that the Anchor of Peace can be dropped with the certainty that the storms of tomorrow will not drag its chain and dash the Barque into atoms. . . .
>
> But I should welcome the return of my natal day with rapture, as each return but brings me nearer home, nearer a union with my Angel

Mother, Brothers and Sisters, who have interrupted the flight of their years of probation in this naked world—who have to commemorate through eternity the great birthday—known to us as death. What a misnomer! To call that death which is in reality life, and indeed what only is life. For can we call that life which is only a pathway to the grave. A passport to the tomb. We fade only to bloom in eternity.[44]

He grasped the complexity and brevity of an earthly existence and seemed to have no fear of death, viewing it as a freeing from life's struggles and a chance to be reunited with loved ones in a peaceful, beautiful eternity. In his prophetic poem titled "Death," he wrote,

> Let me die young, while the hearts free & light
> While the genial Sun glows—ere the shades of might
> Fall o'er my soul, and darken the day
> When happily Death, shall steal life away.[45]

Perhaps this thinking allowed him to be adventurous, to take risks, to enjoy the luxuries and modesties of life, to see the good and the bad, and to continue to seek out a purposeful and meaningful existence.

By 1860, he was living in Atchison, Kansas, near his uncle James, who had invested in property there. Working as a barber, he shared a residence with a fellow barber from Ohio.[46] Despite his employment, he was restless and expressed his discontent at being unsettled.[47] Always with an ear to current events and a desire for a better life, he again contemplated leaving the country, this time for Haiti. Haiti was a symbol of racial independence and freedom in antebellum America. A slave rebellion in 1791 started a revolution in the country that resulted in the establishment of a republic dominated by Black people. The success of the revolution instilled a sense of racial independence and power in the Black Haitian population and made Haiti an attractive place to immigrate. The new Black-run government, in an effort to attract Black Americans, began to collaborate with the American Colonization Society, boasting of the new economic opportunities open to people of color in Haiti.[48]

Attracted by the idea of living and working in a place that welcomed Black people, John Jr. traveled to New Orleans in mid-November 1860 and sailed for the Caribbean the following month with $100 in his pocket. The voyage was long but "tolerable agreeable" and "as monotonous as anything well can be. You see the sun rise, you see the sun set, and you hear the Captain and his

Mate give their orders for working the vessel, and you feel seasick and this is all."[49] After the eighteen-day voyage, he arrived in Haiti. "I have the pleasure of informing you that I reached this Island safely, on the 27th ult," he wrote the *Leavenworth Conservative*. "I suffered some little from sea-sickness, but not seriously." His first days in Haiti were spent in the village of St. Marc, forty miles from the capital of Port-au-Prince. Although he could not speak the native language, he got by with hand gestures and admitted to having trouble figuring out the currency.[50] After a short time in St. Marc he left for Port-au-Prince, where he sought work as an English teacher, but he was unsuccessful in securing a teaching position.[51] Finding himself without employment, he spent time traveling around the country visiting several cities and towns.

As a self-identified "quadroon," born and raised in the South, Rapier was well aware of the effect of skin complexion on one's social and economic opportunities.[52] His desire to travel to the Caribbean was based partly on a belief that his color would be less of a hindrance to his success there than in the United States. Although he had left the divisiveness and segregation of race in America, the issue of color, status, and class were clearly evident to him in Haiti. He described Port-au-Prince as a city with a population of thirty-five thousand, "about two-thirds . . . mixed-bloods and whites," with the majority living in large towns and cities near the coast. Most were of the professional class of lawyers, merchants, and businessmen. People of darker complexions, referred to as Blacks or "negroes," were found most often in the country's interior and were the "pure and unadulterated brethren" of the "mixed-bloods and colored."[53] This distinction of color and complexion by Rapier's terminology hints at both his own biased attitudes and the stereotypes of race and race relations in Haiti at the time.

Race, complexion, and class were issues Rapier observed and experienced throughout his travels in Haiti and Jamaica and brought his own prejudices to the surface. He considered the behavior of the local Black Haitian population as erratic and undignified, giving him an impression that the country was chaotic and disorderly. He commented on Black Haitians to his uncle James, saying, "The Negro race removed from the presence and influences of the white race is incapable of self-government. And today the Haytiens are more barbaric and primitive in their habits and customs and far less intellectual then they were when they achieved their independence." Advising his uncle James, he said that if he was to go to any country, it should be one where "the negro race" is not predominant: "If you wish to emigrate from the United States let me give you as my candid opinion, that it is altogether unjust to yourself to go to any country where the negro race, predominate in ruling numbers. . . . I came here considerably tinctured and spotted with abolitionism and universal freedom but I am now entirely cured of these symptoms of insanity . . . and if I ever make my permanent home, in a country where negroes live in any considerable quantities, it will be where they are slaves."[54] Although Rapier self-identified as a "quadroon," he often separated himself from those identified as "Black" or "negro" whom he considered to be less refined with no ambition. He explained his thoughts to his uncle James, saying, "To the better and more thorough understanding of my letters, you must always bear in mind when I speak of Negroes, I never include Col'd people for they are as distinct from the Blacks as education, cultivation, refinement, and social position are from ignorance, coarseness and stupidity."[55]

After only four months, he became disillusioned with Haiti and headed to Jamaica. In April 1861, he sailed two days on the steamer *Saladin* bound for Kingston. He fell ill with a fever when he arrived and was housebound for several days. Once Rapier recovered, he went out among the local population and surroundings. His impressions of Kingston were not favorable and he described it as "the most woe begone city in the West Indies . . . with broken and rotten wharves, empty warehouses, deserted harbor, and whole blocks of fine fire proof store houses locked up and unoccupied."[56] As he had observed in Haiti, the impact of color and complexion did not go unnoticed in Jamaica, and the animosity between light- and dark-skinned people was clear. "Kingston is the heaven of the West Indies based upon the color of the skin," he said. "The white shows no prejudice to the mixed bloods, but will never employ," and only "bayonets keep the negro from murdering the mulattoes, who are insolent and overbearing to an insufferable degree."[57]

In Kingston, Rapier once again found himself unemployed. He considered establishing himself as a cotton grower but was dissuaded by the lack of funding. A chance meeting with a Canadian dentist, Dr. Beckett, led him in a new direction.[58] Beckett convinced him that dentistry would be a more reliable and profitable source of income. He bragged about making $200 a week over a three-month period "under the guise of a Dentist" and suggested that Rapier "study the science of 'teeth manipulation' under this tuition offering . . . board and lodging" in Beckett's house.[59] Rapier accepted Beckett's offer and was paid $5 per week for the opportunity to study "surgeon dentistry." He threw himself into his studies, telling his uncle James, "I am pushing along with all speed possible in my new profession of Dentist." He even jokingly boasted, "Aren't you proud of your promising nephew—when I see you, I will just pull out two of your front teeth to show you how it is done." As he progressed in dentistry, he developed pride in his work and expressed his ambitions in this field. "I am learning and already have a fair knowledge of a profession by which I can make an honorable and respectable living without being an 'intelligent darkey'—and still with this determination, I expect one day to see a neatly painted sign hanging over a door . . . that will let the passerby know that there lives 'John H. Rapier, Dentist.'"[60]

He spent the winter months under Beckett's tutelage, but by February 1862 he had decided to switch his studies to medicine under the supervision of a local physician, Dr. James Scott. "A Medical Gentlemen offers to permit me to read medicine under his direction gratis while I am pursuing my duties as a Dentist," he told his uncle, "and also, assures me that in 18 months, I will be fitted to enter McGill University of Montreal or the Queen's College in Toronto."[61] Always ambitious, he believed that a physician held a higher social position and a more enhanced reputation than a dentist. For Rapier, a career as a physician was a better choice of profession, and he immediately took to his medical studies, telling his uncle, "[I] am up to my eyes in the medical nomenclature. . . . While physiology is also receiving attention . . . anatomy is a beautiful study and I take a corresponding interest in it."[62] Though he was fully entrenched in the study of medicine in Jamaica, his sights were set on returning home to attend college in the United States or Canada. He informed his uncle James of his plans, reviewing his anticipated expenses for the first six months of college and asking his uncle to "throw me a rope occasionally for the first term." He believed he could teach school and practice dentistry to provide himself with the means to cover his expenses after the first term of medical school but needed assistance from his uncle to get started.[63] John Jr. entertained the idea of delivering lectures on Haiti and Jamaica to earn extra money. With a large enough audience, he felt he could secure sufficient funds to sustain his college education, and he enlisted his uncle's help in deciding the wisdom of such an idea.

By this time, civil war had broken out in the United States, and Rapier quickly became aware of its effects on his family. He kept abreast of the situation through family letters and the occasional newspaper from New York. The safety and well-being of his family was at the forefront of his mind. "I think a great deal of you and father," he wrote his uncle, "and the children in dark clouds that are hovering around the political horizon of the United States." His concerns were mitigated to some degree by the confidence he had in his uncle James to come to his father's aid "in any emergency that may arise in which your aid can serve him and them." He even considered immediately returning to the United States, telling his uncle that the steamer that took his letter "came near taking me." His grave concerns for his family ran deep. "I am ill at ease," he told his uncle, "when I remember that everything that I hold dear in the world, and without whose presence I would not care to live, are surrounded by dangers and probably destruction." He reiterated his reliance on his uncle to aid his father and siblings and knew his own ability to assist was limited due to the distance between himself and his family. Still, Rapier was determined to be of whatever help he could. He believed it was his "solemn duty to do so, at all and every hazard."[64] His concern for his father's ability to support the family especially during this period of civil war was clear. "Father pecuniary speaking," he expressed to his uncle, "will be stripped of nearly every dollar that he possesses. All his means are in the hands of the secessionists." Rapier knew his father was at a low point and described him "as bankrupt in spirit and energy as he is in pocket," making it impossible for him to support his family. His father would need to rely on him "to perform these sacred duties towards this family which . . . time and misfortune ally to prevent his [John Sr.] accomplishing."[65] His younger brother James offered a glimmer of hope when he told John Jr. that the Union troops were "making good heading down south. They have been to Florence and every body Unionists there."[66] Rapier was dedicated and devoted to his father, stepmother, and five younger stepsiblings. He believed it was his responsibility along with his uncle's to provide for them, and his decision to become a physician was partly influenced by this belief. As a physician, he knew his salary would be enough to support himself and his family. "The surest and the cheapest way to do this," he said, "is to educate me for the duties and responsibilities of teacher and guardian to this large family. Now if I graduate as a Physician as I sure will, I shall by my social and cultivated position be able to assume these responsibilities which will be an act of humanity and justice to them and honour and pleasure to myself."[67]

In late May 1862, Rapier finally headed back home, sailing to New York on the schooner *Dolphin*. He made his way to Ohio and enrolled in Oberlin College. Rapier was listed in the college catalog as a resident of Kingston, Jamaica, identifying himself as a foreigner rather than an American, fully understanding the advantages his identification as a foreigner provided him.[68] Oberlin had a reputation as a center for abolitionist activities and perhaps was the reason it attracted Black students, including Alpheus W. Tucker, a member of the "junior class" for 1863, and Charles B. Purvis, who attended from 1860 to 1863. Tucker and Purvis would later serve as surgeons during the Civil War.

Rapier left Oberlin in July 1863 to enroll at the University of Michigan in Ann Arbor and study medicine. As a person of color identified as a foreigner in the school's catalog, he likely faced less controversy being admitted and attending classes.[69] The university perceived him first as a foreigner and then as a person of color. This seemingly small but significant perception made him more accepted as a Black student and less likely to be subjected to mistreatment. Though he was aware of the advantages he gained by this identification, it did not make him less observant of the treatment of his fellow Black students. "The University has been thrown into convulsions during the last ten days," he reported to his cousin Sarah, "because an 'American of African descent' dared to present himself as a candidate for admission to the medical class."[70] That classmate was Alpheus W. Tucker, with whom he had been an undergraduate at Oberlin College. Tucker and Rapier followed a similar educational path, going from undergraduate studies at Oberlin College to pursuing a medical degree at both the University of Michigan in Ann Arbor and then at Keokuk Medical College in Iowa, but their experiences were different. When Tucker arrived at the university, Rapier made note that Tucker had come to the university based on the knowledge that "a col'd gentleman from the West Indies had been admitted to the Med Dept." But despite this fact, Tucker was forced out of the medical school, making it clear that "col'd men are not admitted here." Tucker's friends were furious at Rapier when the university removed Tucker but retained Rapier as a student. "They say I pretend to be a white man when I am nothing but a 'Nigger,'" he told his cousin, making note of Tucker's darker skin tone.[71] He understood how complexion could influence a person's ability to receive an education and advance in society. His own light complexion and perceived origins from the West Indies allowed him to continue his medical studies with little disturbance, while Tucker, who had a darker complexion, was refused the opportunity. Although Rapier was not "passing" as white to obtain an education, his lighter complexion aided him in achieving his goal.

Eager to complete his formal medical education as soon as possible, he left Michigan for Keokuk, Iowa, in February 1864 to attend the medical school of Iowa State University, also known as Keokuk Medical College. By beginning classes immediately when he arrived in Keokuk, he would be able to graduate by early summer of 1864 rather than March 1865, if he remained in Michigan. He anticipated a smooth transition because he self-identified as a man from Jamaica in Iowa: "What a blessed thing for me, that I was born in Jamaica, it enables me to enter any college without questions of lineage. Though my cuticle may be dingied by the heat of an intertropical sun," he quipped, "I am not of the tribe of Ham —Ah! Me. I pity poor col'd persons born in America."[72]

Keokuk is located in the far southeastern corner of Iowa at the junction of the Mississippi River and the Des Moines River. It was a center of commerce, transportation, and military activity during the Civil War, serving as a hub for the departure of Iowa regiments to join with U.S. forces in the East and South. Several hospitals were established during the war to attend to sick and wounded soldiers, including the U.S. Army General Hospital with sixteen wards, 1,350 beds, and a medical college unit.[73] Thousands of soldiers from the South were brought to the city for care and treatment, transported on hospital ships up the Mississippi River. Keokuk Medical College was a midsize school and offered the usual course of study for the mid-1800s, including anatomy, materia medica, physiology, chemistry, medical jurisprudence, obstetrics, and pathology. A course of study in military surgery was also offered where after successful completion of the course, students could qualify for medical staff positions with the army. The school catalog boasted of a new building with "a City Dispensary, where the poor receive gratuitous advice and attention . . . a large lecture room, chemical laboratory and apparatus room." It had a library, study rooms for practical anatomy, and an amphitheater for anatomical and surgical demonstrations.[74]

As a student at the college, Rapier paid a fee of forty dollars for a four-month course of instruction, including six lectures each day. There was a five-dollar matriculation fee, a five-dollar demonstrator's fee, and a thirty-dollar graduation fee. Candidates for graduation needed to be at least twenty-one years old, be of good moral character, have attended two full courses of lectures, and have studied for three years under the direction of a respectable medical practitioner. In addition, they were required to pass an examination given by the faculty and submit a satisfactory medical thesis on an original topic in their own handwriting. Rapier completed all the necessary requirements for graduation by the summer of 1864, including the submission of his thesis, "The True Physician." Of the eighty-two theses that were submitted, John Jr.'s was the only one that did not directly relate to a disease, illness, or treatment but likely was focused more on the inner qualities required to be a physician. It is interesting to note that in addition to Rapier's attendance at the medical school, three other men of color were enrolled at the medical college at the same time—J. D. Harris of Cleveland, Ohio, graduating the same year as Rapier, and Alpheus W. Tucker of Washington, D.C., and Charles H. Taylor of Kingston, Jamaica, both graduating the following year.[75]

The influence of his medical training at Keokuk and his desire to serve during the war led Rapier to request a position in the army as a medical officer in April 1864. "I am desirous of entering the Medical of the Gov.," he wrote; "I will graduate in June, and would beg of you the knowledge of the proper method of making application." In this case, Rapier identified himself as "a native of Alabama and of *African descent*," a requirement to gain a position in the U.S. Army.[76] In June, he made a second request for a position as acting assistant surgeon. Rapier described his education and made it clear that he was a person of color describing himself as "a quadroon of southern birth."[77] A note in his army medical personnel file remarked, "Proper testimonials of professional acquaintances and character, a contract will be made with him."[78] A contract for service as an acting assistant surgeon was issued to him on June 29, 1864. He would enter the army with an officer's rank of lieutenant and be paid $100 per month. Rapier was instructed to report for duty to acting assistant surgeon William P. Powell Jr., surgeon-in-charge of Contraband Camp Hospital in Washington, D.C.[79]

When Rapier arrived, the hospital was under Powell's direction, but by late 1864 Powell had resigned and Anderson R. Abbott had replaced him as director. Rapier was well acquainted with Abbott, having been friends with him when they were students at the Buxton Mission School in Canada.

With his appointment as a contract acting assistant surgeon at the hospital, now known as Freedmen's Hospital, Rapier was provided with a uniform befitting his new position, though he was at first reluctant to wear it. But he was quick to notice the respect shown a Black man in an army officer's uniform and changed his mind about wearing his: "I must tell you coloured men in the U.S. Uniform are much respected here, and in visiting the various Departments if the dress is that of an Officer, you receive the military salute from the ground as promptly as if your blood was a Howard or Plantagenet instead of a Pompey or Cuffee's. I had decided not to wear the uniform but I have altered my mind—and I shall appear hereafter in full dress gold lace, pointed hat, straps and all."[80]

Having a well-paying job and a position that was respected in society was always at the forefront of his mind. While in Haiti and Jamaica, he had expressed his aspirations and desires "to see a neatly painted sign hanging over a door . . . that will let the passerby know that there lives 'John H. Rapier,

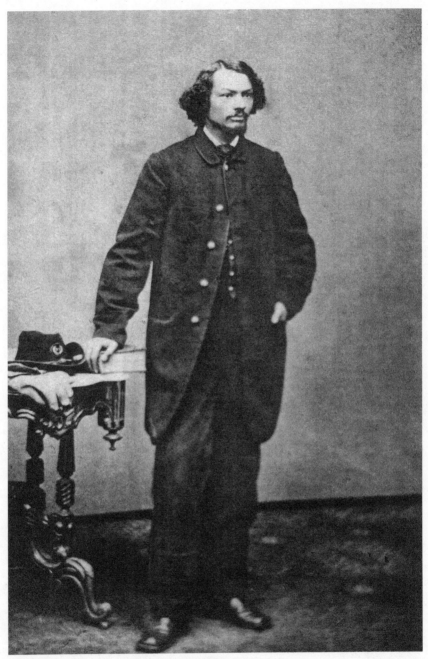

John H. Rapier Jr., c. 1864. *Courtesy Anne Straith Jamieson Fonds, The J. J. Talman Regional Collection, Western University Archives and Special Collections, London, Ont.*

Dentist.'" He articulated this same desire in Washington when he wrote, "On the 14th the most eventful event of my life occurred, I drew $100 less war tax two dollars and fifty cents for Medical Services rendered the U.S. Government. My draft was in favour of 'Acting Asst. Surgeon Rank 1st Lieut. U.S.A.' . . . In the spring I want my drafts payable to Maj. John H. Rapier Surg. U.S.A."[81]

During his service at Freedmen's Hospital, he took on the myriad responsibilities of an army surgeon, from treating patients to performing hospital administrative duties. Typical medical cases included war wounds and sicknesses suffered by Black soldiers and ailments and injuries of civilians such as intestinal disorders, frostbite, respiratory illnesses, tuberculosis, and other conditions.[82] Rapier felt great pride in his work and position as an acting assistant surgeon but felt the strain of the long hours and hard work. "I never worked so hard, and had so little rest, and felt so tired at night as I do now," he wrote to his uncle. He confessed that he had little time to write because he was so tired from hospital work, including daily, weekly, and monthly reports he was required to make to the medical director. Rapier gained a great respect and admiration for the women who volunteered at the hospital. "They are as a class the most indefatigable and earnest-laborers . . . these Angels of Mercy."[83] After spending a full day at the hospital, Rapier would often go out into the community in the evenings to visit homes and treat Black residents of the city who were sick or needed medical attention. "Through summer's heat and winter's cold," said a friend, "I have seen him wending his way among the homes of the lowly, who needed his professional services."[84] The work was demanding and the hours long, but Rapier was committed to providing the best possible care to his patients.

Never failing to recognize the influence his new position had on his professional and social advancement, he took advantage of new opportunities that were offered him. He often socialized and dined with notable visitors to the city, such as famed abolitionist and orator Frederick Douglass. Even though he was in a prominent and visible position as a surgeon at Freedmen's Hospital, Rapier did not have a false sense of equity about how he or any person of color would be accepted or treated, even in the seat of the Union. Excited about a possible visit by his uncle James, he told his uncle that "in all Washington there is not an a number one place for a col. Gentleman to stop," but he was confident that with enough advance notice, he could "fix" him up with decent and respectable housing.[85]

Above and right: Third and fourth pages of a four-page letter from John H. Rapier Jr. to his uncle James Thomas, August 19, 1864, from Freedmen's Hospital, Washington, D.C. *Courtesy Rapier Family Papers, MS 62–4283, series A, box 84–1, Moorland-Spingarn Research Center, Howard University, Washington, D.C.*

Rapier spent what little free time he had socializing with his childhood friend Anderson R. Abbott. Together they attended a celebration of "Free Maryland" in November 1864, held at the Fifteenth Street Presbyterian Church in Washington that commemorated the passing of Article 24 of the Maryland Constitution that freed all enslaved Black people in the state.[86] Rapier and Abbott both served on the organizing committee for the celebration.

I had decided not to wear the uniform but I have altered my mind — and I shall appear hereafter in full dress gold lace, pointed hat Straps and all! Mr Fred Douglass spoke here last night to an immense audience — and to day the <u>Prest</u> sent for him to visit him in the Capitol — Did you ever hear such nonsense the President of the U.S. Sending for a "Nigger" to confer with him on the State of Country — I have been invited to take supper with Mr Douglass to night — I am proud of it — He visited the Hospital to day — He is a fine looking gentle-man. He made a fine impression on the public. I exceedingly regret to hear of Miss Virginia's ill health and hope she may be well soon — I shall write to Miss Pauline in a few days to whom make my apologies for not writing sooner — I have an opening here for Lady Teacher — Pay depends on her qualification. it may be $50 or $30 per Month — If I had the money I would send for Sarah — I believe she could get $50 — If you go to New York come by Washington if you can — I am sorry I have not money in my pocket to offer you a big time — But wait until September 30th and I will do the "clean thing" by you — In all Washington there is not an a number one place for a Col'd Gentleman to stop — But I will fix you up — if you give "due and timely" notice — write to me — Direct my letters John H Rapier M. D. Actg Asst Surg. U.S.A. Tell Mrs Barly I have written to her — Remember me to Mr Clomorgan and the Johnsons Mrs Pritchard & Mr Pritchard write soon I am as usual Yours John A

As a surgeon in Washington, he often treated soldiers of the USCT and gained a better understanding of the conditions under which they served. He became keenly aware of the inequities they faced and the lack of Black officers among their ranks. In January 1865, he joined nearly two hundred others, including Anderson R. Abbott and William B. Ellis, in a letter to Secretary of War Edwin M. Stanton urging him to authorize the raising of "a number of colored regiments, to be officered exclusively by colored men." The signatories believed that offering regiments with Black officers "would result in an uprising of the colored people, unsurpassed even by the enthusiastic response for the

President's first call [for the enlistment of Black soldiers]." They emphasized the hundreds of commissioned Black men currently serving in regiments who were "amply qualified for these positions, both by education and experience."[87] He personally sought the endorsement of the petition from Brigadier General William Birney. Birney responded, saying, "Although specious arguments may be used for it, I sincerely believe your plan to be wrong. Separatism will only deepen and strengthen the guilty prejudice now existing. . . . The best thing is to put the black and white men side by side."[88]

Rapier's dedication to his work at the hospital never ceased, but the long hours and hard work took their toll on his health. In early 1866, he fell ill with bilious fever and succumbed to his illness on May 17 at the age of thirty.[89] His obituary in the *Christian Recorder* recounted a resolution made by the Reunion Literary Club, of which Rapier was a member: "In the death of Dr. Rapier," wrote Mr. W. J. Wilson, "we mourn the loss of one of our most distinguished members, whose gentle, manly deportment, unexceptionable moral character and literary attainments, had secured for himself the esteem and respect of every member of this club, and his premature death, in the full vigor of his faculties, which gave promise of so much usefulness, is the occasion of deep and abiding regret."[90]

John H. Rapier Jr. died at the age of thirty having lived with purposeful adventure and great ambition. He faced the obstacles and barriers of racial discrimination with persistence, intelligence, and humor, navigating through his life with an observant eye and an eloquent expression of his experiences. His adventurous spirit and desire for advancement and freedom motivated him as he paved the way for African Americans through his service as a Black physician and military surgeon.

7. ❦ From Ivy League to U.S. Navy: Richard Henry Greene (1833–1877)

> While surgeons are scarce and I can be of service to my country, I shall remain, when suitable men are plenty I shall resign.
> —Richard H. Greene

Aboard the USS *Ohio* docked in Boston in early November 1863, a young medical officer waited for his orders that would assign him to a ship in the naval fleet. Like other naval officers who had recently received a commission, he wrote home about his arrival and described life on board ship. But when Richard Henry Greene joined the navy, his experience as the only known African American naval officer to serve during the Civil War gave his letters home a unique perspective.[1] Though Greene was identified as a Black man early in his life, his race may have been concealed at the time of his entry into the navy by either benign omission or deliberate action, and it appears to have remained hidden throughout his naval service and his life after the war.

Freeborn in New Haven, Connecticut, on November 14, 1833, Richard Henry Greene was the son of Esther and Richard Greene.[2] His early life was spent a few blocks from Yale College in what was known as Negro Lane, an area of town populated by affluent Black people. Greene's father had established himself in the city in the 1830s as a boot maker coming from North Carolina to pursue his trade. With a friend and coworker, he began his own boot-making business, which he operated successfully for over forty years.[3] The elder Greene became a prominent member of the Black community and a founder of St. Luke's Episcopal Church, an African American place of worship in the city.

New Haven's Black population averaged only 5 to 7 percent of the city's overall population between 1820 and 1861, but compared with other cities like New York (2.7 percent), Boston (1.7 percent), and Baltimore (1.5 percent), it seemed large.[4] Despite the relatively small numbers, a flourishing Black community existed in the mid-1800s, including skilled workers, artisans, and laborers along with preachers, educators, and at least one physician, Cortlandt

Van Rensselaer Creed, who would also serve as a surgeon during the war. At a state convention of Black people in 1854, Amos Beman, a Black New Haven minister and activist, reported that in New Haven, in addition to Black churches and schools, there was "a literary society, a circulating library, and about $200,000 worth of real estate owned by colored people."[5]

By all accounts, Greene's father was considered a man of color. He was identified as either "mulatto" or "colored" in several city directories as well as in the U.S. Federal Census records. As the son of a prominent member of the Black community, the younger Greene would likely have been identified as a man of color like his father during his time in New Haven. One exception occurred in the 1850 census, when the younger Greene was counted twice—once with the Greene family, where he was identified as "mulatto," and a second time with the family of Lucius Wooster Fitch, a white bookstore owner and his tutor, where he was identified as white.[6] It is not clear whether Greene was residing with the Fitch family or merely just visiting on the day of the census taker's visit, but when the family's information was recorded, Greene was given the same racial designation as the rest of the Fitch family.

He received his early education in one of three public schools that was established for Black students in the city. As a teenager, he worked as a clerk in a bookstore owned by Fitch and set his sights on attending Yale College. Greene prepared for admission with private college preparatory instruction from Fitch, who was also an employee of Yale and the son of the Yale College pastor. Greene's employment as a bookstore clerk may have enabled him to pay Fitch, who instructed him in courses required for undergraduate admission, including Latin and mathematics.

Greene was admitted to Yale in the fall of 1853 and began attending classes. His admission was likely based on his educational qualifications and the influence of his association with Fitch. As a freshman, he was subjected to the standard six months' residency requirement before matriculating in July 1854. A typical day for Greene started with prayers in the college chapel followed by class study in Greek, Latin, English grammar, algebra, and geography.[7] He led an active life on campus and in his freshman year became a member of Sigma Delta fraternity and the literary society the Brothers in Unity. Although civil and government records identified Greene as Black, he seems to have been admitted to these collegiate organizations without question. It is interesting to note that the objective of the Brothers in Unity, according to an 1841 description, was "to give the hand of friendship to those who had before met nothing but indignities on their entrance to College."[8] If Greene faced any indignities upon admission due to his color, the Brothers in Unity might have been a welcome group to join. No records from this society make any reference to race, so it is not clear whether other Black students were among the more than fifty members.[9] In general, Yale student records at the time made no note of a student's racial identity. When Greene graduated with a bachelor of arts degree in July 1857, he was among 107 members of the graduating class and became, intentionally or not, the first Black graduate from Yale College. That year, Yale achieved another first when Cortlandt Van Rensselaer Creed became the first Black graduate of the medical college. These two men would both follow a path to service as surgeons during the war.

Greene's racial identity while a student at Yale is difficult to determine. There is no evidence that the university made any reference to a student's color, and Greene's acceptance as a member of several student organizations seems to have occurred without incident. Was he perceived as white, and therefore his attendance at the university was accepted without controversy? Perhaps Greene did not self-identify as Black and assumed a white racial identity by choice or omission. It is also possible that he did identify as Black and may have been recognized as a Black man, but white students and faculty

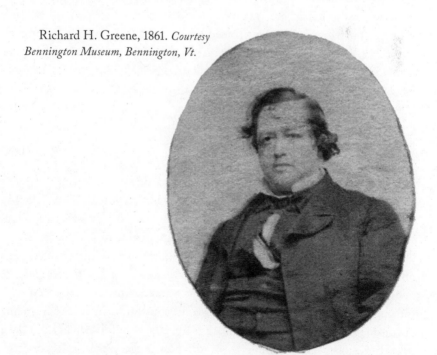

Richard H. Greene, 1861. *Courtesy Bennington Museum, Bennington, Vt.*

overlooked or ignored his color because of his academic prowess and light complexion.

Greene's admission to Yale was primarily based on his academic ability and perhaps on the influence of his white tutor who was a Yale employee, Lucius Fitch. If Greene was perceived as white, there likely would have been no further need for concern or for persuasion in his admission. On the other hand, if he was seen as a Black man, the influence of Fitch may have been critical in his admission. What complicates the question of whether he was perceived as Black or white during his years at Yale are two separate mentions of Greene—in the *Friends' Review: A Religious, Literary and Miscellaneous Journal* in 1874 and in the *American Educational Annual* in 1875. In both publications, Greene is recognized as "the first colored graduate of the academical department of Yale" and among "five colored men" graduated from Yale.[10] This public acknowledgment of Greene as "colored" seems to imply that there was some recognition of his race during the time he attended the university. It seems clear that Yale admitted Black students, but it is difficult to determine whether Greene was considered among them while an undergraduate.

He began teaching after graduation, first at a school in Milford, Connecticut, and then at the Bennington Seminary in Vermont. While living in Vermont he met Charlotte A. Caldwell, a young white schoolteacher. They began a courtship that eventually led to their engagement. His interest in becoming a physician began while in Bennington, and in 1860 he started studying medicine as an apprentice to a local physician. After three years, he moved to Hanover to begin attending lectures at Dartmouth Medical College. He felt "well situated, but lonely," telling Charlotte that in six months he would have a profession that he could "fall back on anytime."[11]

While a medical student, he contemplated joining the navy. He believed his graduation from medical school would provide him with a profession but was not convinced it would make him wealthy, which seemed to be of great concern to him. In September 1863 he told Charlotte, "If you're going to wait until I get rich you may have to wait forever." A navy salary, though, seemed a good prospect for Greene as it would provide him a steady, decent income, and he pointed out to Charlotte that "positions in the navy have been offered to graduates by the government in Washington." The monthly salary of $113 plus rations as a navy surgeon was attractive to him, and even with the uncertainty about the conditions of a naval position, he placed his name in consideration. Prior to his graduation from Dartmouth Medical College in early October 1863, Greene received a partial examination by the navy and was recommended to the naval authorities in Washington, D.C. He was accepted and ordered to appear before the Naval Medical Board in Boston on November 1. He expressed great anxiety about the examination and about his future, asking that Charlotte not mention his navy application to anyone.[12]

Immediately following his graduation, he made a formal application for a position in the U.S. Navy. In a short biography he included with his application letter, he provided information on himself and his medical education. A handwritten note at the bottom of the letter, presumably by a member of the examining board, refers to him as "fresh from school; no practical experience, sprightly and tolerably well booked."[13] Greene received glowing recommendations from two physicians who had known him in Vermont and New Hampshire. Both verified his medical studies and stated that "he is a man of unblemished moral character" and "would make a good and reliable physician, and a good member of society."[14] He completed the required medical board examination on November 2, where he answered questions on the diagnostic symptoms of dysentery, the preparation and dosage of opium, and the definitions of specific gravity, temperature, and latent heat.[15] After successfully passing the exam, he was ordered on board the USS *Ohio*, a receiving ship docked in Boston, to await further orders from Washington. Along with Greene, other newly commissioned naval officers and enlisted seamen were on board awaiting their crew assignments to other ships. Greene found the *Ohio* surprisingly comfortable with a dining hall for officers and a sufficient number of waitstaff. He received his formal appointment as assistant surgeon on November 5 and was assigned to the USS *State of Georgia*.[16] Once aboard his new ship, a 1,200-ton side-wheel steamer, he found a crew of over one hundred men, including sailors and officers. The *State of Georgia* was assigned to the blockade of the North Carolina and Virginia coasts and was soon headed south.

African Americans had previously served in the U.S. Navy on ships with white sailors, and their numbers during the Civil War reached to nearly eighteen thousand. This represented 20 percent of the entire naval forces during the war and a larger percentage than those African Americans who served in the army.[17] A majority of Black Civil War sailors were formerly enslaved people who, after escaping enslavement, joined the navy. Although the army initially barred Black men from service following the federal Militia Act of 1792, the navy did not follow that tradition and allowed Black men to serve in limited numbers.[18] While no formal mandate existed for the separation of white and Black men on Civil War ships, Secretary of the Navy Gideon

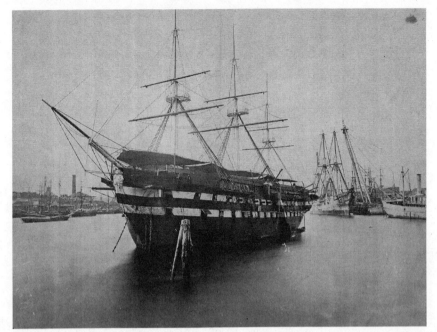

The USS *Ohio*, Boston Navy Yard, Charlestown, c. 1860. *Courtesy Boston Pictorial Archive, Arts Department, Boston Public Library.*

Welles provided guidelines for the recruitment and service of Black men. The guidelines essentially enforced existing prejudices of white naval officers and sailors that perpetuated the stereotype that Black men were inferior, lazy, and lacked intelligence. Welles permitted Black enlistment but restricted the classification of formerly enslaved recruits to "boys," the lowest rank on the rating and pay scales, although some Black sailors did rate as petty officers and served as cooks, laborers, waiters, boat hands, and barbers and occasionally as carpenters.

The perception of Greene as a white man was a significant factor in his ability to be appointed and serve as an acting assistant surgeon and officer on board a naval vessel. His appointment would have been unlikely if he was perceived as a Black man. His rank and assignment were based on his medical education and examination, but his acceptance as a navy surgeon on board a ship with a predominantly white crew would have been possible only if he was perceived and accepted as a white man. All but one Black surgeon in the U.S. Army served at Black-only hospitals or examined Black recruits at recruiting stations, because white officers would not work alongside them and most white soldiers would not allow a Black surgeon to treat them. John

Van Surly DeGrasse was the exception, but he was subjected to constant prejudicial treatment.

No clear identification of Greene as a man of color appears in his naval application or any other available naval records. This is in contrast to the cases of other Black surgeons who served in the army where at least one reference to race can be found in their federal military service records. Until the beginning of his naval career, his racial identity was a Black man, but that seems to have changed with his acceptance as a ship's acting assistant surgeon. Did the navy assume Greene was a white Ivy League medical school graduate, or did it recognize him as a Black man and overlook his color because of its immediate need for surgeons and his ability to "pass" as white? These questions remain unanswered.

For Greene, fresh out of medical school, serving as an assistant surgeon in the navy gave him practical experience as a physician, which would help prepare him for private practice after the war. He treated a myriad of illnesses and injuries on a navy ship, as recorded in the medical log he was required to maintain. It listed information about each patient, including illnesses, injuries, treatments, medications administered, and patients' current condition, with each entry signed "R. H. Greene, A.A. Surgeon." His medical log provides insight into the types and extent of illness and disease that affected the ship's crew. Common ailments included boils, fever, pain, chills, catarrh, cholera, hemorrhoids, nephritis, contusions, burns, gonorrhea, syphilis, and diarrhea. Most patients suffered from illness or disease rather than wounds of war. On average, Greene attended 5 to 18 patients each day, treating all personnel on the ship irrespective of color or allegiance, even occasionally treating Confederate prisoners. By January 1864, Greene had recorded some statistical information. During the first quarter of 1864, he treated 580 patients; in the second quarter, 645 patients. He made notes for patients who were transferred to onshore hospitals and remarked about the outbreak of particular illnesses such as smallpox and measles. Sometimes a medical survey was conducted to assess patients whom he believed required additional treatment not available on board ship; on several occasions, patients were recommended for transfer to onshore hospitals as a result of these surveys.[19]

Greene himself sometimes treated patients onshore. In December 1863, he was called upon to examine the son of a marine commander who had suddenly become ill. Apprehensive about taking on "so important a job," he called upon a fellow surgeon and friend on board another vessel to join him. Greene and his colleague examined the commander's son and reassured him that he did not have a "disorder of the heart," as the young man believed. They made him as comfortable as possible, which pleased his father, and were treated "very courteously" during their visit.[20]

In early January 1864, Greene made a special note about a patient who complained of catarrh but soon showed signs of variola, a form of smallpox. The patient had just arrived from Washington, D.C., where a large number of smallpox cases had been reported. Fearing an outbreak, Greene fumigated the ship by burning chloroform and alcohol and proceeded to vaccinate all wardroom officers and prisoners. The ship was put under quarantine.[21] A large number of the USS *State of Georgia* crew were sick at the time, and the presence of smallpox on board restricted communication with those onshore, keeping the ship from replenishing its supplies and joining the blockade. In mid-January, Greene told Charlotte that as a result of the quarantined status of the ship, his supply of wine and other medicines was depleted. "I have had thus far this month a terrible time," he told her, "smallpox in its most malignant form on the ship and 25 others on their backs at the same time with serious bronchial symptoms, the ship in quarantine and no medicine to be got."[22] He was eventually able to get all his smallpox patients safely off the ship, where they all recovered. The ship was now permitted to leave port to join the blockade. The health of the ship's crew continued to improve, and by the beginning of March 1864 most were healthy except for some cases of measles that developed later that month. Greene believed that the measles would quickly spread among the crew and took whatever measures he could to minimize an outbreak.[23]

Greene served aboard the *State of Georgia* through September 1864, writing many letters to his fiancée and his mother. He often spoke of his indecisiveness about a future in the navy and what his life might be like after his naval service. In January 1864, he wrote Charlotte that "in two years at the most it is my intention to leave the navy and engage in the work of the ministry." Several months later, he expressed his commitment to the navy, saying, "While surgeons are scarce and I can be of service to my country, I shall remain, when suitable men are plenty, I will resign."[24] He was concerned about his future and his ability to support a family, complaining that although the salary was "tolerable . . . between taxes and traveling expenses, mess bills and uniform we cannot save much."[25] "We get some salary it is true," he remarked a few months later, "but the expense is so great that very little is made out of it and nothing done towards a permanent settlement in life."[26]

Life in the navy during the war was fraught with uncertainty, boredom, and loneliness. Greene longed for letters from home and often complained to Charlotte about the lack of letters he received from her. "We are lonely down there," he said, "and I would be very glad to hear from home and particularly from you even if you do write two or three before you receive an answer." Letters from home were a welcome distraction from daily navy life, and he counted on them, telling Charlotte that she was "the long reliever of the tardiness of the blockade."[27] "News from home," he said, "is always interesting and a word or two of remembrance and affection from those we love always encouraging and gratifying." Greene's correspondence with Charlotte described his surroundings and his experience on board ship. As his vessel traveled along the Virginia and North Carolina coasts, he described the calm evenings at sea as well as the tempestuous rocking of the ship during a storm. "It is a beautiful moonlight evening, not a cloud in the sky and most delightful sailing. The cabins are lighted up, a few writing, but most officers and men crowding the deck and enjoying the soft air and beautiful scenery."[28] In contrast, his experience during a stormy evening was somewhat different as the ship "rolled sometimes fearfully and the wind fairly yelled through the rigging. Most of the time one could not stand without a support rope. I fell flat on the deck once the vessel rolled so suddenly."[29]

He was not shy to share his personal feelings about the war and his less-than-enthusiastic opinion on the nation becoming reunited, as "words can hardly express the bitterness the southerners have towards the north."[30] "We may conquer by arms," he said, "but their hatred towards us can hardly be expressed and there will be no sympathy of feelings."[31] In May 1864, he made note that Confederate soldiers were "vigorous and brave," but by September, he believed that "things look now a little like conquering the rebs, and I hope the war may soon come to a speedy close."[32]

The ravages of war and the human toll did not go unnoticed by Greene. He wrote that "the slaughter in these late battles has been beyond your conception—the forts shipping and hospitals literally crowded with wounded. . . . I hope for the best, and God grant that there may soon be an end of these scenes."[33] He was clearly moved by the sight of wounded and dying soldiers when he described a visit to one hospital while docked in Norfolk, Virginia: "One day's walk through the hospital, one day's view of the sick and wounded and dying will fully satisfy any ordinary person's longing for war. It is a very easy thing to be patriotic at home, attend enthusiastic meetings for mutual

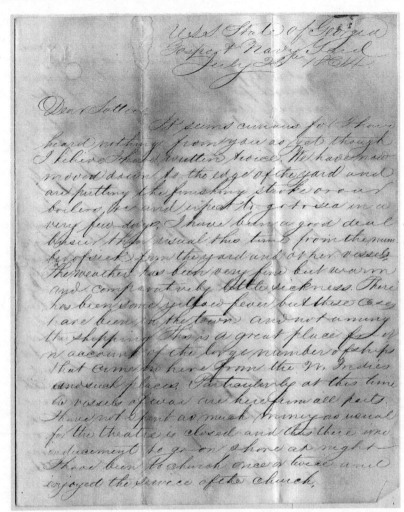

Above and right, first and second pages of a four-page letter from Richard H. Greene to his fiancée, Charlotte Caldwell, July 26, 1864, from aboard the USS *State of Georgia. Courtesy Richard Henry Green Papers, MS 2005, Manuscripts and Archives, Yale University Library, https://archives.yale.edu/repositories/12/resources/5241.*

admiration, and to devise means to forward enlistments and say to others go, it is not so easy to say come."[34]

Greene visited other hospitals, including one in Portsmouth, Virginia, where he found the visit "interesting . . . but sad as the fellow man of the sufferers." He described one patient who had sustained a wound from a minié ball that tore through the hip joint and exited his thigh and how he realized

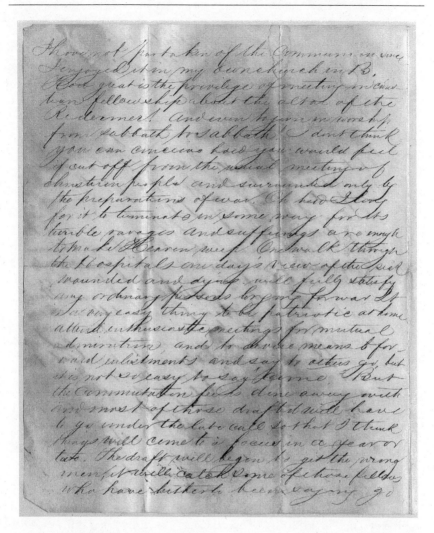

there was no hope for this man's survival. The soldier died the next morning. "This is the sad history of thousands," he wrote Charlotte.[35]

The letters he exchanged with his fiancée got him through each day and kept him focused on the future. He often discussed their wedding plans and what their life together might be like after the war. "Not a day passes but I think of you many times and look forward trustfully and with hope to our coming union." Navy life was difficult for Greene. He felt lonely for home, isolated from his religious community, and fearful of the war's outcome. His indecisiveness about remaining in the navy continued. In May 1864, he entertained the idea of continuing with military service but thought it would be necessary for him and Charlotte to relocate to Baltimore or Philadelphia, where they could live comfortably and still save money from his navy income. By September, he changed his mind: "I am getting pretty well tired of naval life and if I do not get home this time I shall in all probability resign at the end of the next cruise."[36]

In early September 1864, the USS *State of Georgia* was taken out of commission. While Greene awaited his new orders, he was granted leave to return home to Bennington, where he married Charlotte Caldwell in a small ceremony at St. Peter's Episcopal Church. He returned to duty and by the beginning of October was reassigned to the USS *Seneca*, a 691-ton Unadilla-class gunboat with over eighty crew members. At the end of that month, he wrote to his wife telling her how "very lonesome and depressed" he had been since leaving home. "No amount of money," he says, "is sufficient compensation for being separated from home and from you. . . . It does not seem now as I can endure it long. . . . I shall remain a while longer and then resign that we may take some real enjoyment of our lives. I feel the upmost confidence at being able to make a good living at something. The only thing that prevents me now is, that I want to do my share and discharge, as far as possible, my duty to my country."[37]

His new ship participated in several naval attacks on Confederate targets, including Wilmington Port, North Carolina, in January 1865. Greene described life on board ship as the "same routine of Naval life" of which he was "heartily tired" and how he longed for the day of his "liberation."[38] Greene resigned his commission on May 18, 1865, mustering out of the navy at Norfolk. He was now free to resume a quiet civilian life with his wife.

After returning from the war, Greene and Charlotte settled in the small community of Hoosick in upstate New York, where he established a successful medical practice. The 1870 U.S. Federal Census identified the family as white with one child, named Charlotte, born earlier that year. Greene was described by many as an amiable and genial man with interests in natural history and collecting plants. He was a member of the County Medical Society and a "practical" Christian.[39] It appears he was a thoughtful and caring physician. While in Portsmouth, Virginia, he had attended to a pregnant woman, Mrs. A. M. Bissell, recommending a remedy to improve her discomfort. She and her husband had previously lost a child, which had left them distraught and grief-stricken. Mrs. Bissell spoke kindly of Greene's support and comfort to her husband after the loss of their first child. She expressed her deepest thanks for the advice he provided her during her pregnancy and his continued support after seeing her in Portsmouth. "I feel under many obligations to you," she told him, "for the delicate and brotherly attentions shown one at Portsmouth and equally so for your advice and interest in us since. I felt a confidence in you . . . , which I do not entertain towards any physician near us and hence the reason for our troubling you." Greene would later receive a letter from her husband thanking him for his "watchful kindness during my wife's illness" in which he enclosed ten dollars as a token of their gratitude.[40]

By 1875, Greene and Charlotte were living a comfortable life in Hoosick with property worth $3,000.[41] He maintained a well-established medical practice in town and kept abreast of the latest medical advances through his membership in the County Medical Society, his subscription to medical journals, and his acquisition of the latest medical technology.[42]

On March 23, 1877, Richard Henry Greene died of heart disease at his home at the age of forty-three, leaving behind his wife and young daughter. He was interred in his family burial plot in Bennington with a headstone provided by the U.S. government as a veteran of the Civil War.[43] Greene left an estate worth $2,129.85, which included a piece of property from which Charlotte earned a small income.

Richard H. Greene's dual racial identities had a significant impact on his life, his opportunities, and his ability to serve as a navy surgeon during the Civil War. How he chose to identify himself is unclear, but the fact remains that as a Black man with a light complexion, he was able to serve on a naval vessel during the war and treat both Black and white patients without question. His qualifications and his performance on the Navy Medical Board examination secured his position, and his ability to "pass" as white, whether deliberate or not, ensured his rank and position in the navy and helped secure his future as a practicing physician after the war. It is possible that the navy may have overlooked his race because of a demand for surgeons. Being perceived as white changed how people saw and interacted with Greene, how he functioned in society, and the opportunities that were available to him then and in the future. Whether his racial identity as white was his personal choice or a simple omission, his service in the U.S. Navy nonetheless broke the color barrier. Greene's journey from an Ivy League student to an officer and a surgeon during the Civil War reveals the complexity of living and working as an educated Black person in nineteenth-century America. It is an example of the racial disparities that existed and how some overcame them.

8. ❀ Preacher and Physician: Willis Richardson Revels (c. 1817–1879)

> Whether as Doctor or Preacher, Willis R. Revels stands high in every community he goes, and among men of all colors.
> —Benjamin T. Tanner

As a minister of the African Methodist Episcopal (AME) Church, Willis Richardson Revels was a highly respected man. Well known for his religious and community leadership, for his steadfast commitment to abolition, and as a recruiter for the USCT, he is rarely recognized for his service as a surgeon to Black troops during the American Civil War. But though his service was short, he was an important source of care and comfort for Indiana's Black soldiers.

Revels's life began in Fayetteville, North Carolina, where he was born free around 1817 to parents Mary and Rhodes.[1] The Revels family had been free as long as anyone could remember.[2] Willis grew up with several siblings, including younger brother Hiram, who would later become the first African American United States senator. The family's ancestry was believed to be Choctaw Indian through their father, Rhodes Revels, and African and European through their mother, Mary.

Information on the family's Native American ancestry was mentioned in the *Clarion-Ledger* of Jackson, Mississippi, in 1870, which noted that Willis Revels "boasts the blood of Pocahontas in his veins . . . his grandfather having been a full-blooded Choctaw." The *Christian Recorder* corroborated the *Clarion-Ledger*'s claim, referring to a biographical sketch that appeared in the *Baltimore American* that said "his paternal grandfather was a full-blooded Indian of the Choctaw tribe, who married a woman of African descent.[3]

Though their Choctaw lineage cannot be definitively determined, the family held stock in their oral family history. Two of Hiram Revels's daughters, Dora Leonard and Ida Redmond, believed they had Native American ancestry based on their father's claims and sought enrollment in the Choctaw Tribe in 1901 before the Commission to the Five Civilized Tribes of the Department of the Interior. This commission, known as the Dawes Commission, was established by Congress in 1893 to persuade Native Americans to relinquish their title to community tribal lands and have that land divided into individual allotments, thus abolishing tribal governments and communal ownership of land.[4] The testimony of Hiram Revel's two daughters focused on their father's understanding of his ancestry, but they could not convince the commission, and their claim for recognition as Choctaw was denied.[5] It is interesting to note that a commission member's observation recorded at the end of Dora Leonard's transcribed testimony states that "this applicant has the appearance of being possessed of a mixture of white and negro blood, in which the white blood largely predominates; she shows no indication of being possessed of Indian blood, neither does she speak or understand the Choctaw language."[6] This commission member's reliance on stereotypical physical attributes reveals his prejudices and seems to have influenced the decision to deny the sisters' claims. It is nonetheless possible that Willis Revels had some Native American ancestry in addition to African and European.

In the early 1800s, Rhodes and Mary Revels moved from Mississippi to settle in Fayetteville, North Carolina, before Willis was born. Little is known about them, but it is possible that Rhodes was a religious minister. Willis and Hiram along with one other brother became preachers and perhaps were influenced to pursue the ministry by their father. The family's commitment to learning seems evident by the deep interest that Rhodes and Mary had in providing educational opportunities for their children as best as they were able. Willis was drawn to learning as a young boy, and he, along with his younger brother Hiram, received their early education in a private school run by a free Black woman in their community. The school provided a good education, and as Hiram Revels recalled in his autobiography, he "was early imbued with a love of knowledge" while attending the school.[7]

Willis Revels was among many Black people who headed north sometime in the mid-1830s to escape the oppressive and restrictive conditions of life in North Carolina. Fayetteville, located on the banks of Cape Fear River, had a Black community of both free and enslaved persons. In the agrarian-based community, the enslaved people worked primarily in the fields, while a few were artisans like coopers and cobblers. As the majority of Black people in the state were enslaved during the early 1800s, laws were passed and enforced that curtailed any gains once held by free Black people and put more restrictions on enslaved people. In 1826, North Carolina enacted a law that prohibited free Black people from entering the state. By 1835, they lost the right to vote, own property, and earn their own wages. Other restrictive laws soon followed that prohibited them from preaching in public or in the presence of enslaved people, possessing a gun, buying and selling liquor, or attending a public school.[8] These changes in the laws compelled many free Black people to move themselves and their families north to Ohio and Indiana.

As a young man, Willis left his home to further his education and seek a better life. His interest in becoming a physician led him to Hartford, Connecticut, where he studied for two years with a local physician. After leaving Hartford, Revels headed to Indiana. By the time he arrived in Indianapolis, laws had already been enacted in the state limiting free Black people from entering and restricting their settlement in the city. The pervasive racist attitudes of the white population toward Black people affected all aspects of their daily lives. Laws were in place that prevented Black people from voting, serving on juries, and being educated in the public schools. They were subjected to indiscriminate acts of violence in their homes, businesses, and churches. The Black population in Indianapolis never exceeded 5 percent of the city's total population before the war, and laws that restricted Black people from entering the state clearly caused a decrease in the total Black population. By the mid-1830s, Black people in the city were segregated in an area known as "Colored Town." Though restrictive laws were in place when Revels arrived in Indiana, he was able to settle there.[9] Perhaps his well-educated, articulate manner and appearance gave him an advantage.

When he arrived in Indianapolis, Revels followed his religious calling and became a missionary with the AME Church, the world's oldest independent Protestant denomination founded by people of color. Still in existence today, the church was established in 1793, after Black congregants separated from the Methodist Episcopal Church due to racist attitudes and behaviors of its white members. The church achieved recognized independence from the established church through the efforts of its founder, Richard Allen. In 1807 and 1815, Allen filed lawsuits to legally attain independence for the church and was formally granted that independence in 1816.[10] After this success, Allen called for all other Black Methodists in other communities to meet in Philadelphia and officially establish the African Methodist Episcopal Church. Those involved in the newly formed institution created their own conferences and their own distinctive doctrine. They began a weekly newspaper in 1848, the *Christian Herald*, that became the *Christian Recorder* in 1852. The newspaper was the voice of the AME Church, reporting on the day's news and activities of its members and clergy. It became an important outlet for Black soldiers to communicate about their experiences during the Civil War through published letters to the newspaper's editor.

The life of an AME preacher was demanding. Revels began traveling to many cities and communities in Ohio, Indiana, Kentucky, and Missouri. Eager to learn, he sought out mentors everywhere he visited. "There was a mysterious power within him," said AME bishop Daniel Payne, "which urged him—a deep conviction that he must be somebody; and on he went over the numberless obstacles which ever stand in the way of a poverty-stricken, aspiring youth. . . . He made it a point, in whatever city or town he was called upon to remain, to seek out a teacher."[11] In 1834, Revels married Susanna Jones, and their family would grow to include three sons and three daughters. His missionary ministry took him away from home much of the time, but he managed to find a balance between his work on the church circuit and his family life at home.

Though Revels was fulfilled by his religious life, his interest in medicine was at the forefront of his mind. An opportunity to complete his medical education presented itself in the early 1840s, by way of the American Colonization Society (ACS). He was drawn to the ACS by his interest in the emigration of Black people as a means for a free and better life and also by the organization's recruitment policy that paid for an individual's medical education in exchange for service in Liberia. The ACS, founded in 1816 by a white Presbyterian minister, encouraged and supported free Black people in emigrating from the United States to Africa. Its founder, Robert Finley, saw the increasing population of free and enslaved Black people in the United States as a threat to the nation's well-being. He believed Black people would never be fully integrated into American society and could achieve their full potential as human beings only by moving back to their ancestral homeland. Members of the ACS viewed the establishment of their organization and their support of emigration as an opportunity for Black people to live a free and fulfilled life and at the same time as a way to eliminate racial tensions caused by slavery. Many abolitionists, though, opposed emigration and tried to discredit colonization as a "slaveholder's scheme." After harsh criticism from abolitionist supporters, the ACS attempted to rebrand itself by changing its focus from emigration to one favoring educational and missionary work. The ACS acquired an area off the coast of West Africa known as Cape Mesurado using funds received from the U.S. government. This area eventually became the colony of Liberia, emphasizing the ACS's new focus for its missionary work and emigration.[12]

Some Black people were hesitant to leave America for Liberia because they believed doing so would expose them to a greater chance of death in Africa. An increased mortality in Liberia had resulted from "local pathogens, inappropriate immunity, and accidents associated with emigration." In an attempt to assuage their fears and make emigration more appealing, the ACS sent white physicians to provide medical care to the Liberian colonists. Those in the society knew that without the emigration of Black people from the United States, the success of the colony was unlikely. After three white physicians died in Liberia, ACS organizers assumed that "the intense beams of the African sun" made the white physicians more susceptible to disease and death. As a result, they developed a strategy for replacing white physicians with Black physicians based on the belief that Black people could better sustain the harsher conditions in Africa. Their plan offered to fund the medical education of Black men in exchange for the emigration of these new Black physicians to Liberia to practice medicine.[13]

Revels took advantage of the ACS's offer and relocated to New Orleans, where he studied under the tutelage of Dr. Warren Stone, one of the founders of the Medical College of Louisiana, later Tulane University. Stone was a staunch Democrat and during the Civil War served as the Confederate surgeon general for the state of Louisiana. It is possible that he would have had the proclivity to deny a medical education to a Black man but may have extended his teaching services to Revels because his education was under the sponsorship of the ACS. Stone probably believed that this sponsorship would eventually result in Revels's emigration, thus supporting the cause to relocate Black people to Africa. After Revels completed his schooling, he intended to fulfill his responsibilities to relocate to Africa, but his wife, Susanna, refused to leave the country. Unwilling to leave his wife and children behind, Revels withdrew from the arrangements he had made with the ACS and, without hesitation, refunded all the money the organization had provided for his medical training.[14]

Revels returned to Indiana and became a fully ordained AME minister. He continued to preach to communities in Indiana, Illinois, Missouri, Louisiana, Tennessee, and Kentucky and started a small medical practice treating Black patients. As a preacher, he was captivating and inspiring. His voice was described as "eloquent," and he was "known to be one of the ablest orators of the West."[15] After hearing him preach a Thanksgiving Day sermon, an observer remarked, "He held the audience almost spell bound for about forty minutes. I think it was one of the best Thanksgiving Sermons I have ever had the pleasure of listening to."[16]

Though his ministry took him to many cities in neighboring states, he remained connected to Indianapolis. He gained a reputation as a respected member of the local community by both Black and white people and became associated with influential people in the city, including Calvin Fletcher, a prominent white lawyer, landowner, and businessman. Fletcher, who lived a relatively simple life on a farm with his family, supported many civic causes and organizations, including educational development, religious institutions, community service, and benevolent groups. As an abolitionist, he focused his attention on support for freedmen, widows, and orphans, as well as on organizing Black troops during the Civil War. Although he considered himself an antislavery man, he was among the few abolitionists who supported the colonization movement and the ACS. Revels's ties to the ACS may have aided in the development of his friendship with Fletcher, which proved to be an important and influential relationship.

Revels's involvement with the ACS extended beyond the educational advantages he received to include working with the state-organized Indiana Colonization Society (ICS), which had formed in 1829 with the support of the national ACS. The ICS, made up of mostly white members, including Fletcher, organized local groups, raised money, and recruited people to emigrate to Liberia. From its earliest formation, the ACS and ICS believed that "white racial animosity amounted to an insurmountable barrier for free blacks" and that colonization was "the only human way to spare free Black Americans the pain of racial prejudice in Indiana and the rest of the nation."[17] In early 1842, a meeting was held at Revels's Bethel AME Church, where members of the Black community voiced their opposition to colonization. The idea of colonization remained at the forefront of the ICS, though, and in 1846 the group decided that a Black citizen of Indiana should be appointed to visit Liberia. The chosen man would make a full investigation of the condition of the country's citizens and make a report of his visit to the people of Indiana upon his return; ICS members hoped a favorable report would encourage more Black people to emigrate. In choosing their representative, they sought a "worthy" man of "piety and talent, possessing the confidence of the colored people and the agent of this Society," and solicited the services of Revels because of his "great influence" among the Black population.[18] Both the ICS members and the Black citizens approved of Revels's selection, but relentless pressure from abolitionists forced him to withdraw from the appointment.

The Black population of Indianapolis during the mid-1800s was considered small but "eminently decent, industrious and respectable." Revels gained a good reputation both inside and outside his community and was considered to be "well esteemed by whites as his own race."[19] He was not shy to express his religious and political views through public engagement from the pulpit, through active participation in community groups, and in letters to prominent individuals and newspapers, both local and national. By 1850, he was well established in the city, living a comfortable life with his wife, Susanna, and their children. Despite his personal successes in the community, the environment in the city was far from favorable for Black people. Beginning in 1850, contentious debates were held regarding an amendment to the Indiana Constitution that would severely curtail Black settlements in the state. The amendment was ratified statewide by 60 percent of voters, all of whom were

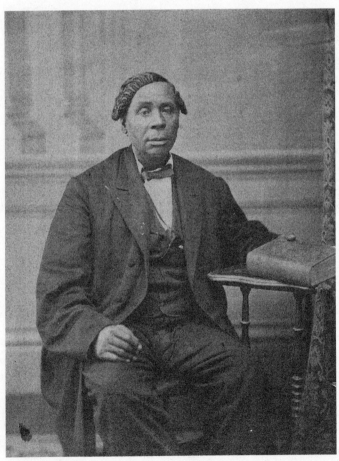

Willis R. Revels, c. 1870. *Courtesy Indiana Historical Society, P0491, Indianapolis, photo cropped.*

white, since Black people had no right to vote. Several other laws were enacted putting further constraints on the Black population. With the establishment and enforcement of these "Black laws," Indiana possessed the most restrictive Black settlement laws in the North, resulting in very little increase in the population after 1850.[20]

Revels's main focus was on his religious life. He proved to be a great success in his ministry, helping his church grow on both the local and national levels. In the mid-1850s, he was assigned to the Quinn Chapel African Episcopal Church in Louisville, Kentucky. The church had been established in the 1840s with services first held in the homes of its members and then in a room above a stable. The congregation eventually moved to a partially finished brick building in 1854 until a new church building was completed. After he arrived, Revels began soliciting funds from donors in the North for the new sanctuary, completed in 1858. The church gained a reputation as an "abolitionist" church because of its large free Black congregation and active educational programs. This reputation led many enslavers to restrict enslaved persons from attending services there.[21]

Revels became involved in a dramatic confrontation over the issue of slaveholding church members in the AME Church during the 1856 general conference held in Ohio. A resolution was put forth to expel all church members who were enslavers, regardless of the circumstances. Revels took a more conservative opinion, reminding the opposition that some enslaved people were purchased by relatives with the intention of setting them free. He told the conference members that "he would not have a rule created here which would hinder such acts of mercy." Debate ensued on whether the church was truly antislavery. In defending the church, Revels said it had "always prohibited slavery" since its formation. He went on to challenge Northern ministers "to pick up 'rifles and field pieces . . . and go down South and fight the enemy on their own ground.'"[22]

In 1858, Revels was transferred to Chicago, where he remained for three years. His ministry work and medical practice kept him very busy. A visitor from Indianapolis commented that he had "found Rev. W. R. Revels at the parsonage, and looking as well as I ever saw him. I had but little of his company, as he was engaged in practicing medicine, in connexion with the labors of his charge."[23] As pastor of the church, Revels was a community leader, often organizing and chairing civic meetings. In the midst of a continued push to have Black people emigrate from the United States to Africa and Haiti, he presided over a meeting of Black citizens where an agent of Haiti presented a proposition from Haiti's president to provide a refuge for Black Americans from "a life of degradation and slavery in the United States."[24] Revels participated on a committee that considered and debated the proposition. Committee members planned to open communication with Haiti in relation to the offer and "the inducements held out to the colored emigrants from the United States."[25] After much consideration, Revels determined that the proposal was not advantageous to Black Americans. He believed the "vile spirit of Negro hate" motivated white people to encourage and support the white Haitian "scheme" to relocate Black Americans to Haiti without consideration of and without representation from the majority Black Haitian population. He spoke of the "impracticality of sending native-born Americans to a foreign land with a different language, culture, and religion" and noted that Black Americans showed "evidence of vitality, of self-appreciation, of progress, in all elements of American civilization."[26] He firmly believed that staying in America was the best choice. "God's providence designs . . . ," he said, "to provide for them an ample home in conjunction, and neighborly association, with the numerous other races of men to be found here."[27]

Returning to Indianapolis after the start of the Civil War in 1861, he became pastor of the Bethel AME Church. Founded in 1836, it became known as an abolitionist church, often harboring escaping enslaved people on their way to Canada via the Underground Railroad. Built on the small but recurring monetary contributions from the Black community in the city, the church played an important part in the lives of its members and the community. As pastor, Revels preached at regular Sunday church services, officiated at weddings and baptisms, and provided spiritual support and comfort to the congregation. He was well respected and admired by church members.[28] Those outside the congregation made note of the success of Revels's ministry. A visitor to the church commented that "Dr. Revels has been pretty successful here this year." The visitor remarked how Revels had been able to bring improvements to the church, including a much-needed new roof. Indianapolis had become a more appealing place for Black people to settle in Indiana, despite the state's restrictive laws, due in part to Revels's reputation.[29]

Strong sentiments about the Civil War extended throughout the United States, including among the Black population in Indiana. Many were eager to participate in the war, but few opportunities were available to Black people. Some people called for the official acceptance of Black men in the military, but the idea was met with resistance. Revels wanted to do his part and expressed this desire in a letter to his friend Calvin Fletcher in July 1862. He told Fletcher that "he and others of his race would fight if they had permission to do so."[30]

Black men were prevented from joining the U.S. Army until 1863, although some served in state-organized Black troops. Since Indiana was not yet authorized to form a Black regiment, Revels actively participated in recruiting Black soldiers for troops being formed in Massachusetts. At the same time, he and his family continued supporting formerly enslaved people who were escaping from the South by opening their home and providing food and shelter. Fletcher observed Revels's efforts and said he had "a great flow of contrabands to his house and is eat out much by the refuges and others that flee to him."[31] Revels's support extended to the families of Black soldiers during the war. The *Christian Recorder* noted that "the Doctor [Revels] has also made arrangements with the sanitary commission in this city for a portion of the sanitary funds, to be shared among the colored soldiers' wives. The Doctor has been indefatigable in his efforts, during the war, in forwarding the interests of our people."[32]

In early 1863, the federal government began a systematic approach to recruit Black troops, and in the spring, the U.S. War Department issued General Order Number 143, authorizing the formation of the Bureau of United States Colored Troops to coordinate and organize the efforts of Black regiments for the United States.[33] Thousands of Black men had already joined regiments formed under the coordination of individual states but now would become part of the officially recognized USCT.

Indiana governor Oliver P. Morton supported the organization of Black troops only as a means to spare white men from the draft: "I am in favor of using anything to put down the rebellion," he said, "even dogs and tomcats. . . . The use of negro troops is simply a question of expediency . . . [and] . . . will do away with the necessity of drafting so many white men." In a speech in July, Morton's support was more palpable when he said, "Let us make what use of them we can, but you all know that they have been tried, and have fought with distinguished valor. . . . If the rebels against the Government can use them for its destruction, shall we not be permitted to use them for our national preservation?"[34]

On November 30, 1863, Secretary of War Edwin M. Stanton sanctioned the recruitment of African Americans in Indiana for a single regiment. General orders were issued in December by Indiana's adjutant general to begin accepting recruits, leading Morton to approve the establishment of a Black regiment in Indianapolis. Anxious to participate, Revels called upon his friend Calvin Fletcher to arrange a meeting with the governor. On December 7, 1863, Revels and Fletcher met with Morton, resulting in the appointment of Revels as a recruiting officer to the newly formed 28th Regiment. The *Indianapolis*

Daily Journal reported on the appointment the next day, noting that Revels would be a recruiter for the new battalion. A broadside was immediately issued by Revels and fellow recruiting officer Silas Shurcraft appealing to Black men to answer the call of their country and to "let your moral sensibility and patriotism respond." A location in the city was needed to serve as a camp for the newly recruited soldiers, and Fletcher offered his own land on the outskirts of the city for the mustering and training of the new regiment.[35]

Revels began actively recruiting Black men for the regiment and made several appeals for volunteers in the daily city newspaper: "The State of Indiana calls upon you to bear a part in the glorious work of putting down the slaveholders' rebellion and saving the Union. Will you not march to the rescue of your suffering brethren, and give to them in fact the freedom which is now declared to be theirs of right?" Interested Black men were directed to apply to the commandant at the courthouse and send any inquiries to the recruiting officers about pay and benefits.[36] Garland White, a fellow AME minister, was also a recruiter for the regiment and would become its regimental chaplain.

By early December, 50 Black men had enlisted, and by the end of the month that number increased to 265. As the regiment formed, a physician was needed to serve as surgeon. Eager to be of service, Revels volunteered. After passing the medical board's examination, he was appointed acting assistant surgeon in January 1864. In a letter to the *Christian Recorder*, a minister proudly announced, "Our venerable esteemed Elder Dr. Revels passed an examination before the Medical Board of Examiners . . . and received an appointment of assistant surgeon from his Honor the Governor. The Dr. exerts a powerful influence here, among our people."[37]

Organizing a regiment in the middle of winter came with many challenges. In early January, Indianapolis faced record cold temperatures and snowfall. The *Indianapolis Daily Journal* reported that "at the Colored Camp many of the men were injured, some with frozen ears and noses, which actually burst open with the cold. We heard of a great many cases of injuries to persons who were in the open air." Revels administered medical care to soldiers who had fallen ill from the frigid winter camp conditions while continuing to examine new recruits. "Dr. Revels was in camp treating forty-nine cases of serious illness," the *Indianapolis Daily Journal* reported, "of which one man had already died from congestion of the brain, brought on by rushing out in the snow in the night while delirious."[38] By the end of the month, 163 additional men had entered the regiment. During his three months as acting assistant surgeon, Revels examined over 1,000 recruits.[39] The few federal records found for Revels confirm his service and make note that "pro-tem Assistant Surgeon W. R. Revels, 28th USCT was on duty with his regiment at Camp Fremont (Camp of Rendezvous) in Indianapolis, Indiana from January 8, 1864 to March 24, 1864."[40]

Revels fulfilled an important role as physician to the 28th Regiment, providing much-needed medical care to sick and ailing soldiers. As the regiment acquired a full contingent of soldiers and officers, the soldiers marched through the streets of Indianapolis as they prepared to leave for Washington, D.C., where they would provide military support in defense of the nation's capital. In April 1864, the regiment joined several other Black regiments of the Army of the Potomac in the siege of Petersburg and the Battle of the Crater in Virginia. The 28th's participation in these battles, along with several other Black regiments, was crucial to the success of the U.S. Army. Revels did not join his regiment on its journey east but remained behind in Indianapolis, continuing to support the war and provide for the steady flow of formerly enslaved people who made their way north.

Although much of his attention was focused on the recruitment of Black soldiers, Revels continued leading his church and was described as "indefatigable" in his efforts to raise funds for repairs to both the church building and schoolhouse.[41] While he spent three months in the middle of the winter examining recruits, he still tended to his church duties and assisting formerly enslaved people in his home. By early April the toll of his commitments caught up with him, and he fell ill with bilious pneumonia, which affected his heart. His illness kept him bedridden for several weeks and caused great concern to his church members and his family. Those closest to him believed he would not survive, but by the end of April he had recovered sufficiently from his illness to attend his daughter's wedding.

After his recovery, he faced an incident that tested both his resolve and his faith. The Bethel AME Church was a center of antislavery activity from before the start of the Civil War, and its strong and vocal antislavery stance did not sit well with much of the city's white population. On the morning of July 9, 1864, a fire broke out in the church, burning it to the ground. Revels and the church trustees believed the fire was "the work of an incendiary—one, no doubt, of those who teach negroes are fit only for slaves—that they cannot be elevated, morally or socially, and that, if they try, they shall not succeed."[42] Though the church was insured, the trustees had failed to collect money toward the insurance premium, instead taking up a collection for the relief of freedmen. Occurring at the height of the war, the church's resources to rebuild were limited. Many of the congregation's men were serving in the

U.S. Army, and those remaining, mostly women and formerly enslaved people, had fewer resources and less ability to contribute to church reconstruction. Revels started a campaign to raise the necessary funds to rebuild. He appealed to the large readership of the *Christian Recorder* for monetary contributions, saying, "We ask you to lend as liberally as possible, remembering that he who soweth bountifully, shall reap also bountifully."[43] His lifelong friendship with Calvin Fletcher proved beneficial after the fire. In an effort to assist, Fletcher rented a local building, Fuquai Hall, for use as a temporary church for Revels and his congregation until a permanent structure could be built.

Keeping busy with fundraising to rebuild, Revels continued his ministry and his active medical practice. While unwavering in his commitment to his local church, he took on a more active role in the AME Church on a national level. He attended several church conferences throughout the United States and accepted a leadership role as an elder statesman. Revels was described as "one of our ablest and oldest preachers, known throughout the West as one of the strong towers in Zion."[44]

In 1865, he was transferred from his church in Indianapolis and appointed pastor at St. Paul's Chapel in St. Louis, Missouri. Leaving behind his family, he traveled to St. Louis and reestablished himself at his new church. During his second term at St. Paul's, he was equally admired and proved to be successful in growing its membership. Revels would often travel back to Indiana by train to visit his family. One day in early 1866, the train on which he was traveling ran off the tracks. He sustained severe injuries to his ribs and breastbone as a result of the accident and was confined to his bed for more than a month. His injuries would plague him for the rest of his life. Revels's attending physicians were not hopeful for his recovery.[45] Calvin Fletcher often visited Revels while he was confined. They were among the last visits these two friends would have. Fletcher died only a few months later, in June 1866. Revels suffered another great loss in September when his beloved daughter, Henrietta, known as Nettie, died from consumption.

He recovered from his injuries and returned to St. Louis to resume his pastoral duties. Though he was quite successful in his efforts to increase church membership, the building could not sustain the increased number of attendees, so he began a fundraising campaign for the construction of a new church. He remained in St. Louis through 1869.

By the late 1860s, Revels had reached middle age, but his devotion to the ministry and medicine were steadfast. Though his work within the AME Church as a minister is well documented, his career as a physician is not, since his larger-than-life image as a preacher overshadowed his medical career. What little we know of his career as a physician comes from small references made in the *Christian Recorder* and in records of the federal government. He maintained a successful medical practice and "by his skill in medicine and industry, gained a respectable competency, and established a patronage bringing in an abundant income."[46] Those who praised him for his ecclesiastical skill also remarked on his "medical services to mankind" and considered him a "physician of more than ordinary ability."[47] His patients praised him and were not shy to say how "he had saved their lives by his medical skill." Revels was described as "encouraging" in providing advice and possessing "a tone of voice so assuring, that your heart bounds and opens quickly to his confidence."[48]

His deep interest in education led to his contributions to the *Repository of Religion and Literature*, a publication of the Indiana Annual Conference of the AME Church,[49] and he was part of a team of ministers who managed the publication.[50] He was revered as a man of "universal respect . . . with so many ardent personal admirers"; the *Christian Recorder* noted his "hospitable generosity, and the power with which he at once inspires your confidence and respect."[51] As a physician and a moral leader, Revels took up causes that appealed to both physical health and spiritual well-being. In 1867, he championed the cause against the use of tobacco from the perspective of a physician and a spiritual leader. He pleaded his case in a series of articles in the *Christian Recorder*, basing his claim on both the detrimental health effects of tobacco use, the enormous cost to obtain it, and the consequences on the soul and spirit. Referring to tobacco as an "obnoxious weed" and a "wicked expenditure," he used his own personal experience with tobacco and a scientific approach as a physician to discourage its use.[52]

By his mid-fifties, Revels had become a revered elder of the church. Still plagued by pain from injuries sustained in the train accident, he considered retirement. "I am suffering so much from an injury I received by a railroad accident, four years ago," he said, "that I fear I shall be compelled, after the present year, to retire from the field."[53] Though he had concerns for his health, his commitment to continue his ministry outweighed his consideration of retirement, and he accepted an appointment at the Bethel AME Church in Baltimore in 1870. He was described as "an easy and fluent speaker, and has all the outward indications of an earnest, sincere and zealous Christian."[54] By this time, Revels's brother Hiram had been elected to the U.S. Senate, representing Mississippi, and the two often shared the pulpit during Sunday services. He remained in Baltimore for a few years before returning west to Indiana.[55]

The last years of Revels's life were spent in Indianapolis. He was stricken with a lung infection in the winter of 1875 that confined him to his bed. Revels believed that the injuries he had sustained in the 1866 train accident had made him more susceptible to lung infections and respiratory illnesses. While convalescing, his pastoral duties were handled by a junior minister. He returned to his duties by the early part of 1876, including baptizing eleven new converts in a canal in the city.[56] But Revels never fully recovered from his injuries. Over the next year he continued to preach although his health was failing. By early 1877, he was again confined to his bed. Visitors noted that "he is certainly a very sick man and dangerously so. His affection is of the left lung and acute rheumatism. He is but a skeleton of his former self."[57] Throughout the spring and into the summer, he remained at his home and received numerous visitors asking after his health. His prominence within the AME Church brought local parishioners to his bedside as well as clergy from out of town.[58]

His health continued to decline, and a stroke in early 1878 left him partially paralyzed on his left side. Many grieved for him when they learned of his precarious condition. Revels remained lucid during his illness, and "anyone in conversation with him would not think that he is bad off as he is. He entertains company as though nothing was the matter with him." But his family admitted that Revels had finally acknowledged the severity of his condition: "He cannot bear it much longer."[59] He was much diminished in his capabilities and, when discussing his inability to attend an upcoming conference, wanted attendees to know that he was "a wounded soldier—not whipped, but wounded. Yes, tell the brethren," he said, "I retire from the field of battle a conquered conqueror."[60] No longer able to fulfill his pastoral duties, he spent his days at home with his family and often took carriage rides around town. He knew the end of his life was near and told those close to him that he was "only waiting the Master's call."[61] On March 6, 1879, he died at his home in Indianapolis.

Willis R. Revels was the only African American preacher-physician to serve during the Civil War. His devotion to uplifting the Black community, providing medical care, and advocating for emancipation was unwavering. Rising from humble roots, Revels became an influential leader in his community and his church. He holds a unique place in Civil War history as a physician, preacher, and military recruiter who provided both physical and spiritual healing to soldiers during the war.

9. ❦ Physician, Politician, Postmaster: Benjamin Antonius Boseman Jr. (1840–1881)

I know him to be a young man of excellent character and attainments.
—Charles E. Simmons, MD

On July 30, 1864, Secretary of War Edwin M. Stanton placed his signature on a letter authorizing the employment of Benjamin A. Boseman Jr. as a contract surgeon with the U.S. Army. Boseman had already achieved more than society expected of a Black man in the nineteenth century by obtaining a medical degree and becoming a physician. Now he would serve his country during the Civil War and go on to become a prominent citizen of Charleston, South Carolina.

Born free in 1840, Benjamin Antonius Boseman Jr. was the oldest of five children born to Annuretta Livingston and Benjamin Boseman Sr. of Troy, New York.[1] By the time of Boseman's birth, slavery had been abolished in New York State for thirteen years, making it an appealing place for African Americans to settle in the mid-1800s. Situated on the eastern bank of the Hudson River, less than ten miles from the state capital of Albany, Troy's proximity to the river made it a center of commerce and industry. The city had several grist and sawmills, a cotton factory, carriage and gun factories, three breweries, and a steamboat ferry business that made regular trips across the river. Boseman's father had made his way to New York State from Florida, where he was born, arriving sometime in the early 1830s. He was an enterprising man who took advantage of the growing city and became a steward on sailing vessels in the mid-to-late 1800s. The city had an active antislavery community, and Boseman Sr. took a prominent role in abolition and suffrage activities.[2] During the Civil War, he worked as a merchant selling provisions to the U.S. Army and eventually became a caterer. Boseman Jr.'s mother, Annuretta, was born in Jamaica and traveled to New York on the *Orbit*, on which she was employed as a stewardess.[3] Both parents worked hard to provide their family with the best life possible. They had a keen interest in the education of their children, all of whom received formal schooling.

Boseman Jr.'s early education was obtained at the city's segregated public schools. At the age of fourteen, he was admitted to New York Central College in McGrawville. Attending college exposed him to a new, more egalitarian environment. The college was considered progressive for the mid-1850s, opening admissions to "both sexes and all classes." Founded in 1849 by the American Free Baptist Free Mission Society, the school held that "all, rich and poor, black and white, male and female, may stand on one common platform with the fixed belief of the equality and brotherhood of the whole human family." Catering to its students' physical, mental, and moral well-being, the school boasted that "no pains will be spared in guarding the habits and moral character of pupils; they will be kept under the most wholesome rules, none of which will infringe on freedom of thought, or freedom of speech." For both women and Black students, this unique and more open environment was a welcome change.[4]

The school offered three courses of study—classical, scientific, and university. Boseman likely chose the scientific course, which included classes in French, philosophy, mathematics, history, natural history, German, rhetoric, and physics. The school schedule was rigorous with fall, winter, and summer terms, exams at the end of each term, and two- to four-week vacations between terms. Yearly tuition was twenty-four dollars per year plus room and board, in addition to fees for incidentals, wood, and washing.[5]

Boseman showed an early interest in becoming a physician. At the age of sixteen, he began an eight-year apprenticeship in the office of prominent Troy physician Thomas C. Brinsmade, who held an honorary medical degree from Yale College and served as president of the New York State Medical Society. His apprenticeship with Brinsmade continued while he attended New York Central College, from which he graduated in 1858. Medical education in the nineteenth century consisted of both an apprenticeship with a physician and attendance at medical school lectures. An apprenticeship was the usual and most common path taken by those seeking a career as a physician and generally consisted of book study and practical experience. It often included compounding medicines and assisting in the treatment of patients as well as daily menial tasks for the physician.

With an established apprenticeship, Boseman now pursued a formal medical education at the Medical School of Maine at Bowdoin College in Brunswick. He was provided with comprehensive instruction in medicine including lectures in anatomy, physiology, materia medica, chemistry, pharmacy, theory and practice of medicine, surgery, obstetrics, and medical jurisprudence. He paid an admission fee of fifty-five dollars and graduation and matriculation fees of twenty-three dollars. Boseman had access to the school's extensive medical library of over 3,500 volumes, a French anatomical cabinet with its varied collection of specimens, a chemistry department with demonstrating apparatuses, and a surgery department with its extensive collection of surgical instruments. The school boasted that "no efforts will be spared by the Professors, which may tend to render these means beneficial, and to promote the instruction of pupils in Medical Sciences." Candidates for graduation were required to have spent at least three years in professional studies with a regular practitioner of medicine, in addition to passing all course exams, a final examination by the medical school faculty, and the submission and defense of a senior thesis.[6]

Boseman graduated in 1864, having successfully completed all his requirements, including his thesis, "The Importance of Medical Statistics," which argued that the use of statistics in the study and treatment of diseases was an overlooked but essential element in medical practice. He believed that statistics provided "more correct and reliable data upon which to establish certain facts and evidence" and, in cooperation with knowledge, observation, and experience, greatly served patients and the profession.[7] His younger siblings all received formal educations also and after completing their studies were employed in professional positions: two public school teachers, a bookkeeper, and an attorney with a law degree from Howard University.

By the time of Boseman's graduation from medical school, the Civil War had been raging for three years. He followed the war's progress and was now ready to do his part, turning his efforts toward applying for a position as surgeon with the U.S. Army. In his application, he said, "I am a colored young man, a resident of this city [Troy]. . . . Seeing your advertisements for surgeons and assistant surgeons for colored regiments and being unaware that there was any law prohibiting the employment of colored men, (providing of course, they were competent) to such a capacity and knowing also that there were several in the service, I have written to obtain permission to appear before the Examining Board in New York City."[8] He detailed his medical education and experience and enclosed several letters of support from three prominent Troy citizens. His mentor and instructor, Dr. Thomas Brinsmade, had already sent several letters to the surgeon general in support of his application. He described Boseman as "a young gentleman of unexceptional habits and great general worth." Brinsmade believed that Boseman's preliminary education was "better than that recommended by the American Medical Association."[9] All of his supporters praised him for his education and his character. Congressman John Griswold declared that this "colored young man . . . in all respects education, respectability of character, etc.—is entitled to consideration."[10] William Seymour, MD, professor of obstetrics at Berkshire Medical College, said Boseman was "well informed for a graduate of his years and particularly well fitted as a surgeon in one of the colored regiments."[11] Prominent Troy physician Charles E. Simmons noted that he had known Boseman for several years and that he was "a young man of excellent character and attainments," recently graduated from medical school, and "fully qualified for the position which he desires to assume."[12] Boseman had established his qualifications and credibility and now only needed to pass the Army Medical Board examination.

In June 1864, he received official authorization from Secretary of War Edwin M. Stanton to be employed as a contract surgeon with the U.S. Army and appeared before the Army Medical Board of Examiners. After passing the

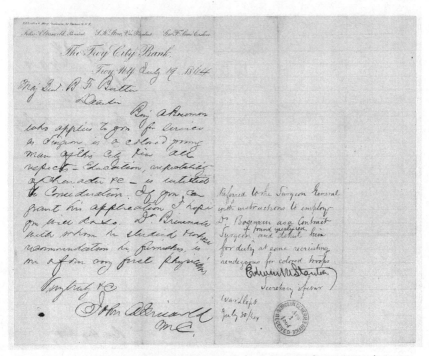

Letter acknowledging Benjamin A. Boseman Jr.'s application for a surgeon's position with the signature and approval of Secretary of War Edwin M. Stanton. *Courtesy National Archives and Records Administration, Washington, D.C.*

exam, he was recommended for an appointment as a contract acting assistant surgeon. With a rank of captain and pay of $100 per month, Boseman received his first assignment examining Black recruits at the recruiting rendezvous at Camp Foster in Hilton Head, South Carolina. A recruiting rendezvous was an enlistment and mustering location for Black soldiers joining the USCT. The camps generally consisted of wooden structures and tents that functioned as housing, food service, supply warehouses, administrative offices, and medical services for troops.

After seven months, he tired of the routine examinations and desired a transfer to a hospital where his skills could be challenged and improved. Writing to Congressman John Griswold on March 13, 1865, he asked for Griswold's assistance in obtaining a transfer to "one of the colored hospitals at Washington or Alexandria or even Norfolk or Portsmouth." Griswold had been of assistance to him when he made his initial application for an army position, and now he hoped the congressman could exert some influence to secure him a transfer. "My medical knowledge and experience," Boseman wrote, "will hardly be added to if I am to continue in this position for any length of time."[13] It is not clear whether Griswold intervened on his behalf, but by May 1865, Boseman was transferred to Mount Pleasant, South Carolina, for a short time before he returned to Hilton Head, where he tended to sick and wounded soldiers of the 21st Regiment of the USCT. Organized in South Carolina, the 21st Regiment served in Jacksonville, Florida, and then returned to South Carolina, where it served at Hilton Head and Folly Island. Although not officially the regimental surgeon, Boseman was assigned to provide medical care to soldiers of the regiment. He continued in this position until September 16, 1865, when his contract was annulled at his own request.

Boseman's presence as a Black surgeon among the soldiers of the 21st Regiment would have been a positive and empowering influence. Black soldiers were regularly subjected to racial discrimination that adversely affected their health and well-being. They suffered from inadequate access to medical care due to a lack of available and competent surgeons, fewer and poorer quality of medical and general supplies, and a lack of decent army-issued clothing and food rations. The presence of Black surgeons was rare but important, as they could advocate for improved medical care and better services for Black soldiers.

After the war Boseman remained in South Carolina, taking up residence in Charleston, where he established a successful medical practice. His arrival in town was announced in the local newspaper, and his new medical practice advertised office hours from 8 to 11 AM and 4 to 7 PM.[14] Boseman's hometown newspaper, the *Troy Times*, reported that "a young colored medical student, who served as Assistant Surgeon in a colored regiment, has commenced a practice in Charleston, and his success exceeds his most sanguine expectations."[15]

As a medical doctor, Boseman was described as "very successful with patients, and displays a great deal of skill, in his treatments."[16] He had "the family practice of the most influential and respectable members of the colored population in the city."[17] By January 1866, he had married Virginia Montgomery and started a family that included three children.[18]

As a contract army surgeon during the war, Boseman was an advocate for Black soldiers under his care. After the war, he continued to advocate for the progress of African Americans through activism and participation in the political system with a keen interest in his own personal advancement. In November 1865, the Colored People's Convention of the State of South Carolina convened at Zion Church in Charleston. Boseman's attendance at the convention provided him with good exposure to Black politicians in the state. The convention's purpose was to deliberate "upon the plans best calculated to advance the interests of our people, to devise means for our mutual protections, and to encourage the industrial interests of the State."[19] He took his experience at the state convention and considered his options for the future. He was not content serving only as a physician and sought other positions of leadership, power, and influence. After the enactment of the Reconstruction Acts of 1867 that gave Black men the right to vote three years before the passage of the Fifteenth Amendment to the U.S. Constitution, Boseman seized the opportunity to be at the center of political power in South Carolina. Setting his sights on a seat in the South Carolina House of Representatives, his name was placed on the ballot, and he succeeded in becoming a representative of Charleston in 1868.

He served in the House from 1868 to 1873 and was among several Black men elected at the time. Boseman became the only politician, Black or white, to be elected to three consecutive terms during Reconstruction.[20] But the election of Black men to political positions in South Carolina was not without controversy and protest. Charleston had become a prosperous city dominated by the white elite who were resistant to relinquish the power and positions they had long held. The *New Hampshire Patriot* echoed the discontent that was felt: "What a progress we shall make in the South with 'Cuffee' and 'Sambo' thus leading the van in its principal cities—dishonored and degraded vagrants, who have crawled into the places that were once filled by genius, worth and

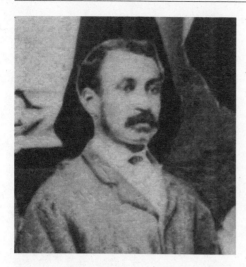

Benjamin A. Boseman Jr. as a representative in the South Carolina Legislature, pictured among the "Radical Members of the First South Carolina Legislature after the War," c. 1870. *Courtesy Library of Congress, LC-DIG-ppmsca-30572, Washington, D.C.*

talent? Who will not vote at the North, to brush away, as we would the web of the spider of this shameful and infamous burlesque upon government in the South?"[21]

As a member of the House of Representatives, Boseman was considered a "consistent and conservative Republican."[22] He was described as having "acquired considerable polish, and an amount of information which he can communicate in a very agreeable way. His conservative efforts . . . [which] so often stemmed the tide of corruption, are well known to all our taxpayers."[23] He served on several committees, including the Committee on Public Printing and the Medical Committee, making regular reports on committee resolutions and participating in debates on various bills under consideration. In July 1868, Boseman introduced civil rights legislation that would "prevent discrimination between persons by those carrying on business under license on account of race, color, or previous condition." Public opinion against the legislation was expressed in the local newspapers. Charleston's *Tri-Weekly Mercury* claimed, "It will be a sorry day when the Radicals of South Carolina attempt to enforce their odious social equality doctrine. . . . The bogus carpet-bag and negro Legislature insists upon depriving hotel keepers, railroad and steamship companies from making a distinction between the races. We presume the next step will be to invade the sanctuary."[24] The *Charleston Daily News* believed that the Radical members were attempting to force the new law through the legislature.[25] The legislation eventually passed after changes were made to the bill in the Senate, but the final law did little to change or reduce discrimination.

In addition to his public service as a state legislator, Boseman held several other positions in Charleston. He was appointed physician to the Charleston City Jail in 1869 by South Carolina governor Robert Scott, served on the Board of Regents of the state lunatic asylum, and held a position as a vestryman at St. Mark's Episcopal Church. He was also appointed to the Board of Trustees of the University of South Carolina in 1869 by a majority vote of the state legislature and was the board's Secretary. During this time, he served in the Second Division of the National Guard of South Carolina as inspector under the leadership of fellow Black legislator Robert Smalls, who served as major general. Smalls was well-known in the country for his courageous capture of a Confederate supply ship on which he worked as a deckhand, steering it into U.S. waters as a means to gain his freedom and that of Black men on board ship.[26]

Boseman also involved himself in several business ventures as a means to move himself up the social and economic ladder. He owned shares in the South Carolina Loan and Trust Company and in 1870 helped establish the Black-owned Enterprise Railroad, Inc., taking on the prestigious position of vice president.[27] He hoped it would advance his own personal position while providing transportation for the Black community. After the company received authorization from the state legislature to incorporate, it began construction that was completed in 1874. The railroad's horse-drawn carriages carried passengers and freight throughout the city, connecting Charleston docks with the city's railroad stations. The railroad continued under Black leadership for nearly a decade until white people gained a majority control of its management and ownership.

After completing his third term as a state representative in 1873, he resigned his seat to become the first Black postmaster of Charleston. Appointed by President Ulysses S. Grant, he held this position for eight years and was the highest paid postmaster in South Carolina with a salary of $4,000 per year.[28] However, reaction to the newly appointed Black postmaster was disapproving. Eliza Holmes, wife of Charleston physician Henry McCall Holmes, was appalled at Boseman's appointment and wrote to a friend, "Surely our humiliation has been great when a Black Postmaster is established here at Headquarters and our Gentlemens Son's to work under his biddings."[29] The *Charleston Daily News* held a contrary opinion that "the new appointee is an intelligent, courteous and educated colored man" who had served his country in the war and was the physician to the Charleston jail. "In all relations," the article said, "he commanded a good share of the respect of citizens of all shades of political complexion, and it is expected that in the important post to which he has now been appointed, he will prove a conscientious, trustworthy and competent officer."[30] He was described in his postmaster position as "civil and accommodating . . . and an excellent officer. . . . A more acceptable colored man could not have been placed in such a position."[31]

Boseman led a relatively quiet but prosperous life, occasionally voicing his opinion on political issues and candidates running for public office. In mid-January 1881, he fell ill with Bright's disease and died one month later on February 25 at the age of forty. At the time of his death, his estate was valued at $11,375.06 and included property in Charleston, a horse and buggy, life insurance policies, cash, stocks, and other assets. His obituary remembered him as "a faithful and efficient officer, a sterling man," and "an honor to his race."[32]

10. ✤ A Family Affair: Charles Burleigh Purvis (1842–1929)

American manhood must know of no color.
—Charles B. Purvis

Charles Burleigh Purvis was born in Philadelphia on April 14, 1842, to famed abolitionists Harriet Forten and Robert Purvis. Reared in an affluent and influential Black family, Purvis was surrounded by well-educated, politically savvy, and intellectual antislavery activists. His family's home was a center of abolitionist activities in Philadelphia and a stop on the Underground Railroad. Charles B. Purvis carried the activist torch lit by his parents and grandparents as he served his country as a nurse and surgeon during the Civil War and as a physician, educator, and activist after the war.

The greatest influences on Purvis's life were his parents and the legacy of his grandfather James Forten, who set the stage for the activism and social consciousness that would be a central tenet for generations of their family. James Forten was born free in Philadelphia in 1766 and educated in a Quaker school. After his father died, he was forced to quit school to help support his family. As a teenager he served during the American Revolution and after the war was an apprentice to a white sailmaker, from whom he learned the trade. His skill and hard work gained him promotions and led to his ownership of the company by the age of thirty-two. As his business and reputation grew, so did his wealth. Although Forten was freeborn, he identified with the struggle of enslaved people and considered it his struggle too. He was one of the nation's most outspoken Black critics of enslavement.[1] Forten and his wife, Charlotte Vandine, were founders and leaders of several antislavery groups. Hosting many abolitionist gatherings in their home, the Fortens also supported antislavery journals and newspapers and provided refuge for formerly enslaved people. They spoke out about freedom and equality at every opportunity, which brought them a level of celebrity that attracted antislavery activists to Philadelphia from all over the country.

James and Charlotte had nine children, including Harriet, the mother of Charles Purvis. The Forten home was filled with intellectual discourse, political activism, and a progressive social consciousness that fueled the family's cause and encouraged the next generation in continuing the effort. Harriet and her eight siblings were taught to live honest, respectable, and responsible lives centered on abolition and equality. With the influence and encouragement of their parents, the Forten children were educated in private interracial schools and by private tutors. They participated with their parents in antislavery activities and were vocal proponents of abolition. Harriet joined her sisters and mother in founding the Philadelphia Female Anti-Slavery Society in 1833.[2]

Robert Purvis, Charles's father, was no less an influence on Charles than his mother. Robert was born free in South Carolina, the son of a white naturalized British cotton broker, William Purvis, and a free "mulatto" mother, Harriet Judah, of German and Jewish ancestry. Harriet Judah had been enslaved when she arrived in South Carolina in 1766 but was freed through a provision in her enslaver's will.[3] After the death of Robert's father, he and his mother along with his two brothers lived off the wealthy inheritance from his father's estate, enabling him to be educated by private tutors and attend Amherst Academy, a private preparatory school in Massachusetts, later Amherst College. Purvis's wealth and his light complexion offered him a certain amount of freedom that most Black men in nineteenth-century America did not experience. Despite these advantages, he chose to live and identify as a man of color, accepting the fact that he would be subjected to all the prejudices and discrimination that identity held. He became an outspoken proponent of education and an ardent abolitionist who considered himself "bound with those in chains."[4] It is no wonder that James Forten took an immediate liking to Robert Purvis and welcomed him into the family as a son when he married Forten's daughter Harriet in 1831.

Robert Purvis and Harriet Forten Purvis settled in Philadelphia, where they started a family and led an active and socially conscious life. Like the generation before them, they were devoted to social justice, serving as an example of activism and service to the next generation. Keeping in the tradition with the Forten and Purvis families, they participated in the antislavery movement, opened their home to formerly enslaved people as a stop on the Underground Railroad, and were vocal in their support of women's rights. Together with Harriet's father, they established the Vigilant Association of Philadelphia and the Female Vigilant Association, which raised funds and supported those escaping enslavement. In the Purvis home, formerly enslaved people found a safe haven on their journey to freedom. Robert was referred to as the "President of the Underground Railroad" whose house "was a well-known station where his horses and carriages and his personal attendance were ever at the service of the travelers upon that road."[5]

Robert approached social issues from a human rights perspective rather than a singularly Black person's or women's rights view. He believed Black people born in the United States were not African American but native American and as such were due the same rights and privileges as any white American. When referring to the rights of Black people, he said, "There is not a single African in the United States. We are to the manner born; we are native Americans."[6] His view on women's suffrage was similar: both men and women should have the right to vote equally. He and Harriet gave their unwavering support to the suffrage movement, often attending women's rights meetings and publicly expressing their advocacy for a woman's right to vote. He once said, "I would prefer to bide my time for twenty years before I shall deposit a ballot, if at that time I may be allowed to take my wife and daughter with me to the ballot-box."[7] Although he desired the right to vote as an American-born citizen, he felt that right should be extended to women and was willing to wait for his right to vote until his wife and daughter could also exercise that same right.

Establishing a home in Philadelphia, their family grew, including son Charles Burleigh, the fifth of eight children. They were an affluent Black family living a comfortable life with several servants, including an English governess for their children. By 1834, their peaceful life was threatened by riots and attacks that were being made on Black businesses and homes. They became a target, not only because of the family's vocal and public statements on abolition but because they were suspected of harboring formerly enslaved people. These threats against the Black community continued to grow, reaching a peak by 1842. Historian Margaret Hope Bacon described one incident that year when, after giving an antislavery speech, Robert Purvis was met by the "English governess of his children who pleaded with him not to go home because the mob had surrounded his house and intended to kill him." Despite the governess's pleas, Purvis "rushed home where he found his terrified wife and children." Though safe, "he sent them . . . upstairs, and took a seat on the stairs, with his rifle across his knees," intent on protecting his family at all costs.[8]

As a result of the increasing threats, Robert and Harriet decided to move their family to a farm in Byberry, Pennsylvania, about twelve miles outside

Philadelphia. They believed relocating would provide a safer and more peaceful life for their children, despite the fact that as the only Black family in Byberry, they were still confronted with racism and discrimination. The farm had a large house with over one hundred acres of land and was situated across from the Quaker Friends Meeting House and Friends school. They raised livestock, kept horses, and grew fruit trees, flowers, and vegetables. Their home was called Harmony Hall, and it included a separate room used as a schoolroom for the children.[9] After they arrived at the farm, Purvis began construction of a room in the basement to hide formerly enslaved people. Charlotte Forten, the niece of Harriet Forten Purvis, was a schoolteacher and lived with the Purvis family for a time in 1858 and 1859. She was not only a cherished family member but also the tutor for the younger Purvis children. In her diary, Charlotte described the Purvis home as always elegant and orderly.[10]

Their home, like that of James Forten, became a center of abolitionist activities with a constant influx of guests. William Lloyd Garrison, white editor of the antislavery newspaper the *Liberator*, was a frequent guest of the Purvises and commented that Robert and Harriet were gracious and hospitable hosts who welcomed not only their friends and family but also those escaping enslavement "en route to Canada."[11] Their progressive ideas and abolitionist activities, like those of the generation before them, were a great influence on their children, including their son Charles and their niece Charlotte Forten.

Charles B. Purvis seemed destined from birth to carry the torch of activism and abolition thanks to the legacy of his grandfather and the example set by his parents and perhaps also by his namesake, Charles Burleigh, a fiery, red-haired abolitionist, known for his intellect, dedication, and impassioned eloquent words.[12] His family's affluence allowed him to receive his early education from private tutors as well as from the Quaker school across from the family's farm. He reminisced about his school days, describing how his first teacher found "pleasure in arousing me from my delightful slumber by squeezing water from a sponge in my ear."[13]

Education was an essential part of the upbringing of every member of the Purvis and Forten families. Robert Purvis was a strong proponent of education and fought for nondiscriminatory public schools in Philadelphia. After attending the Friends School in Byberry, the Purvis children were required to attend the public schools alongside white students, where they were subjected to discrimination and poor treatment. In 1853, after the county established segregated schools and excluded the Purvis children from the mainstream public schools, Robert protested by refusing to pay the school tax as part of his property taxes because he believed his "rights as a citizen . . . have been grossly outraged in depriving me, in violation of law and justice, of the benefits of the school system which this tax was designed to sustain." He said the proscription and exclusion of his children from the public school system was illegal, and he believed it an "unjustifiable usurpation" of his rights. Because of this exclusion, Purvis felt compelled to "obtain the services of private teachers" to instruct his children. His protest was eventually successful; the school board voted to no longer exclude Black children from public schools.[14]

After completing his early education, Charles gained admission to Oberlin College in Ohio, where he was an undergraduate from 1860 to 1863, studying in the teachers' course of the preparatory department. Oberlin College had a reputation as a center for abolitionist activities and was one of the only colleges, at that time, to admit students without respect to race or gender.[15] In the 1862–63 academic year, the school had 401 female and 457 male students.[16] Perhaps this more open admission policy attracted Purvis to the college. Oberlin professor Reverend Henry Cowles, when asked whether Black and white students were required to associate with one another, replied,

> The white and colored students associate together in this college very much as they choose. Our doctrine is that *mind* and *heart*, not *color*, make the man and the woman too. We hold that neither men or women are much the better or much the worse for their *skin* color. Our great business here is to educate mind and heart, and we should deem ourselves to have small cause to be proud of our success if we should fail to eradicate, in no long time, the notion that nature had made any such difference between the colored and the white classes that it would be wrong for either to associate with the other as beings of common origin and a common nature. . . . If you are a young gentleman of color, you may expect to be treated here according to your real merit; and if white, you need not expect to fare better than this.[17]

Admission requirements included testimonials of good character in addition to an excellent academic record. To be accepted as a full member of the student body, it was necessary to complete a six-month probation period. Purvis paid a school fee of $15.00 per year with incidental expenses of $2.25 per year. Various living accommodations were offered to students, including a room at the college that came with a stove for heating. The teachers' course in which Purvis was enrolled included studies in mathematics, languages, and history as well as physical, biological, and psychological sciences, literature, economics, social and political science, and civics. Students were also required to participate in the teachers' institute for instruction in the theory and practice of teaching.

Purvis spent three years at Oberlin before he turned his interest to studying medicine at Cleveland Medical College in 1863, later the medical department of Western Reserve College. Medical school acceptance required evidence of a student-teacher relationship with an established physician. In the list of medical students for the year 1862–63, he is recorded as hailing from Philadelphia with Dr. Bunce as his "preceptor."[18] This is likely Hiram A. Bunce, a graduate of Yale and a respected physician in Cleveland. Though he is listed as Purvis's preceptor, it is unclear whether Purvis actually studied under Bunce's tutelage.

The school's annual medical course of lectures was conducted over a four-month period with six lectures daily, including medical and surgical clinics held each Wednesday. Purvis had access to the medical museum with a large collection of paintings and illustrations of anatomy, diseases of the skin, circulation, and other medical subjects as well as a one-thousand-volume library. In addition to standard medical subjects such as anatomy and materia medica, students were required to take the chemical course to gain an understanding of chemistry, electricity, galvanism, pneumatics, magnetism, and toxicology. A large collection of instruments and apparatuses were made available to demonstrate the principles of surgery, and students observed a variety of surgical operations. Purvis successfully fulfilled the requirements for graduation, which included medical studies for three years, attending two full courses at the medical college, submission of a thesis on an acceptable medical subject, and payment of a twenty-dollar graduation fee. Testimonials of good moral character and achieving a passing grade on the faculty-administered examination were also mandatory.[19] Purvis submitted a thesis titled "Variola," on smallpox, in which he describes three varieties of the disease with their diagnoses and treatments.[20] In March 1865, he was one of fourteen graduates to receive a medical degree and the first documented Black graduate of the medical school.

While still a medical student, he volunteered as a nurse at Freedmen's Hospital in Washington, D.C., from June to October 1864. The hospital was established in 1862 by the U.S. Army and was one of the few in Washington that treated Black civilians and soldiers. By the time of his arrival, the hospital had a Black surgeon-in-charge and a staff of mostly African Americans. When the war began, the majority of nurses at most hospitals were male, often convalescing soldiers. Women were not considered physically

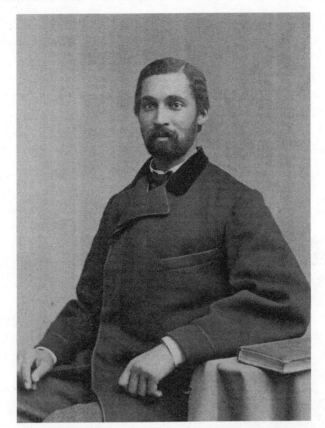

Charles B. Purvis, c. 1860. *Courtesy Weld Grimké Family Papers, William L. Clements Library, University of Michigan, Ann Arbor.*

or mentally equipped to manage nursing duties, but when fewer men were available, women were hired to take on those responsibilities. His work as a nurse at the facility would be the start of an enduring relationship with the hospital that lasted more than fifty years. Like his cousin Charlotte Forten, who offered her services as a teacher and nurse during the war, Charles was inspired by a shared family tradition of social activism, service, and a strong desire to work for freedom.[21]

In June 1865, Purvis took a position as contract acting assistant surgeon at Freedmen's Hospital working alongside surgeons Anderson R. Abbott, John H. Rapier Jr., and William B. Ellis. His position provided a monthly salary of $100, and he remained a contract surgeon until October of that year. After the war, he assisted with the transition of Freedmen's Hospital from the control of the U.S. Army to the Bureau of Refugees, Freedmen, and Abandoned

Lands. He remained there as it further transitioned to the teaching hospital for the newly formed Howard University medical department in 1868. Purvis accepted a teaching position at the university in early 1869, the second Black medical school faculty member, following Alexander T. Augusta, who had been appointed the previous year. Purvis's commitment to the medical program is evident by his long association with the university as an educator, faculty leader, administrator, and member of the board of trustees. He was described as laboring "indefatigably for the progress of the institution."[22] During his tenure as a professor, he taught materia medica, medical jurisprudence, obstetrics, diseases of women and children, and midwifery. In 1871, he received an honorary degree from the university's board of trustees and by 1883 was the surgeon-in-chief of Freedmen's Hospital, a position he held for ten years. In addition to his administrative and teaching responsibilities, he continued to practice medicine and served as the hospital's ward physician.

Just as his professional relationship with Howard University began, his personal life changed when he met Ann Hathaway, a white woman who had traveled south from Maine to teach freedmen. She came to Washington, D.C., to direct the facility established by the National Association for the Relief of Destitute Colored Women and Children. Charles and Ann were

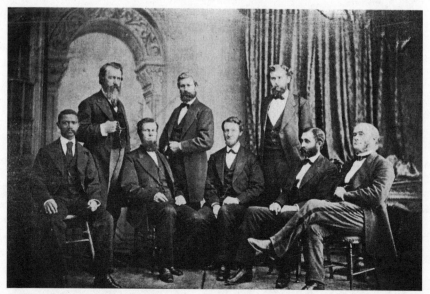

The faculty of Howard University Medical Department, 1869–70, including Alexander T. Augusta (*far left*) and Charles B. Purvis (*second from right*). *Courtesy National Library of Medicine, Bethesda, Md.*

married in 1871 and had two children. His interracial marriage was controversial as many saw it as a betrayal of the Black community. He was viewed
as classist, "advancing his own interests by claiming to be Negro at the same
time disdaining any association with the Black people."[23] The *Washington
Bee* commented that "Dr. C. B. Purvis and his wife never go to society of
any kind, the white people won't take them and the colored don't like her." A
differing opinion noted that "Dr. Charles B. Purvis's society and that of his
wife are eagerly sought."[24]

He continued to encounter difficulties because of his personal circumstances. When he decided to send his two children to private schools while
at the same time advocating for the education of Black children in public
schools, many saw this as hypocritical and elitist. The struggle between private and public school attendance for his children was reminiscent of his own
experience during childhood when he attended both a private and a public
school. His interracial marriage would continue to cause him difficulties as
he established himself in leadership positions within the community.

In 1873, the country suffered a financial crisis that impacted Howard University. Medical department faculty were asked to resign, after which the
university's trustees reappointed the same instructors at the same salaries with
the understanding that they would be paid only if the necessary funds could
be raised. There were only three medical school faculty—Charles B. Purvis,
Alexander T. Augusta, and Gideon S. Palmer—who accepted the conditions
and continued to work without pay. "While I regret the University will not be
able to pay me for my services," he wrote Howard University president O. O.
Howard, "I feel the importance of every effort being made to carry forward the
institution and make it a success."[25] During this time, he was instrumental in
keeping the medical department afloat and enlisted the help of several other
physicians who agreed to assist him. He assumed an administrative role in
the department beginning in 1873 and was elected secretary of the faculty, a
position he held for twenty-three years.

His dedication to the university's medical department was only one example of the influence of his family's legacy of advocacy for education and
social justice. While managing his medical career and training new medical
students, he served as a trustee of the Colored Women's Relief Association
and advocated in favor of home rule for the District of Columbia. He was
among 1,300 citizens of Washington, D.C., who in 1877 signed a petition
to newly elected president Rutherford B. Hayes commending his inaugural
address that supported local self-government. The letter also requested the

extension of that support to the District of Columbia and the selection of three commissioners for the District "from our own citizens, fully assured that the happiness and prosperity of our people will be greatly promoted thereby."[26] Purvis was among a committee of four individuals tasked with presenting the petition to the president.

Purvis was often in a position to report on Freedmen's Hospital and its management. In testimony before a government appropriations subcommittee convened in the U.S. Senate in 1878, he provided testimony on the history of the hospital and patient statistics. His policy was to accept and treat all people who needed medical care regardless of color. He noted that during an outbreak of the flu or "la grippe" that caused overcrowding in all city hospitals, the facility was "always pretty full, especially in wet winters like this. We always try and have room for one more, but during the 'grip' we were at our wits' ends, but we did not turn any away. . . . We never refuse anybody who is sick." He described the hospital as having three hundred beds and being "by far the largest hospital in the city" with "many cases of rheumatism and lung trouble" as well as typhoid fever. He said, "Our hospital is not exclusively what its name, 'The Freedmen's,' indicates. Out of 3,279 patients last year, 525 were white."[27]

Purvis served as surgeon-in-chief of Freedmen's Hospital from 1883 to 1893, though his tenure was not always met with favor from the public. In 1883, the *Washington Bee* claimed that he had "no identity with the colored race" and was being "kept in a position against the will of the people."[28] Three years later, it was reported that a petition was circulating demanding the secretary of the Interior make a change to the administration of Freedmen's Hospital. Five hundred signatures were secured supporting the removal of Purvis as surgeon-in-chief, and a search for a replacement was initiated. A short list of candidates who could replace Purvis included Alexander T. Augusta, who was described as having a "reputation of being a first-class physician and surgeon . . . very conservative in his views and will no doubt make a fine Surgeon in charge of Freedmen's Hospital."[29]

Support for Purvis and Augusta was divided with strong opinions on both sides. Despite any opposition he faced, Purvis maintained his position for a few more years until Daniel Hale Williams was appointed as the hospital's chief administrator in 1894, replacing Purvis. Williams was the founder of Provident Hospital and Training School in Chicago, the first Black-owned and Black-operated hospital in the United States. He had served as Provident's administrator since its founding in 1891 before assuming the position of surgeon-in-chief at Freedmen's Hospital. There was some controversy surrounding the circumstances of Purvis's departure. It was reported that he had resigned, but he believed his removal as surgeon-in-chief was politically motivated since he was a Republican and Williams was a Democrat. He did not think highly of Williams: "The new surgeon-in-chief caused much trouble as he persistently sought to force himself into the faculty of the college to be a professor of surgery and made it quite clear that unless his ambition was gratified the college could not expect very many advantages or favors from the hospital."[30] Despite his removal, Purvis continued his relationship with the university.

His activism was extended to his own profession when in 1869, along with Alexander T. Augusta and Alpheus W. Tucker, he sought membership and access to the Medical Society of the District of Columbia, an affiliate of the American Medical Society. The society was the local medical organization that licensed physicians in Washington and through membership enabled physicians to hold consultations with one another and participate in discourse on medical cases for the benefit of their profession. In early 1869, Purvis and Augusta had their names submitted for membership (Tucker applied three months later), but they were denied. Without membership, they could not consult with other physicians or participate in discussions of current medical cases and treatments. In some instances, white physicians stole patients from Purvis and Augusta. "It is not an uncommon experience of mine," said Purvis, "to have physicians take my patients, they knowing I had not been dismissed, doing me great injury."[31]

It was suggested by a local newspaper that their desire for membership was a way to force themselves into a social relationship with white physicians and that the society was a private social organization. Purvis argued that social organizations were never granted charters and that the charter of the Medical Society "sets forth that the object of the Society is to advance medical science, which science, as we understand it, belongs to the world and not to the Medical Society of this District." He pointed out that one of the charter's provision made it "a punishable offence for any member of the Society to hold consultation with a physician who is not a member" and noted that this provision "acted as a great stumbling block to our practice." He believed that this provision denied them the practice of medicine as "those who otherwise would have employed us, refused on the ground that if consultation should ever be required in the case at hand, that they preferred employing those who could be consulted with." He went on to state that "nothing is more surprising to us than to find men who derive a large share of their support from the colored people of the city so bitter in their opposition to us." His understanding of the obstacles and his resolve to fight for justice and equality were clear when he stated that "such opposition is not new to us. We met it when we attempted to enter the medical college; we met it when we applied to enter medical college; we met it when we applied, in common with other students, for our diplomas; we have been at war with it ever since we commenced the practice of our profession and we expect to do so until we conquer it."[32] Undeterred by this setback, Purvis and Augusta helped formed the National Medical Society of the District of Columbia, declaring it a racially integrated organization.

Never one to shrink from action in the fight against discrimination, Purvis often acted upon his support for equal rights and Black representation in civic and political arenas. In September 1874, he and his friend John Mercer Langston, a Black attorney, were refused service in a Washington, D.C., restaurant and filed a lawsuit. The presiding judge in the case ruled in their favor, imposing a $109 fine against the restaurant after determining that the restaurant violated an 1872 legislative act that made it a misdemeanor to refuse to serve a person based on "race, color or previous condition of servitude."[33]

Purvis continued to break barriers, sometimes due to unexpected circumstances. On the morning of July 2, 1881, President James Garfield was waiting for a train at the Baltimore and Potomac Railroad Station in Washington, D.C., when an assassin's bullet struck him in the back and the arm. As fate would have it, Purvis was at the station and came to the president's aid. He was given an "honorable mention" along with several other physicians in a federal report of the incident, which noted that he "did all that science and skill could accomplish towards the patient's relief."[34] His treatment of the wounded Garfield that day gave him the distinction of being the first Black physician to attend to a sitting president.

In 1898, Purvis suffered the loss of his beloved wife, Ann, whose miniature portrait he wore on his watch chain. After her death he lived alone in their home for three years before marrying Jennie C. Proctor Butman, a white woman from New England. His two children, Alice and Robert, were adults and practicing medicine and dentistry in Boston and Philadelphia, respectively. As he entered his sixties, he suffered from some physical disabilities and decided to apply for a military pension. In his application of 1905, he claimed his "permanent disability . . . from chorodites of both eyes, [and] neurasthenia . . . from typhoid fever" were contracted while working at Freedmen's Hospital during the war. Though this would have qualified him for a service-related disability, his application was rejected by the Pension Bureau, which claimed he was ineligible because he was "employed in the Civil branch of the U.S.

Service only" as a contract surgeon.[35] This was a common reason for rejection, especially among applying Black surgeons, including William P. Powell Jr. and Anderson R. Abbott.

Purvis officially retired from Howard University in 1905, but his connection to the school continued with his election to the university's board of trustees three years later, and he served in that position for the next eighteen years. He maintained a regular correspondence with the university president, often discussing current events and issues related to the university and the medical department. After relocating to Boston in 1908 to be closer to his daughter, he established a medical practice after passing the state medical examination and became a member of the Massachusetts Medical Society. Though he enjoyed his practice, he decided to retire from medicine a few years later.

Retirement gave Purvis and his wife time to travel to Europe, spend time in the mountains of New Hampshire, and enjoy the winter months in California. He told his friends that he was "employed as most idlers employ time. I read some, talk a plenty, dance occasionally. One meets all sorts of people in a place such as this."[36] Purvis maintained a social consciousness and concern for social justice. Commenting on World War I, he said, "It is strange to see how blind the people are to their own short-comings. Racial prejudice is the most unreasonable of all prejudices, those who have it seem to enjoy having it. The great war has opened our eyes to the fact that the prejudice of race, against race, is responsible for the ill feeling & prejudice existing. What terrible times we live in! Civilized man has departed."[37]

As the years went by, he became keenly aware of his own failing health, noting his many ailments: "There are too many pains playing hide and seek amidst my bones, muscles, and nerves, to indulge in brag." Despite this acknowledgment, he still felt he could contribute to society. "While I have passed the four score mark," he wrote, "I am insouciant to the fact that men older than I have played an active part in the affairs of life," making reference to Michelangelo, "who drew plans of St. Peter's when he was 89"; Sophocles, who "wrote his Oedipus at 99"; and Dandola, "who stormed Constantinople at 90."[38]

Purvis's health continued to decline. He understood that he was in his twilight years, saying, "I am here in spite of an urgent invitation to make a long visit to the land of mystery."[39] On January 30, 1929, at the age of eighty-six, Charles Burleigh Purvis died while on his yearly visit to California. His enduring legacy of activism and advocacy is a testament to his commitment to freedom, justice, and equality.

11. ❀ The Black Ivy League: Cortlandt Van Rensselaer Creed (1833–1900) and William Baldwin Ellis (1833–1866)

> I had my fears and doubts as to whether I would be admitted at "Yale."
> Knowing the prejudice against color was somewhat apparent, in time
> past, I, however, felt nerved for a trial.
>
> —Cortlandt Van Rensselaer Creed

Cortlandt Van Rensselaer Creed and William Baldwin Ellis share a common achievement: they were among the first Black graduates of Ivy League medical schools—Creed, a graduate of the Medical Institution of Yale College, and Ellis, a graduate of Dartmouth Medical College. Born free in the East Coast communities of New Haven, Connecticut, and New York City, both set their sights on an advanced education, a career in medicine, and service to their country as surgeons during the Civil War.

The journey toward a medical education for Black people in the United States was challenging. Prior to 1847, no African American had been trained at a U.S. medical school, let alone an Ivy League school. But in 1850, three Black students, Daniel Laing Jr., Isaac H. Snowden, and Martin Delaney, were accepted to Harvard Medical School. Their admission was adamantly protested by white students. Despite Harvard's policy to accept Black applicants on the merit of their qualifying examinations, the school capitulated to the pressure of white students and expelled the Black students.[1] Though some Blacks were admitted to medical schools like the Medical School of Maine at Bowdoin College and the Medical Institution of Yale College, this policy did not represent an accepted or common practice in the mid-nineteenth century. Admission did not mean acceptance. Black people who pursued a medical education found little encouragement and faced many obstacles and discrimination along the way. Even with exemplary academic credentials, acceptance into a medical school for African Americans was rarely achieved.

Creed and Ellis were raised in families that emphasized education as a means for advancement. The comprehensive schooling their parents were able to provide for them and the influence and inspiration they received from prominent Black members of their communities made it easier for Creed and Ellis to consider careers as physicians and instilled in them the vision to see their potential, the confidence to believe in their abilities, and the strength to pursue careers that were nearly out of reach because of their color.

Cortlandt Van Rensselaer Creed

Cortlandt Van Rensselaer Creed was born free in 1833 in New Haven, Connecticut, the son of Vashti Duplex, a teacher, and John Creed, a steward and caterer. Vashti was the daughter of a successful landowner and Revolutionary War veteran, Prince Duplex. A strong advocate of education, Prince Duplex raised seven children, all of whom received an education, including Vashti, who would become the first Black schoolteacher in New Haven. Vashti tutored her son Cortlandt at home before he began his formal schooling. Creed's father, John, was born in the Virgin Islands and immigrated to New Haven sometime in 1820. He was involved in both religious and political activities in the city. He and Vashti married in 1830 and welcomed the birth of their first son, Cortlandt Van Rensselaer Creed, a few years later.

John worked as a janitor at Yale College and served as a steward for the literary group the Calliopean Society, a group of students predominantly from the South. He later became a successful caterer, preparing and serving meals to Yale alumni for nearly forty years.[2] John Creed's ambition and work ethic allowed him to amass enough wealth to move his family into a house in a traditionally white neighborhood in the late 1840s. His estate at the time of his death in 1864 was worth $13,468 and included a library, furniture, and several pieces of property.[3]

John's contacts and connections with Yale alumni and administrators included the wealthy and influential Cortlandt Van Rensselaer. Rensselaer, an 1827 graduate of Yale and the son of a wealthy New York landowner, was a Presbyterian minister who served as a missionary to enslaved people in Virginia in the early 1830s. It is likely that John developed a personal relationship with Rensselaer while working at Yale and may have received guidance from him as he developed his catering business. John Creed's high regard for Rensselaer is evidenced by his choosing the name Cortlandt Van Rensselaer Creed for his firstborn son. This connection may have influenced Cortlandt's admission to the medical college, similar to the way Richard Greene was admitted as an undergraduate. Greene, one of the first Black graduates of Yale College, was tutored by Lucius Fitch, a white Yale employee, who likely influenced his undergraduate admission in 1854.[4] Regardless of the impact that white men may have had on their admissions, acceptance at the school would not have been possible without their exemplary academic records.

Cortlandt Creed's parents were intent on providing a stellar education for all of their children. After being homeschooled by his mother, Cortlandt was sent to the progressive New Haven Lancasterian School for a more formal education. The Lancasterian School was a public school founded on the ideas of John Lancaster, where more advanced students taught less advanced ones. This system claimed to reduce the number of adult teachers required, thus lowering costs, but provided more instructors to students through the use of student teachers. The school's philosophy enabled it to offer an education to working-class families that was previously unavailable to them. At the Lancasterian School, Creed received instruction in spelling, reading, writing, and arithmetic along with geography, astronomy, history, English grammar, ornamental penmanship, and the drawing of pictures and maps.[5] This comprehensive education provided a good foundation to further his studies in medicine.

After graduating from the Lancasterian School, he began his medical education in December 1853, under the tutelage of respected white New Haven physician George E. Buddington. Creed referred to himself as an "office student" who applied himself closely to his studies and "was not long in unravelling the delicate network which surrounds the study of medicine." Under the instruction of Buddington, he attended to the doctor's patients, and as he remembered, "The doctor generally would send me to look after his patients, until at last he seldom operated without my assistance or presence."[6] His success at the Lancasterian School and his medical apprenticeship with Buddington encouraged him to apply to Yale's medical school. He was accepted in September 1854. Writing to famed Black abolitionist and statesman Frederick Douglass, Creed said of his acceptance, "I had my fears and doubts as to whether I would be admitted at 'Yale.' Knowing that prejudice against color was somewhat apparent, in time past, I, however, felt nerved for a trial." He admitted that as a student at Yale, he "never experienced anything other than the most polite treatment from my fellow classmates."[7] One year earlier, Richard Greene had been admitted as an undergraduate at Yale, and his attendance seemed little affected by his color. Although both Creed and

Greene were identified as Black, "mulatto," or "colored" in federal records, Yale student records made no note of the racial identity of students. Whether Creed and Greene experienced mistreatment while attending Yale cannot be definitively determined, but their presence was unusual and controversial.

The Medical Institution of Yale College was the nation's sixth medical school when Creed was admitted. It offered a rigorous course of study, including the principles and practice of surgery, anatomy and physiology, materia medica and therapeutics, chemistry, theory and practice of physic, and obstetrics. A medical and surgical clinic was held each week at the Connecticut Hospital, where students could gain experience in clinical care of a variety of cases. Creed had access to an anatomical museum, a cabinet of materia medica, the Museum of the Yale Natural History Society, a cabinet of minerals, and the libraries of the medical and academical departments. He paid a fee of $12.50 for each course with a $5.00 matriculation fee in addition to a graduation fee and a fee for a license and diploma. The requirements for a degree of doctor of medicine were three years of study for those without a bachelor of arts degree and two years for those with a degree, plus attendance at two full courses of lectures. In addition, each graduate was expected to have attained the age of twenty-one, had a good moral character, and successfully completed a formal oral examination before the State Board of Examinations, which included a dissertation presented on a medical sciences subject.[8]

Creed fulfilled all the requirements for a medical degree, including his "Dissertation on the Blood." He received his medical degree on January 19, 1857, along with ten other medical school graduates.[9] Although the ceremony marked the first time an African American received a medical degree from Yale, this achievement was not mentioned by either the college or the local newspapers. In that same year, Yale conferred the first bachelor of arts degree to another Black student, Richard H. Greene—another achievement that went unmentioned. Recognition of Yale's Black graduates was made seventeen years later in two publications that acknowledged "the first colored graduate of the academical department of Yale . . . among five colored men" who graduated from the school.[10] It appears there was some knowledge of the graduation of Black students at Yale, even though no racial designations appear in the school's student records. Greene would go on to attend Dartmouth Medical College and serve as a surgeon in the navy during the Civil War.[11]

After graduation, Creed intended to spend time in Europe and then settle down in Jamaica or Liberia, following in the path of supporters of Black emigration.[12] This idea may have been influenced by his relationship with his namesake, Cortlandt Van Rensselaer, who was a member of the American Colonization Society, which advocated for Black emigration. Creed eventually decided against emigrating and remained in New Haven, where he established a medical office in his father's home. By this time, he had married Drucilla Wright, a young woman from North Carolina with whom he had four sons.[13]

Creed gained a reputation as a caring and attentive physician and was often recognized in local newspapers. A letter from a patient to the *Weekly Anglo-African* in November 1859 expressed his "obligations to Dr. C. V. R. Creed . . . for the very successful and professional services that I received from him." Stricken with scrofula (a tuberculosis infection of the lymph nodes), the writer was referred to Dr. Creed for treatment. A longtime sufferer of the disease, he had little expectation of improvement under Creed's care, but after treatment, the patient believed that "to the best of my knowledge, I am now entirely free from my old enemy, the scrofula, and enjoying what I have not done before for nearly sixteen years—the blessings of health." Creed's success as a physician was a result not only of his compassionate and professional care but also of his "untiring industry and skill." His success created for him "an enduring niche in the temple of fame."[14] Though the majority of his patients were Black women and men, he treated some white patients.

His dedication to both medicine and education inspired him to pass his knowledge and skills on to a younger generation of medical doctors. In 1860, he took on a young medical student from Liberia as his apprentice. William Henry Ealbeck studied under Creed and went on to complete a medical degree at the Medical School of Maine.[15] Creed's desire to share his knowledge continued throughout his life and did not exclude female students. Women in the nineteenth century were often discouraged from advancement and denied an education, so it was unusual when Nellie Van Wyck, a young white woman from Glen Falls, New York, began studying medicine under Creed's tutelage.[16]

Creed was living a relatively comfortable life with his wife, children, and parents in New Haven when the outbreak of the Civil War in April 1861 roused his desire to participate in the fight for freedom. He was anxious to put his medical skills to use in service to his country and wrote to Connecticut governor William Buckingham requesting a position but was told that all the appointments had been made.[17] He continued to follow the war effort and found other ways to participate, including work with the Colored Freedmen's Aid Society.

Two years later, in 1863, when the recruitment of Black soldiers officially began, Creed registered for the draft and was listed as a physician from New

Haven.[18] He once again requested a surgeon's position with a regiment of Colored Volunteers in a letter to Governor Buckingham: "I beg the privilege of going out with the regiment, as surgeon. I was examined last summer, before the 'Massachusetts Medical Commission' for the U.S. Army, and passed my examination with credit, and should have long since been in the field, had it not been for the alarming illness of my wife, who is now slowly convalescing."[19] He had received an appointment as assistant surgeon with the 55th Massachusetts Colored Infantry that June, but he was unable to accept the position because of his wife's illness.

In a show of support for Creed's application, Dr. P. A. Jewett, Creed's former instructor at the Medical Institution of Yale College, wrote to Governor Buckingham describing Creed as "a young man of good ability and first-rate education. I know of nothing against his moral character. I have no doubt he would perform the duties of Asst. Surgeon satisfactorily."[20] Creed secured an interview with Buckingham that took place sometime between December 7 and December 18, 1863, perhaps as a result of Jewett's letter. Following up on his interview, Creed wrote to the governor and reminded him of their conversation: "[You] wished me not to engage my services in any other direction until I heard from you which would be in a few days. I have therefore resorted to this medium, hoping that I may hear from you, by return mail." He appealed to the governor for a "position in a regiment from my own state" and provided a list of twenty-four individuals as references, including the president of Yale College, Theodore Dwight Woolsey; Yale professor Reverend Leonard Bacon; and Civil War naval officer and New Haven native Admiral Andrew Hull Foote.[21]

His wife's declining health caused Creed to again put off military service until after her death in late January 1864. He reapplied for a position as acting assistant surgeon, but as he came late to the recruitment, positions in the 29th Regiment of the Connecticut Colored Volunteers had already been filled. Instead, he accepted a position with the 30th Regiment, where he served for nearly two years, from January 1864 until November 1865. As an army surgeon, he was remembered for "his valuable service" and the "remarkably good care" he provided to his patients. He was "universally respected and beloved by the men for his courtesy and unwearied interest in their welfare."[22]

The 30th Regiment to which Creed was appointed was described as "a very excellent class in morals, drill and efficiency . . . with a marked degree of intelligence."[23] He examined recruits and tended to their illnesses. In the summer of 1864, the regiment was sent south to Virginia, where it joined other

Black regiments to form the 31st Regiment of the USCT. Creed did not accompany his regiment to Virginia but instead was detached to the Department of the East. It was standard procedure for Black surgeons to be reassigned to hospitals or recruiting stations rather than serve with their regiments in the field, where white surgeons would not work alongside them.

Following the end of the war, in the summer of 1865, Creed was still a surgeon with the Connecticut Colored Volunteers. He married his second wife, Mary A. Paul, in New York City in July, and they had four daughters and two sons. The family lived in New Haven, where Creed resumed his medical practice and provided care to the city's residents.

In his later years, he continued to practice medicine, and his prominent reputation was often referenced in the local newspapers. In 1881, his involvement in a local murder case made national news. Jennie Cramer was a young woman admired for her beauty and known to most residents of the city. On the morning of August 6, her lifeless body was found lying face down on a beach, a bruise on her forehead and shoulder.[24] Creed was asked to participate in the woman's autopsy as a medical expert. The case garnered national attention, and Creed's involvement was often mentioned. The *New York Times* reported that "Dr. Creed is a colored man, and a graduate of the Yale Medical College, having been the first of his race to graduate in any department of the college. . . . He has been a great reader, and is a polished and interesting talker upon almost any subject. His standing in the medical profession of the city is excellent, and he assisted at the autopsy of the Cramer girl."[25] The article went on to present Dr. Creed's view on the murder and his opinion on the unanswered questions in the case, including the origin of the bruise on Cramer's forehead. The focus on a Black physician's participation and opinion in such a prominent murder case was unusual and a testament to Creed's reputation as a physician.

In December 1879, he joined the Connecticut National Guard as assistant surgeon in the all-Black 5th Battalion. After the Civil War, many African Americans who had served during the war wanted to continue their service by joining the National Guard, but they were restricted because of color. Black Civil War veterans in Connecticut decided to form independent guard units in hopes they would eventually receive official acceptance and recognition. The state of Connecticut passed an act permitting the formation of the all-Black 5th Battalion in 1879. The battalion consisted of four companies; Creed belonged to Company A, known as Wilkins Guard of New Haven. It is likely he participated with the 5th Battalion in a public parade in 1880.

Many Black people eagerly awaited the appearance of the battalion and "the utmost interest was manifested by large throngs of colored people as the sound of the drums and band music was heard drawing near, telling that the battalion had started."[26]

Creed was proud of his service during the war and became a member of the Grand Army of the Republic, but after many years with the group his membership came under question.[27] In 1897, he became ill and was receiving aid from the organization during his illness. The GAR, as part of its support of veterans, provided care for sick members. To qualify for this aid, veterans were required to supply proof that they were honorably discharged from the military. When Creed submitted proof of his service, the GAR became aware that he technically had never been in the regular army. He could provide discharge documentation only from the Connecticut National Guard. As proof of military service and an honorable discharge were the prime requisites for admission to the GAR, his membership was revoked and the care he had been receiving withdrawn.

Creed's life took a downward turn beginning with the death of his mother, Vashti, in 1879. After living a relatively affluent lifestyle, legal and funeral

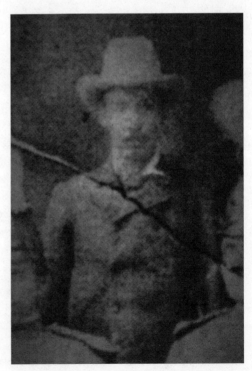

Cortlandt Van Rensselaer Creed, all-Black 5th Battalion, Wilkins Guard, c. 1879. *Courtesy The Ethnic Heritage Center, New Haven, Conn.*

expenses from his mother's death along with other personal matters, including troubles with his wife, led to the depletion of the family's fortune. He was forced to sell family land to cover expenses and move to a small apartment with his son Edward. The financial stability he once knew was gone, but he continued his medical practice in his New Haven community. He became a member of the Connecticut Medical Society in 1885 and was described as "our only colored physician" who is "affable, courteous, talented," and "equal to the task" in any emergency.[28]

The good reputation he had earned was soon tarnished, though, as his impoverishment led to his inability to pay rent or sustain himself. At one point he faced eviction because of his inability to pay his monthly rent. He amicably addressed the issue with his landlord, who eventually abandoned the eviction proceedings.

In his later years, he remained active in alumni activities at Yale and in civic organizations in the city, including the National Afro-American League. He attended the organization's convention in Washington, D.C., and was reported to have "in eloquent terms pledged his support to the League."[29] The status of Creed's marriage during this time is not known, but his wife and daughters had permanently relocated to Brooklyn, New York, while he remained in New Haven.[30] The 1900 U.S. Federal Census revealed that his wife, Mary, and three daughters were living in Brooklyn with her brother and his wife while Creed was a boarder in a home in New Haven.[31] Along with a questionable marriage, he continued to suffer great losses with the tragic deaths of his eighteen-year-old son, Cassius, in 1890 from "congestive chills" and of his twenty-three-year-old daughter, Mary "Addie" Adeline, in 1892.[32] Creed's grief was compounded by the widespread local and national newspaper coverage that resulted from the circumstances and investigation surrounding his daughter's death. He was drawn into the situation not only as a grieving father but also as a respected physician.

Creed lived eighty miles away from his wife and their daughters in Brooklyn, but when daughter Addie fell ill in late November 1892, he rushed to be by her side and tend to her illness. Addie, the second of his four daughters, was described as a "fashionable dresser" with a beautiful soprano voice who sang in the St. Augustine Episcopal Church choir. She was known in her community as "not only pretty, but intellectually above the average and vivacious to a marked degree."[33] Addie and her mother operated a dressmaking business from their home, but to help make ends meet, they often hosted boarders. Henry F. Downing, an African American novelist and editor of the *Brooklyn Messenger*, was one such boarder. Downing was generally well respected and had served as the U.S. minister to São Paulo da Assunção de Loanda in Portuguese West Africa.[34] Although Downing was married, he had lived apart from his wife for several years and now resided in the Creed home in Brooklyn. It was no secret that the forty-year-old Downing was attracted to Creed's daughter, and it was said that he paid "assiduous court to Addie." While in church each Sunday, Addie was "attended by Downing," and this circumstance was met with adverse comments by the congregation.[35] The scandalous nature of the apparent intimate relationship between Downing and the twenty-three-year-old was uncomfortable and shocking to those in the community.

During a Sunday church service in October 1892, Addie collapsed. She was examined by Black physician Dr. Charles E. Barton and found to have a weak heart, but some thought otherwise. Suspicion grew about the nature of her condition, and later that month Barton was summoned to the Creed home, where he found Addie had a "much more serious complication for an unmarried woman": Addie was pregnant, and as an unmarried woman, pressure was brought to bear upon her and her family for what was considered a scandalous and shameful condition.[36] Mary Creed, in an effort to protect her daughter's reputation, informed Barton that Addie was married to Henry Downing, who boarded in their home. Downing's obsession with Addie was well known in the community, and he was believed to be the father of her unborn child. When Downing approached Barton about Addie's condition, he admitted his responsibility and, according to Barton, "was afraid the girl might injure herself through desperation and wanted me to warn her against resorting to violence."[37] Addie was quite distressed by her condition. Her family had deep concerns for her safety. Mary believed her daughter had fallen into a "despairing mood and often said that she would rather die than face disgrace." Barton advised Mary to "watch Addie carefully, to comfort and cheer her as best as they could and advise her to keep cool and do nothing rash."[38]

But on November 29, 1892, Addie died in her home surrounded by her family. They called on Barton to examine her and confirm her death. When he arrived, Addie's body was laid out on the bed, and he was informed by Creed that she had died from "organic heart disease." Barton had no reason to question this assessment based on his own previous determination of a weak heart and the good reputation of Creed as a physician.[39] The family assured Barton that she had died suddenly in their presence and no malpractice or improprieties were involved. Barton observed empty medicine vials in the room that apparently had been administered to Addie during her illness and believed the family was truthful about the circumstances of her death. Since Creed was unable to issue a death certificate for his daughter because he was not a registered physician in New York, Barton extended a professional courtesy to Creed by completing the certificate based on Creed's assessment of the cause of death—heart disease. Yet the submitted death certificate was questioned by the authorities and an investigation of the circumstances surrounding Addie's death was initiated, including exhuming her body. After the coroner's examination, it was determined that she died from "hemorrhage consequent upon interference with embryonic development."[40]

Addie had an abortion, but it was unclear whether it was self-inflicted or aided by someone, perhaps her physician father desperate to spare his daughter's reputation. Mary believed her daughter never attempted a "remedy" for her pregnancy, although she had "threatened to do so."[41] When Creed had learned of "Addie's troubles" from his wife and of the threats his daughter made regarding herself and her pregnancy, he begged Mary "to leave the case to him and not to attempt any remedy of her own." In his testimony given at hearings held to investigate his daughter's death, Creed stated that he was "absolutely ignorant of the fact that Addie had been a victim of malpractice, although he believed afterward that she had killed herself by doing what physicians had declined to do for her. She was my favorite daughter," he told the court, "and I had great expectations of her future."[42] It is not unreasonable to think Addie may have attempted to abort her unborn child to avoid disgrace. It may also be possible that her father, a trained and respected physician, aided his daughter in terminating her pregnancy, either by administering medicines or by performing an abortion as a means to protect her reputation. Creed may have felt responsible for Addie's pregnancy, as his absence from her daily life left him unable to protect her from the advances of an older man. No matter how Addie died, the circumstances of her pregnancy and her death devastated Creed. It weighed heavily on him for the rest of his life.

By 1897, Creed had lost two children, his home, and his entire life's fortune. His personal belongings were put on public auction, and he was drinking heavily. He was found wandering the streets of the city one day and brought to the police station before being transferred to the almshouse. The *New Haven Register* described him as "decrepit and friendless" and noted that "liquor caused his downfall." He was "so infirmed . . . that he could not walk from his cell to the wagon without assistance."[43] Creed's diminished condition saddened his community. In a letter to the editor of the *New Haven Register*, a writer and longtime New Haven resident described him as "the poor old man" who roamed about the city, "broken-down, poor, and neglected. He was always kind and gentle and never forgot to act like a gentleman . . . and to see a fellow reduced to poverty and neglect is certainly to be regretted." The writer hoped that the "good people who have found the old man and know of his wants will see to it that his remaining days are made as comfortable as possible."[44] Creed was hospitalized with kidney problems and edema. Once released from the hospital, he found a small room for himself in a boardinghouse. His illness and impoverishment left him a diminished man.

There is no doubt that the loss of his son and the circumstances surrounding the death of his daughter contributed to his downfall. In 1899, he suffered a fractured arm in a streetcar accident, adding to his ailments. Despite these difficulties, he continued to practice medicine as best as he could. His reputation as a decent and knowledgeable physician remained with him. While walking the streets of New Haven, he was often called upon to attend to injured persons and never hesitated to provide medical care to those in need. In October 1899, while passing a grocery store, he was asked to see to a store employee who had received several lacerations on his hand from an exploding soda bottle. Creed evaluated the man's injuries and dressed his wounds successfully.[45] In another incident, after a patrolman found a lifeless body lying in the street in front of a grocery store, the officer stopped Creed to ask him to see whether the man was still alive. Creed confirmed the man was dead.[46]

After many years as a prominent physician who had provided medical care to the Black community of New Haven, Creed died a pauper of Bright's disease on August 8, 1900, at the age of sixty-seven. He was buried in Grove Street Cemetery in New Haven. Creed's legacy remained strong in his community. As a testament to his contributions, a school in New Haven, the Dr. Cortlandt Van Rensselaer Creed Health and Sports Sciences High School, was named in his honor.

William Baldwin Ellis

Born free in New York City in 1833, William Baldwin Ellis spent his early life in Newark, New Jersey, where his father, Jefferson, was a barber and his mother, Serena, worked at home raising eight children, of whom William was the oldest. Newark's Black community was well established by the mid-1800s with an AME Church that had ties to the Underground Railroad and the education of Black children. Through the church's efforts, a school was established, where it is likely Ellis and his siblings received their early education.[47]

Living near New York City in the mid-nineteenth century would have exposed him to the social, political, and cultural environment of a large metropolis. He likely had contact with the community of Black elite who had established themselves in the city in the mid-1800s, including physicians, businessmen, and entrepreneurs. New York had become a haven for formerly enslaved people after slavery was abolished in the state in 1827 and was a place where free Black people could find new opportunities. Among its prominent citizens was James McCune Smith, the first African American to hold a university medical degree and own a pharmacy in the United States, and William P. Powell Sr., a staunch abolitionist, businessman, and father of William P. Powell Jr. Access to this group of accomplished and successful African Americans would have been an inspiration to any young Black man and may have influenced Ellis's decision to pursue a medical education.

Although much of his early life is a mystery, a short autobiography written as part of his application for a surgeon's position during the war provides some insight into his interest in medicine and the beginning of his medical studies. In 1848, at the age of fifteen, he began studying medicine with John Grimes, a white physician in Boontown, New Jersey, where he learned "the compounding of drugs and medicines as well as medicine proper."[48] Grimes was an abolitionist who published Boontown's first newspaper. His home was a stop on the Underground Railroad, which he operated with the help of his brother. New Jerseyites were divided on their views on slavery, and Grimes was often harassed at his home because of his public opposition to enslavement.[49] With his staunch abolitionist leanings, he was an ideal mentor and teacher for Ellis, who studied with him for one year before beginning another year-long study with Dr. Ira Nichols in Newark. Following his time with Nichols, Ellis traveled to the British West Indies, where he was employed in a pharmacy in Kingston, Jamaica, dispensing medicines and putting his knowledge to work. He visited the wards of the Penitentiary Hospital in Kingston, presumably to dispense medications and where he likely gained hands-on experience with patients. After returning to the United States in 1850, he worked in a local drugstore while resuming his study of medicine and surgery under the tutelage of prominent Black physician Peter W. Ray in Brooklyn, New York.[50] Ray had earned his medical degree from the Medical School of Maine at Bowdoin College. He owned and operated his own medical practice and pharmacy.

Ellis remained under Ray's tutelage through 1855, when he enrolled in the medical school at Dartmouth College.[51]

The annual course of lectures at Dartmouth lasted three months and consisted of four lectures each day. Ellis paid a fee of fifty dollars plus a three-dollar matriculation fee and a fee of fifty cents to check out books from the library. Surgical operations were performed before the medical class during lectures at no additional cost to the students. He had access to an anatomical cabinet for study with a collection of French osteological preparations as well as veins, arteries, nerves, and pathological specimens. To qualify for graduation, Ellis needed to be at least twenty-one years old, to possess a good moral character, and to have knowledge of experimental philosophy and Latin. Completion of a three-year study of medicine with a practitioner was required along with attendance at two courses of public lectures in all branches of the profession at a regularly organized medical institution. In addition, he was obliged to pass a private examination before the medical faculty and defend a dissertation on a medical subject.[52] His dissertation, "General Diseases (in the Male) Gonorrhea and Syphilis," discussed the theories on the cause of the diseases, the commonalities and differences between syphilis and gonorrhea, and the symptoms and treatments.[53] Ellis successfully completed all requirements and graduated in 1858, becoming one of Dartmouth's earliest Black medical graduates.

After graduation, Ellis returned to Brooklyn and practiced as a physician while working in a pharmacy at Gold and Plymouth Streets, likely the Black-owned establishment of his former teacher Dr. Peter W. Ray or perhaps Black pharmacist Philip A. White. Although he kept a low profile, he participated in public discourse on issues of the day while attending local meetings. In 1860, the *Weekly Anglo-African* reported on a debate that ensued at a meeting organized by local scholars to discuss the question, "Which has sustained the most injustice at the hands of the American people, the American Indian or the Anglo African?" Ellis attended this meeting and "spoke with much power and force, setting forth" his opinion on the advantages that American Indians had over the Anglo-Africans. He said that "from the landing of the Pilgrims . . . they have had arms placed in their hands wherewith to defend themselves, and had courted the hostility of which the opposition complained. They have retreated voluntarily before the march of civilization, and are by no means to be compared in point or moral and social susceptibility to the Anglo-African."[54] He also attended a public meeting of young men from the Williamsburg area of Brooklyn in May 1860 that was advertised as "Free Suffrage! Free Men!" The meeting's purpose was to form an organization in support of voting rights. His attendance attests to his interest in and support for the fight for equality.[55]

In 1861, Ellis married Priscilla Madeline Matthews in New York, and sometime thereafter they relocated to Philadelphia, where he set up a medical practice.[56] They remained there for several years, during which time they had two children. The family eventually moved back to New York, where their third child was born.

Ellis made his first request for a position as a surgeon in the U.S. Army while in Philadelphia. Writing to Edward C. Mauran, the adjutant general of Rhode Island, in August 1862, he said he was seeking a position in one of the "colored regiments" being organized in the state. I am "a colored man," he wrote, "and therefore, better fitted by nature to attend to the medical wants of colored men." He provided his medical education credentials and remarked that he was "capable of performing the necessary surgical duties."[57] Though it is not known what response Ellis received from Mauran, he did not receive a position.

With the establishment of the USCT in 1863, Ellis wrote to Major George Stearns, a well-known recruiter of Black soldiers, requesting a position as "surgeon in one of the regiments of colored men now being raised in Pennsylvania under your supervision."[58] Several letters of recommendation were included with his application, including one from a professor at Dartmouth College who described Ellis as "correct and gentlemanly in the greatest degree . . . and from his standing as a scholar, I have no hesitation in recommending him as a proper person to fill the office of Surgeon of the 54th Regt." He went on to say that "I should regard the appointment as eminently fit under the circumstances."[59] Another letter from a physician certified that Ellis was indeed a graduate of Dartmouth and that he was "qualified for the post of Asst. Surgeon to the colored Massachusetts Regiment (54th) to which he desires to be appointed."[60] The supervisory committee for recruiting for the USCT in Philadelphia recommended Ellis to Secretary of War Edwin M. Stanton, and as a result, he was invited to take the required Army Medical Board examination in Washington, D.C.[61]

Arriving in Washington in mid-July, he signed a certificate for "candidates for appointment into the medical staff" of the army, stating his qualifications and educational credentials for a position as surgeon.[62] Over a three-day period, he was tested by the Army Medical Board on anatomy, the practice of medicine, surgery, and hygiene as well as on literature and science.[63] Ellis followed up his examination with a visit to the surgeon general's office on

Aug. 13th 1862

Mr. Edward C. Mauran Adjt. Gen.
of Rhode Island

Dear Sir

I hereby submit to you my application for the Surgeoncy of the regiment of colored men called for in your state by the proclamation of Governor Sprague.

I am myself a colored man, and therefore I think the better fitted by nature to attend to the medical wants of colored men. Being also a graduate in Medicine and Surgery of Dartmouth College, I am of course capable of performing the necessary surgical duties also. A reply is respectfully requested.

Above and right, letter from William B. Ellis to Rhode Island adjutant general Edward C. Mauran, August 13, 1862. *Courtesy Rhode Island State Archives, Providence.*

July 27 to determine if he had passed. No one in authority was available to speak with him, but a messenger informed him that he had received a "favorable" report. Still unsure about successfully passing the exam, he wrote to Hammond for a more definitive answer.[64] On November 26, 1864, he signed a contract and took an oath of office to serve as a contract acting assistant surgeon with the U.S. Army in "Washington or somewhere" for pay of $100

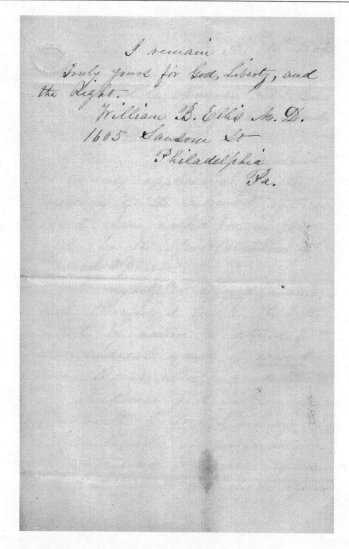

per month.[65] There is nothing to indicate why there was a delay between his examination in July 1863 and his contract in November 1864. He was assigned to Freedmen's Hospital in Washington, D.C., where he served for two years alongside Anderson R. Abbott and John H. Rapier Jr. Ellis continued to serve at the hospital until his contract ended in August 1865. An entry in the *Military Record of the Sons of Dartmouth in the Union Army and Navy* described him as having a "good reputation as a surgeon."[66]

Among his many patients at Freedmen's Hospital was Sojourner Truth, famed abolitionist and women's rights activist. Truth was a passionate advocate of both racial and gender equality and never shied away from public advocacy in both words and deeds. On September 13, 1865, the sixty-seven-year-old Truth was on an errand "for blackberry wine, and other necessities for the patients at Freedmen's Hospital," where she had been working. Traveling with a white female colleague from the facility, Laura S. Haviland, she entered the platform of a streetcar and was immediately met by the conductor, who pushed her and told her to "go back—get off here." When she refused, he forcibly grabbed her right arm, wrenching it forward, and told her, "I'll put you off." When Haviland was asked by the conductor if Truth "belonged" to her, she responded, "She belongs to humanity." Truth and Haviland recorded the number of the car and the name of the conductor and filed a report of the encounter with the president of the streetcar company. Truth's report resulted in the conductor's arrest for assault and battery.[67]

To support her case, Truth used a recent federal law passed in March 1865 that desegregated streetcars in Washington, D.C., based on the streetcar experience of Alexander T. Augusta in February 1864. In her case against the streetcar conductor, Ellis was called as a medical expert to confirm the extent of her injuries. He testified that "the old woman's shoulder was very much swollen, and he had applied liniment." Her injury was due to the wrenching of her shoulder and not from "rheumatic affection."[68] The judge found in favor of Truth, in part because of Ellis's testimony. He served as an expert witness in a second court case for an incident that occurred in December 1865. On a cold winter's day, an African American baby was found in the woods wrapped in a bag. Ellis was asked to confirm the baby's death and that the infant had been born alive. His testimony aided in convincing the jury that the baby's death was intentional.[69]

As a Black physician, his appearance as a medical expert in a court of law was unusual. Black witnesses, regardless of their positions or professions, were generally considered unreliable and not credible. The accepted testimonies of Ellis, Alexander T. Augusta, and Cortlandt Van Rensselaer Creed in court cases helped break the stereotype of Black witnesses.[70]

Ellis's contract with the government as a surgeon was annulled in August 1865, but he continued to serve at Freedmen's Hospital until his death on December 29, 1866, from typhoid fever.[71] He was survived by his wife and three children, who eventually moved back to their home in Brooklyn, New York. The *Medical and Surgical Reporter* reported on his death, saying, "Dr. William B. Ellis, Assistant Surgeon in the U.S. Army, late of Brooklyn, N.Y. died at the age of 33 years."[72]

* * *

Cortlandt Van Rensselaer Creed and William Baldwin Ellis overcame the challenges of racial discrimination to obtain medical educations at two of America's Ivy League schools. They served their country honorably during the Civil War and demonstrated their commitment to the fight for freedom. Creed and Ellis forged new pathways for Black physicians through their testimony as medical experts in often controversial court cases. Through their military service and their dedication to providing medical care to soldiers and civilians, they demonstrated that Black people's intellect and abilities could make a difference in their communities and their country.

12. ✣ The Iowa Connection: Alpheus W. Tucker (1844–1880), Joseph Dennis Harris (1833–1884), and Charles H. Taylor (1844–1875)

> I would now be glad to serve as Surgeon and Physician, the freed people in and near Savannah, wish to grow up with them and help them to attain the honorable position which I am sure they will speedily secure for themselves.
>
> —J. D. Harris

I n the town of Keokuk, Iowa, situated along the Mississippi River, a midsize medical college stood in the 1860s. The school provided the usual course of study in medicine for the mid-nineteenth century, but what made this institution unique was its four African American students. Alpheus W. Tucker, Joseph Dennis Harris, Charles H. Taylor, and John H. Rapier Jr. (see chapter 6) all found their way to Keokuk Medical College and received medical degrees in 1864 and 1865 before serving as surgeons during the Civil War. What attracted four Black men to a medical school in Iowa? How were they able to gain admission when most schools in the United States refused them on account of color?

African Americans had settled in Iowa during the nineteenth century despite the state's restrictive laws against Black people. In 1839, while still a territory, Iowa passed "an act to regulate blacks and mulattoes" that attempted to prevent them from moving into the territory.[1] When a territorial census was taken the following year, more than 170 people of color were recorded as "free colored persons." The first federal census, taken ten years later when Iowa was granted statehood, reported a small increase of 30 "free colored persons." Despite the enactment of a second restrictive law passed in 1851, the Black population grew from 200 in 1850 to more than 900 in 1860. These restrictive laws were eventually appealed in 1864 and ruled unconstitutional. Though the laws were intended to discourage Black people from entering Iowa, they continued to put down roots in the state.[2]

The city of Keokuk was an appealing place to settle. Its strategic location in the southeastern corner of Iowa along the Mississippi River and its close proximity to several slaveholding states, including Missouri, Arkansas, Kentucky, and Tennessee, made it an attractive refuge for those escaping enslavement. Keokuk was also an important location for commerce and transportation. Its accessibility to a major waterway likely drew a greater diversity of people, products, and services and perhaps encouraged a greater tolerance to a multiplicity of ideas. During the Civil War, it was a city brimming with military activity. In 1861, the first military camp and medical hospital was established in the city, with more hospitals opening during the war to attend to the increasing number of sick and wounded soldiers. Thousands of soldiers from the South were brought to the city for care and treatment, transported on hospital ships up the Mississippi River. The four Black men who attended Keokuk Medical College, also known as the Iowa College of Physicians and Surgeons, may have been drawn to the city for these reasons. Additionally, several of the medical school faculty were army surgeons who taught courses such as military surgery; after completing these classes, students could qualify for medical staff positions with the army. Eager to serve their country during

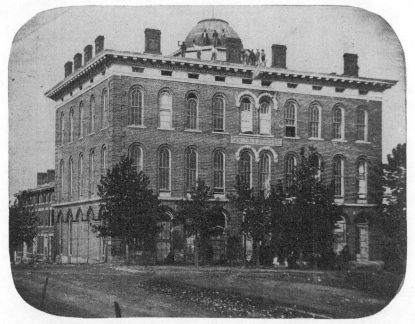

Medical College Hospital, Keokuk Medical College, c. 1865. *Courtesy National Library of Medicine, Bethesda, Md.*

the war, this may have further influenced the decision of these four men to attend the Iowa school.

Keokuk Medical College was a burgeoning educational institution in the mid-1860s. A four-story building had been built in 1858 that served as the school and hospital. Tucker, Harris, Taylor, and Rapier attended classes in the new building and enjoyed large lecture rooms, a chemical laboratory and apparatus room, a library, and a museum. The first floor included a dispensary where the city's indigent population received free medical advice and treatment from the school's faculty. A large surgical amphitheater on the third floor was used for "surgical and anatomical demonstrations . . . arranged so every student may witness the most delicate operation." The building had 248 beds for patients on three floors as well as a dining room, kitchen, and wood room in the basement. Other hospitals in Keokuk provided students the opportunity to observe a large number of diverse clinical cases. Lectures were offered on the standard subjects of practical and surgical anatomy, surgery, pathology, theory and practice of medicine, obstetrics, and materia medica.[3]

The medical college also offered a unique course in military surgery, which likely attracted those interested in serving in the army during the war. Dr. J. C. Hughes, professor of surgery and president of the Army Medical Board of Examiners for Iowa, was the course instructor. "By frequent examination" he could "qualify students for positions with the medical staff of the army." Instruction at the college began on October 20 for the 1864 school session and continued for four months, including six lectures each day. Tucker, Harris, Taylor, and Rapier paid a fee of forty dollars for the entire course in addition to fees for matriculation and a demonstrator's fee. A graduation fee of thirty dollars was also required, and all fees were due one week after the start of the session. The school provided a list of recommended books to be purchased by each student as well as suggestions on lodgings. Candidates eligible for graduation must have attended two full courses of lectures, be at least twenty-one years of age, have a good moral character, and have studied three years under the direction of "a respectable practitioner." In addition, they were required to submit a medical thesis four weeks before the session ended and pass the final examination.[4]

Each of the four Black men who graduated from Keokuk Medical College arrived in Iowa from different circumstances but for the same purpose—to obtain a medical education. John H. Rapier Jr. had attended Oberlin College in Ohio and then enrolled at the University of Michigan medical school in July 1863, eventually transferring to the medical school in Keokuk. Writing to his cousin Sarah Thomas, he told her of his admission to Keokuk and his intention to study medicine there beginning in February 1864 with hopes of graduating in June. Remaining in Michigan, he told her, would have only prolonged his graduation, which he was unwilling to do. His admission to Keokuk seems to have been accomplished with little controversy. He had recently returned from the West Indies and chose to identify as a foreign man of color from Jamaica rather than as American-born. This choice made his admission more acceptable. Rapier made no attempt to deny he was a man of color, but he understood that identifying himself as a foreigner and circumventing his American birth would be advantageous to his acceptance as a medical student.[5]

Alpheus W. Tucker's admission was achieved through a more contentious path. Like Rapier, Tucker had attended Oberlin College, where he graduated in 1863. His interest in medicine led him to the University of Michigan after he learned that another Black man had been admitted, namely Rapier. Tucker arrived in Ann Arbor on October 20, 1863, and presented himself for admission. Corydon L. Ford, secretary of the medical faculty and professor of anatomy and physiology, accepted his matriculation fee and placed his name in the student register as the 296th medical student without expressing the slightest objection.[6] Tucker's acceptance to the medical school program was based on the merits of his academic record and not on his color. The knowledge he had acquired at Oberlin College allowed him to meet the admission requirements, which included an understanding of the natural sciences and Latin.

When Tucker arrived on his first day of classes, he was met with jeers and summarily rejected by his fellow white students. William Byrns, a white medical student, described the incident to his wife the following day. Referring to Tucker as "a full blooded darkey," he said Tucker "came to the second lecture and as he did not enter until after most of the boys had taken their seats his appearance was greeted with some demonstration. Many cried, 'Caw' a manner of expressing disappointment peculiar to the Mich. University. Others cried 'take him out.' The poor negro seemed alarmed. . . . The entrance of the Prof put an end to the confusion. . . . After that lecture the individual was no longer to be seen."[7] Byrns updated his wife on "that negro affair in the University" a week and a half later, telling her that "the negro was informed by one of the Faculty that for the peace & harmony of the institution he had better leave & he left."[8] Rapier, who was also a student at the medical school, described the event:

The University has been thrown into convulsions during the last ten days because an "American of African descent" dared to present himself as a candidate for admission to the medical class. . . . He was permitted to matriculate by the officer in charge of the depart. But when the gentleman showed himself in the lecture it was a signal for commotion among the copperheads and many unprincipled republicans. The faculty willing to pander to this prejudice invited Mr. Tucker to leave the university. He did so after receiving his fees back. So you see Col'd Men are not admitted here.[9]

The white students' protests swayed the faculty, who requested Tucker's immediate departure from the school. Writing to the editor of the *Detroit Advertiser and Tribune*, Tucker questioned the validity of the faculty's decision: "I would like to know, if there be any by law in the State University, to prevent my attendance? I was told that the students objected to sit under the same roof with me! Why did they not object to riding in the same cars with me on my way to Ann Arbor? . . . Supposing that some of the students did object, have they a right to control the University in such matters?" He believed the number of students who opposed his presence was much smaller than the school claimed and instead the faculty were to blame for his forced departure because of their own racist attitudes. "A negro-hating faculty," he wrote, "will soon make negro-hating students." Tucker made clear that he would not be deterred by the treatment he received, which he noted was "more suited to an uneducated than an educated community. Your treatment of me," he said, "will not prevent my continuance of my medical education elsewhere."[10] After Tucker's departure, Rapier encountered Tucker's friends who were furious at Rapier because he was retained as a student by the university while Tucker was asked to leave. Rapier told his cousin Sarah, "They say I pretend to be a white man when I am nothing but a 'Nigger.'"[11] Tucker's rescinded admission to the University of Michigan led him to Keokuk Medical College in 1864, where he attended lectures and received his medical degree in early 1865.

Joseph Dennis Harris, better known as J. D., came to Keokuk after studying with a physician at the U.S. Marine Hospital in Cleveland, Ohio, and at the medical department of Western Reserve College. He decided to transfer to Keokuk because he believed the school's "ideas of Medicine are more modern than those of Western Reserve College and consequently, more correct."[12] He attended in 1863 and 1864 and received his medical degree after completion of his courses. Charles H. Taylor's path to Keokuk began after his arrival in the United States from the West Indies in May 1863. He traveled to Washington, D.C., where he was employed as a hospital steward at Contraband Camp Hospital.[13] After serving for a year there, he made his way to Iowa and received his medical degree a year later in 1864.

To better understand the influences and motivation of Tucker, Harris, and Taylor to pursue a medical degree in Iowa and join the army as surgeons, we need to take a closer look at their life stories.

Alpheus W. Tucker

Alpheus W. Tucker was a native of Detroit, Michigan. He was born free in 1844, the second of three children of an Ohio-born mother, Mary, and a Kentucky-born father, George W., who was employed as a barber. Detroit was a major stop on the Underground Railroad and often the last stop for the formerly enslaved before they reached freedom in Canada. George was an active abolitionist, handling subscriptions for the abolitionist newspaper *The Mystery*, founded by Martin R. Delaney.[14] Alpheus had one older sister, Georgette, and one younger brother, Cassius. It seems his parents were well read, having named their sons after two historical figures—Alpheus, the Greek river god, and Cassius, a character in Shakespeare's *Julius Caesar*. They were determined to provide a good education for their children, as evidenced by Alpheus's academic achievements in college and medical school. The family made their home in Detroit but were separated for a time. Alpheus and Cassius were part of the household of Edward and Emily Hubbard in Detroit in 1850. Emily Hubbard was born in Kentucky and perhaps a relative of their father. Their sister Georgette was living in Lorain, Ohio, with the Almond family, perhaps relatives of their mother.[15]

By 1860, the entire family had moved to Toledo, Ohio, where George continued working as a barber and Mary provided for the family at home. Now a teenager, Alpheus began to contemplate his future. At the age of seventeen, he entered Oberlin College in Ohio, studying in the preparatory department. John H. Rapier Jr. and Charles B. Purvis also attended Oberlin around that time and would later join Tucker as surgeons during the war. The preparatory department was "specially designed to prepare students for College," utilizing student instructors from the theological and higher college classes. Students were obligated to "have pursued the ordinary English branches and have studied Latin for two years" and have "testimonials of good character."[16]

To be accepted as a full member of the student body, successful completion of a six-month probation period was required. As a student, Tucker paid a school fee of $15.00 per year with incidental expenses of $2.25 per year. Various accommodations were offered to students, including a room at the college with a stove for heating. As a junior in the preparatory department during the 1862–63 academic year, he had classes in Latin, Greek, and English, along with elocution, orations, and arithmetic. Courses were varied and included languages, sciences, mathematics, history, and biblical studies, with specified textbooks on each subject. It was mandatory to attend regular church services, daily prayers each morning and evening, and weekly religious lectures. Tucker had access to the college's six-thousand-volume library and specimen cabinets for the natural and earth sciences that contained nearly eight thousand objects. Three academic terms were held in the winter, spring, and summer with one vacation period and exams conducted at the end of each term. Oberlin also had a "Young Ladies' Department" that included courses in mathematics, chemical and natural sciences, philosophy, economics, geography, and languages as well as penmanship, elocution, music, and art. The nearly equal number of women and men attending Oberlin during that year and the diversity of subjects offered to female students seem to indicate a more progressive attitude toward admission than found in other colleges in the nineteenth century, which may have attracted both Tucker and Rapier.[17]

After completing his studies at Oberlin, he was accepted at the University of Michigan medical school but summarily rejected by the white students when he appeared for his first day of class, as discussed above. The uproar of the students and the request for Tucker to leave the school led to his decision to transfer to Keokuk Medical College in 1864, where he graduated the following year. The ongoing Civil War and the military surgery course taught at the college may have encouraged his interest in a position with the U.S. Army. This career path influenced the course of his life both personally and professionally.

Tucker applied for a position with the army, and in March 1865 he passed his Army Medical Board examination and was issued a contract as an acting assistant surgeon. He was assigned to Freedmen's Hospital in Washington, D.C., where he served for six months at a salary of $100 per month. At the end of his contract, he remained in Washington and took up residence in Alexandria, Virginia, where he provided medical care for the newly freed Black population, most likely at L'Ouverture Hospital in Alexandria or Freedmen's Village in Arlington.

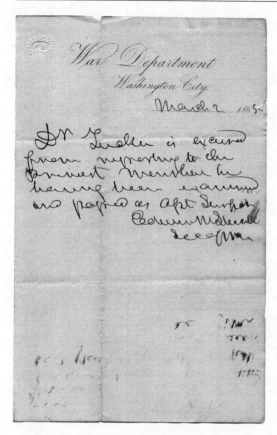

Appointment memo for
Alpheus W. Tucker, signed
by Secretary of War Edwin
M. Stanton, March 2, 1865.
*Courtesy National Archives
and Records Administration,
Washington, D.C.*

Tucker moved back to Washington, D.C., and expanded his opportunities personally and professionally. He met and married Martha E. Wood, a native Washingtonian, in early 1867 and welcomed a daughter the following year. They settled into life as Tucker continued his medical practice and became active in local politics. As a physician, he tended to the medical needs of Black residents in the city. On one occasion, he was called to the home of a woman in labor "and in a short time . . . delivered four children—three lively boys and a girl." The multiple birth was quite newsworthy with an announcement appearing in a local newspaper and reprinted in the *Alton Telegraph* in Illinois on July 25, 1873.[18]

He became involved with local politics facilitated through his association with the Fifth Ward Republicans. In June 1868, he was nominated for the position of Fifth Ward physician and elected by a vote of one hundred to fourteen.[19] Despite the overwhelming vote in his favor, those opposing his nomination thought that "putting colored men in office just at that time would jeopardize the chances of the Republican party in the Presidential election." One member was shocked at the idea of a Black ward physician. "Think of Dr. Tucker attending to my wife," he remarked, to which Tucker replied, "I have attended your wife's betters."[20]

One of the most significant actions taken by Tucker, along with Alexander T. Augusta and Charles B. Purvis, was a move to seek equality in the medical profession. Membership in medical societies was a critical source of professional development and opportunities and often a requirement to maintain a medical practice. The Medical Society of the District of Columbia was the local medical organization that licensed physicians in Washington and through membership enabled physicians to hold consultations with one another. When Tucker, Augusta, and Purvis sought admission to the society in 1869, they were met with resistance and blatant racism that resulted in a vote against their membership, limiting their medical practices. Tucker noted that the inability of Black physicians to consult with other white physicians subjected them "to great disabilities," and he recalled three separate instances when consultations were denied. One physician with whom Tucker wished to consult informed him that if he were to confer with Tucker, the society would "impose a fine . . . for doing so."[21]

After an appeal to the U.S. Congress found that the Medical Society had discriminated against them solely based on the color of their skin, no immediate remedy was offered.[22] Undeterred by this setback, Tucker, Augusta, and Purvis helped establish the National Medical Society of the District of Columbia and declared it racially integrated.[23]

Little else is known about Tucker's life in Washington, D.C. He continued serving as a physician in the Fifth Ward of the city and provided medical care to its residents from his office in the Colonization Building at 450 Pennsylvania Avenue, Northwest, where he kept office hours from 1 to 8 PM each day.[24] He was a member of the Colored Knights Templar and served as the second officer in the commandery.[25] In 1879, Tucker traveled to Detroit to visit his family and spent some time in Canada. He contracted a cold and after traveling back to Detroit died as a result of his illness on January 4, 1880, at the age of thirty-five.[26]

Joseph Dennis Harris

Joseph Dennis Harris was born free in Fayetteville, North Carolina, in 1833 to Charlotte Dismukes and Jacob Harris. His parents were born enslaved, the product of white fathers and Black enslaved mothers, but were free by the time of Joseph's birth. A Black child's status was based on the mother's, regardless of the status of the father. If the mother was enslaved and the father free, the child was considered enslaved. White men in North Carolina who fathered children with enslaved Black women often arranged to free their children and establish apprenticeships for them in trades like blacksmithing and plastering.[27] Perhaps this was how Jacob Harris became free.

Joseph, better known as J. D., spent his early life in Fayetteville. By 1850, his father had died, leaving his mother to raise eight children alone. Harris was employed as a blacksmith while his two older brothers were brickmasons.[28] It is possible that J. D. learned his trade from his father. The family relocated to Cleveland, Ohio, where there was a strong abolitionist community. After a few years in Cleveland, Harris made his way to Delhi, Iowa, where he worked as a plasterer. He lived in a boardinghouse in town where the residents included a physician and a surgeon.[29] Living in close proximity to two medical professionals may have influenced his decision to pursue a medical education. In 1856, while living in Delhi, he published a book, *Love and Law, South and West, a Poem*. The fictionalized story, formatted as a poem, centers on a free Black person in North Carolina seeking freedom in the West without the protection of the law. On the title page of the book, Harris's name appears as "J. D. Harris, M.D. of Delhi, Iowa." The book was published eight years before he received his formal medical degree. Perhaps he had studied or apprenticed with the physician or surgeon at his boardinghouse and now considered himself a medical doctor. A formal medical education was not necessarily a requirement to practice medicine at the time, and some practicing physicians had training only through apprenticeships. He may have identified himself as a medical doctor and desired to boost his reputation.

Harris began to actively participate in the Ohio Anti-Slavery Society with his friend John Mercer Langston. Langston received his education at Oberlin College and went on to obtain a law degree, becoming Virginia's first African American representative in Congress.[30] Harris was a strong proponent of emigration from the United States to Haiti as a means for Black people to have a better life. The Anti-Slavery Society, of which he was a member of the executive board, had its first meeting in 1859. He actively raised funds for the organization as well as recruited for and promoted the emigration and colonization movement. Discontented with life in America, Harris proclaimed, "God grant that I may never die in the United States of America!"[31]

After hearing of U.S. representative from Missouri Frank P. Blair's speech in 1858 favoring emigration, Harris expressed his support of this idea to Blair.

"While it is evident that the white and Black races cannot exist in this country on terms of equality," he wrote, "it is equally certain the latter will not long be content with anything less. . . . The Government drives us to Canada, where we are indeed free, but where it is plain we cannot become a very great people. We want more room, where it is not quite so cold—we want to be identified with the ruling power of a nation."[32]

Harris also wrote to the editor of the *Cleveland Morning Leader* in mid-April 1860 outlining "a proposed visit to Central America" to seek out and purchase property "for the benefit of such free colored persons of African descent as desire to find homes." It was an idea he regarded as "eminently wise and patriotic." Describing the favorable support he received, he suggested that the islands of "Hayti and Dominica" would "offer the most favorable inducements to colored men desiring to emigrate."[33] Published alongside Harris's letter was a letter of introduction from Blair to E. G. Squire, former chargé d'affaires of Central America. Blair described meeting Harris and the "high opinion" he formed of him as a result of "the report of others who are well acquainted with him." Blair encouraged support of Harris's plans to travel to Haiti and believed his visit would "have an excellent effect upon the minds of his own people if he should be able to report favorably. . . . The visit of Harris will prove a forerunner of a numerous colonization."[34] Harris was described a few months later as "a respectable and intelligent colored citizen of Cleveland" who had for several months "been practically engaged in awakening an interest among educated and enterprising men of his race the subject of forming a colony and emigrating to the West India Islands."[35]

Harris embarked on a journey to the Caribbean in May 1860, searching for a suitable location for colonization. He documented his trip in several letters to the *Cleveland Daily Leader*, the first of which was published on July 4, titled "A Summer on the Borders of the Caribbean Sea." The letters culminated in a book of the same title published that year and was described by New York's *Evening Post* as "sensible and agreeable." The article noted that "to those who take an interest in the final destiny of that family of the human species which has been transplanted from Africa to the New World, we can commend this work as having an important bearing on that great question."[36]

Harris boarded the sailing vessel *John Butler* in New York City on May 19 and set sail for Santo Domingo in the West Indies. His time on board ship was spent learning the "Dominican language" with his "afternoons spent in fishing, and catching sea-weed, watching the flying-fish, or in looking simply and silently on the everbounding sea."[37] After sailing for twelve days, the ship arrived and he remarked that "of course, I have not been long enough to know whether it is a fit place for a man to live in, or for a number to colonize . . . lovely, exquisite, and delicious in its vegetable production, I do set it down a perfect paradise."[38] The *Cleveland Daily Leader* suggested that Harris was well "pleased with the climate, productions, people, and prospects of Dominica."[39] He was described by a *New York Herald* correspondent as "quite an intelligent and enterprising slightly colored gentleman . . . and the duly authorized agent of some twenty-five families of said State [Ohio], recently arrived here, intending to select a location and make arrangements for planting a colony, etc." The majority of his time was focused on locating a suitable place for free Black people to move to and settle, but he also developed an interest in studying fevers, which would be the subject of his medical school thesis four years later.

After his return to the United States at the end of the year, he joined forces with James Redpath and the Haytian Emigration Bureau, where he was appointed the "Traveling Agent for Ohio" for emigration and colonization.[40] Redpath was a white abolitionist, journalist, and ardent supporter of the migration of Black people to Haiti and had traveled there several times in 1859 and 1860, assessing the country and its suitability for colonization. He had numerous discussions with Haitian government officials and as a result was asked to direct efforts to attract emigrants from America through the Haytian Emigration Bureau. Harris continued drumming up support for this cause through fundraising, presenting talks, and writing articles defending emigration. He was dismissed from his position in late 1861 by Redpath, who claimed Harris "lacks energy."[41] Despite his dismissal, he maintained his support of emigration to Haiti. In April 1863, at the celebration of emancipation in the District of Columbia, the *Evening Star* reported on his participation, saying, "J. D. Harris (colored) of the Haytian Bureau of Emigration" was among the audience.[42]

During this time, Harris made a decision to pursue a formal medical education and began studying under the tutelage of prominent Cleveland physician Martin L. Brooks at the U.S. Marine Hospital in Cleveland. Brooks's position as surgeon-in-charge at the facility provided Harris with observable medical cases and practical experience.[43] He enrolled in the medical department at Western Reserve College in 1863 but soon headed off to Keokuk, Iowa, to continue his studies. A year later, after completing his requirements, he received his medical degree.

After graduating, Harris traveled to Washington, D.C., seeking a position as a surgeon in the U.S. Army. He presented letters of recommendation to U.S.

senators James Harlan and James W. Grimes and to U.S. representative James F. Wilson from Iowa. Offered a contract acting assistant surgeon position in June 1864, he was assigned to Balfour Hospital in Portsmouth, Virginia. He served as surgeon-in-charge of three wards of Black patients, earned a salary of $100 per month, and was considered a good physician, with one observer noting the "excellent care the colored soldiers received in Balfour Hospital."[44] Not everyone was happy with Harris's presence in Portsmouth, though, despite his good reputation. A letter to the editor of the *Christian Recorder* in early July 1864 said, "Portsmouthians were terribly startled, and with eyes extended, mouth opened, hair on end and hands in pockets, they could be seen in groups, talking very low. 'There's a nigger doctor in Portsmouth, in the capacity of a U.S. Surgeon.' It was too much: A negro M.D. on sacred soil? They could not stand it. Some of them tried to die, others went in search of the last ditch, while Surgeon Harris, with an ability that is second to no surgeon in this department, is rendering invaluable service, to the sick and wounded soldiers."[45]

By February 1865, Harris applied for a regular army surgeon's position in hopes of going south among the freedmen. Writing to Secretary of War Edwin M. Stanton he said, "Having read with great interest—even enthusiasm, your report of the freed people at Savanah [*sic*] . . . I have the honor of serving the Government as Surgeon in Charge of three wards of this Hospital [Balfour Hospital] . . . and I would now be glad to serve, as Surgeon and Physician, the freed people in and near Savanah."[46] The army was not in favor of appointing him. Colonel George Suckley, medical director, responded to Harris's request and suggested that his examination be put off and he continue his duty under W. A. Conover, medical director of the 25th Army Corps, until Conover saw "fit to order him before the board."[47] In May, Harris was examined before the Army Medical Board. He did not receive an army commission but instead remained a contract acting assistant surgeon. He was transferred to the Bureau of Refugees, Freedmen, and Abandoned Lands and by the fall of 1865 was working at Howard's Grove Hospital in Richmond, Virginia, as surgeon-in-charge.

By all accounts, he provided good care to his patients and managed his responsibilities well. Ira Russell, a surgeon with the U.S. Sanitary Commission, in his report on hospitals in Virginia, visited a number of medical facilities including Howard's Grove Hospital. Russell noted that Harris was a "very intelligent colored gentlemen from Cleveland, Ohio." The hospital "was neat, orderly and well located. Dr. Harris has seen a good deal of service, is familiar

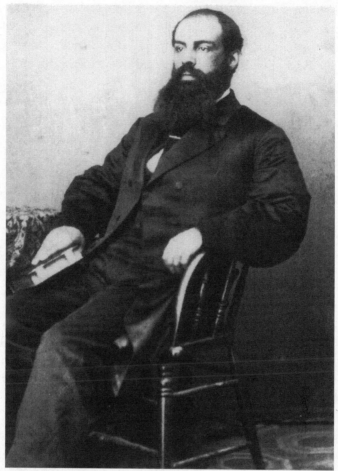

J. D. Harris, c. 1868. *Courtesy Greg Harris and Eureka Springs Historical Museum, Eureka, Ark.*

with the peculiarities of his race, and [is] deeply interested in its elevation and welfare." The Sanitary Commission was a civilian organization tasked by the federal government to provide medical and sanitary assistance to U.S. forces during the war. Russell made assessments of hospitals and evaluated their needs. In his report, he noted Harris's opinion that Black people maintained "vital power" and, contrary to the notions of most white surgeons, were able "to bear disease." Harris believed that many of the white surgeons provided insufficient care to Black patients, using stereotypes of Black people as physically weaker than white people to claim they could not be treated successfully or recover from their ailments. He often overheard white surgeons commenting that "a sick negro will die, do what you will." Harris contended these white surgeons were lazy, indifferent, and ignorant, and their attitude "looks upon sick allegations as an excuse to cover up the results of bad practice."[48]

By 1867, Harris became interested in politics, advocating for greater Black representation. At a public meeting held in Fredericksburg, Virginia, at which Harris presided, he argued for more Black representatives in "one-half the City Council and to have the selection of the Mayor."[49] He took his political agenda and his ambitions to the polls in a run for lieutenant governor of Virginia in 1869. Harris campaigned in the state with his sister and on one occasion attempted to travel by steamer from Norfolk to Richmond. Although possessing two second-class tickets, they were ejected from the steamer by the captain when they refused his request to vacate the saloon, a public seating area.[50] In his nomination, Harris was described as having "a solemnity of tone and earnestness of expression that warmed the colored brethren toward him." Harris's service during the war, where he was seen providing care to wounded soldiers, was compared with that of his opponent, a former surgeon with the Confederate army, who was described as interested only in adding "stars to his collar."[51] Virginia's *Staunton Spectator* described him as "a resident of Hampton, Virginia," and "a physician of high standing in his profession."[52] Harris ran a respectable race but lost the election by a vote of 99,600 to his opponent's 120,068. He made one more attempt at a political career when he was nominated for a Senate seat in the state legislature. He received only three votes out of the twenty-three votes that were cast.[53]

Harris married Elizabeth Worthington in 1868, a Princeton-educated white woman, who had served as a missionary and moved south to be a teacher to freedmen. They had two children, a girl born in South Carolina and a son born in Washington, D.C. Harris took a position as assistant physician, secretary, and treasurer of the South Carolina Lunatic Asylum in Columbia, but by November 1870 he was dismissed from his position, according to Harris, "*solely* and *purely* because of the prejudices which exist against my color and race."[54] He and his family moved to Washington, D.C., where he established a medical practice, was a ward physician at Freedmen's Hospital, and served as a "physician to the poor" with the District of Columbia government, earning fifty dollars a month.[55]

Harris's mental state began to deteriorate, and by 1877 he was committed to the Government Hospital for the Insane, later St. Elizabeths Hospital. Washington's *Evening Star* reported that "a jury empaneled to inquire as to the mental condition of Dr. Joseph D. Harris, on the petition of his wife, represented by Dr. B. A. Lockwood, and, found that he is not of sound mind, capable of managing his estate."[56] He spent the next seven years as a patient at St. Elizabeths until his death on December 25, 1884, the result of "chronic mania and epileptic apoplexy." He was fifty-one years old.[57]

Charles H. Taylor

Charles H. Taylor was born in the West Indies in 1844. At the age of eighteen, he boarded the ship SS *Plantagenet* and sailed to the United States with the intention of becoming "an inhabitant of America."[58] After he arrived in New York City, he made his way to Washington, D.C., where he was employed as a hospital steward and then a nurse at Contraband Camp Hospital.[59] As a hospital steward, Taylor would have been a modern-day pharmacist, compounding prescriptions and managing medications in addition to assisting surgeons. Although his life prior to arriving in America is unclear, he may have acquired some knowledge of chemistry or medicine in the West Indies or perhaps worked in an apothecary there, giving him the experience necessary to secure a job at the hospital. Working with Alexander T. Augusta, William P. Powell Jr., and Anderson R. Abbott, he was likely influenced in his decision to seek a formal medical education. By 1864, he enrolled in Keokuk Medical College, where he attended lectures and received a medical degree in 1865.

Taylor's interest in serving in the army prompted his letter of application for a position to Brigadier General Joseph K. Barnes, surgeon general, in June 1865. He described his medical education and informed Barnes that he was "anxious to be employed among Freedmen, with whom I am identified of race."[60] Although he did not receive an army commission, Taylor was offered a contract with the Bureau of Refugees, Freedmen, and Abandoned Lands in August earning $100 per month.[61]

By September, he was on duty at Lincoln General Hospital for Refugees and Freedmen in Savannah, Georgia, serving under the direction of surgeon-in-charge Alexander T. Augusta. Perhaps his previous connection with Augusta at Contraband Hospital prompted his appointment to Lincoln Hospital. He was joined the following year by Black assistant surgeon T. L. Harris. Among Taylor's responsibilities was administering smallpox vaccinations to freedmen. Difficulty in completing this task developed due to the lack of transportation available to medical staff when conducting hospital business away from the main facility. The hospital was located outside the Savannah city limits, requiring surgeons to travel in order to provide medical care to

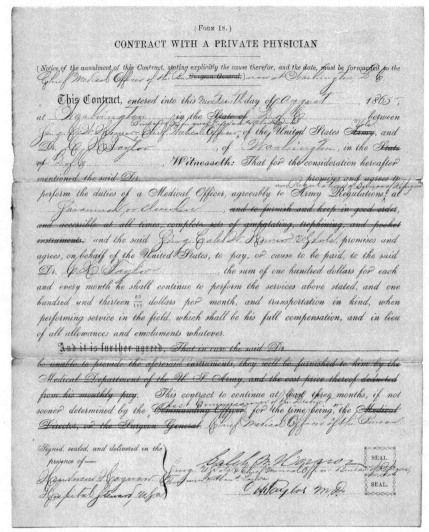

Charles H. Taylor's "Contract with a Private Physician," August 19, 1865. *Courtesy National Archives and Records Administration, Washington, D.C.*

patients. An ambulance was available for transporting the sick, but the army quartermaster who was responsible for the distribution of supplies, including ambulances, refused to allow the hospital staff to use the ambulance except for transporting patients. Augusta expressed his concern about the situation, saying it "puts us to great disadvantages and inconvenience in attending to the official business of the hospital. My assistant [Charles H. Taylor] has to go every afternoon to the office of the bureau to vaccinate the Freedmen and he refuses to do so if he has to walk. Which I confess in the sun or rain is not very pleasant."[62] It is not known if the ambulance situation was ever resolved. Taylor's appointment in Savannah lasted until January 1867, when he transferred to Augusta and then to Brunswick, Georgia, in May of that year.

Physicians with the Bureau of Refugees, Freedmen, and Abandoned Lands worked under difficult circumstances, including limited supplies, limited personnel, and extended work hours. In Georgia, they provided services and care to thousands of freedmen over several counties. Many faced violent opposition by white people who were not favorable to the care that both white and Black physicians were giving to freedmen. White physicians were threatened, and the risks to Black physicians, including Taylor, Augusta, and Harris, were even greater because of racism and bigotry. Taylor's poor treatment began even before he arrived at his post in Brunswick. When he attempted to board the steamer that would take him to his new assignment, the captain of the vessel refused to let him on as a passenger despite the fact that he had already paid his fare. The delay caused him to reach his new post late.[63]

When he finally arrived, Taylor assumed his new responsibilities and served out his contract until late November 1868. He hoped to attain a position in the regular army and wrote again to Surgeon General Barnes, requesting a position. He noted his service with the Freedmen's Bureau for the past three years and his previous employment at Freedmen's Hospital in Washington.[64] From all accounts, Taylor never received a position in the army and instead established a private practice as a physician in Savannah.

Little is known about Taylor's personal life. He married Eveline Cashin, but the marriage ended in divorce in 1872. Three months later he married his second wife, Laura Deveaux. They lived a relatively quiet life in Savannah.[65] Taylor died on May 2, 1875, in Richmond, Virginia, from "congestion of the lungs" at the age of thirty.[66]

* * *

Taylor, Tucker, and Harris, along with John H. Rapier Jr., found an opportunity for education and advancement in the midwest town of Keokuk, Iowa. Perhaps they were attracted by the town's location on the Mississippi River, where a diversity of commerce and people moved through the town. Maybe Taylor and Tucker felt empowered to come to the medical school because of the presence of Rapier and Harris or were drawn by the military surgery classes the school offered. We may never know the precise reasons why four Black men found their way to the same medical school in Iowa.

The impact these Black surgeons made and their contributions during the war can still be felt today. In 2019, the University of Michigan paid homage to one of these surgeons, Alpheus W. Tucker, by establishing a professorship in his honor. Dr. Theodore Iwashyna, the first Alpheus W. Tucker, MD, Collegiate Professor of Internal Medicine, explained that naming the professorship after Tucker recognizes "the University's history of racism and the faculty's complicitness" in that racism. "Naming a professorship in his honor seemed, to me," he said, "to be a way to apologize" for that wrong and "commit to doing better in the future. It is meant to remind us that our institution (as all institutions) is imperfect, and that constant efforts to live up to our democratic ideals are necessary. Progress does not happen by some invisible force. It happens when people make the effort to fight for justice."[67]

Fourteen African American men became physicians and served during the American Civil War, making an important contribution to the fight for freedom and justice. Challenging the prescribed notions of race in America, they played a crucial role in the evolving definition of freedom, citizenship, and patriotism.

Notes

Bibliography

Index of Regiments

Index

Notes

Preface

1. *American Medical Times* 8, no. 2 (January 9, 1864): 24.
2. *Report of the Adjutant General of the State of Illinois*, 391.
3. *American Medical Times*, 24.
4. David O. McCord, Carded Records Showing Military Service of Soldiers Who Fought in Volunteer Organizations during the American Civil War, 1890–1912, documenting the period 1861–1866, Records of the Adjutant General's Office, 1762–1984, Record Group (hereafter RG) 94, National Archives and Records Administration, Washington, D.C. (hereafter NARA).
5. J. B. McPherson, E. M. Pease, Charles C. Topliff, Joel Morse, M. O. Carter, Henry Grange to Abraham Lincoln, February 1864, Letters Received, ser. 360, Colored Troops Division, Records of the Adjutant General's Office, 1762–1984, RG 94 [B-11], NARA.

Introduction

1. Jenkins, *Climbing Up to Glory*, xii–xiv.
2. *Map Showing the Distribution of the Slave Population of the Southern States of the United States*, U.S. Census Bureau, accessed June 21, 2020, https://www.census.gov/history/pdf/1860_slave_distribution.pdf.
3. Long, *Doctoring Freedom*, 44.
4. Bucchianeri, *Brushstrokes of a Gadfly*, 312.
5. "Letter from Little Rock," *Janesville (Wisc.) Daily Gazette*, May 10, 1864.
6. "The Late Outrage upon Surgeon Augusta in Baltimore," *Christian Recorder*, May 30, 1863.
7. J. B. McPherson, E. M. Pease, Charles C. Topliff, Joel Morse, M. O. Carter, Henry Grange to Abraham Lincoln, February 1864, Letters Received, ser. 360, Colored Troops Division, Records of the Adjutant General's Office, 1762–1984, RG 94 [B-11], NARA.
8. Masur, *Example for All the Land*, 46.
9. "With Malice toward None: The Abraham Lincoln Bicentennial Exhibition: Lincoln and Frederick Douglass," Library of Congress, accessed September 14,

2020, https://www.loc.gov/exhibits/lincoln/lincoln-and-frederick-douglass
   .html.

10. "Tender of Colored Regiments," *New York Tribune*, August 5, 1862; Lincoln,
   Collected Works, 356–57.

11. Glatthaar, *Forged in Battle*, 81.

12. Quoted in Glatthaar, 79–80; quoted in Marrs, *Life and History*, 22.

13. Willis, *Black Civil War Soldier*, 6.

14. Rapier Jr. to James P. Thomas, August 19, 1864, Rapier Family Papers,
   MS-4283, Moorland-Spingarn Research Center, Howard University, Washington, D.C.

15. Cowden, *Fifty-Ninth Regiment*, 45.

16. Long, *Doctoring Freedom*, 70.

17. Masur, *Example for All the Land*, 44.

18. Humphreys, *Intensely Human*; Downs, *Sick from Freedom*.

1. Breaking the Color Barrier

1. Rapier Jr. to Sarah Thomas, November 12, 1863, Rapier Family Papers,
   MS 62-4283, Moorland-Spingarn Research Center, Howard University,
   Washington, D.C.

2. Bonner, *Becoming a Physician*, 211–12.

3. Williams, *Self-Taught*, 11, 18.

4. Jay, *American Colonization Society and American Anti-Slavery Societies*,
   130.

5. Span, "Learning in Spite of Opposition," 30.

6. Bonner, *Becoming a Physician*, 8, 203.

7. Bonner, 218, 224.

8. Stauffer, *Works of James McCune Smith*, xxi.

9. Abram, *"Send Us a Lady Physician,"* 110.

10. Rapier Jr. to Sarah Thomas, November 12, 1863, Rapier Family Papers.

11. *Annual Reports of the American Colonization Society*, 10.

12. Quoted in Reid, *African Canadians in Union Blue*, 152.

13. Quoted in Reid, 152.

14. Litwack, *North of Slavery*, 139.

15. Alexander T. Augusta to Abraham Lincoln, January 7, 1863, Records Relating to Medical Officers and Physicians, Alexander T. Augusta, entry
   561, Records of the Adjutant General's Office, 1780s–1917, RG 94, NARA.

16. Creed, "Frederick Douglass, Esq." (letter to the editor), *Frederick Douglass'
   Paper*, August 24, 1855.

17. Rapier Jr. to Sarah Thomas, November 12, 1863, Rapier Family Papers.

18. Alpheus W. Tucker, "To the Editor of the Advertiser," *Detroit Advertiser and Tribune*, November 5, 1863.

19. Reid, *African Canadians in Union Blue*, 148.

20. Andrews, *New York African Free-Schools*, 25.

21. William P. Powell Sr. to Dr. Inman, Liverpool, May 5, 1852, inserted in the Liverpool Royal Infirmary School of Medicine Minutes, 1845–1859, S.3076, at the entry for May 29, 1852, Special Collections and Archives, Sydney Jones Library, University of Liverpool, England.

22. Look In, "A Soldier's Letter," *Christian Recorder*, July 9, 1864.

23. "The Victory and Its Effects," *Christian Recorder*, July 11, 1863.

24. *Indianapolis Daily Journal*, December 8, 1863.

25. Alexander T. Augusta to Abraham Lincoln, January 7, 1863, Records Relating to Medical Officers and Physicians, RG 94, NARA.

26. Anderson R. Abbott to Edwin M. Stanton, February 6, 1863, Records Relating to Medical Officers and Physicians, RG 94, NARA.

27. John H. Rapier Jr. to William A. Hammond, April 21, 1864, Records Relating to Medical Officers and Physicians, RG 94, NARA.

28. John Van Surly DeGrasse and Alexander T. Augusta, Records Relating to Medical Officers and Physicians, RG 94, NARA.

29. Records of the Record and Pension Office, Records Concerning Medical Personnel, 1839–1914, Station Cards, Acting Assistant Surgeons, 1862–68, 1898–1901, entry 567, Records of the Adjutant General's Office, 1780–1917, RG 94, NARA. A review of federal records, including duty station cards, shows that Black surgeons were appointed to facilities that treated only Black patients.

30. Woodward, "Notes on a Trip through Arkansas," quoted in Humphreys, *Intensely Human*, 68.

31. Blanchard, Nayar, and Lurie, "Patient-Provider and Patient-Staff Racial Concordance," 1184–89.

32. Damon Tweedy, "The Case for Black Doctors," *New York Times*, May 15, 2015.

33. Parry, "Elizabeth Fee and Feminist Public Health," 873–74.

34. Humphreys, *Intensely Human*, 57.

35. Humphreys, 57–59.

36. *Christian Recorder*, September 24, 1864.

37. Long, *Doctoring Freedom*, 88.

2. Catalyst for Change

1. *1836 Free African Americans*.

2. Henderson, *Free Negro in Virginia*, 9.

3. Bogger, *Free Blacks in Norfolk*, 139.

4. Bogger, 138.

5. *Matchett's Baltimore Directory for 1847*, 369; both John and Alexander Augusta are listed as barbers.

6. Bristol, *Knights of the Razor*, 107.

7. The Oblate Sisters of Providence was the first religious order of women of color. Established in the United States in 1829, the order's primary mission was the education and care of African American children.

8. Still, *Underground Rail Road*, 110; Smedley, *History of the Underground Railroad*, 223.

9. "1848–1865: Gold Rush, Statehood, and the Western Movement," Calisphere, accessed February 26, 2020, https://calisphere.org/exhibitions/essay/4/gold-rush/.

10. Nell, "Impressions and Gleanings of Canada West," *Liberator*, December 24, 1858.

11. Alexander T. Augusta to Abraham Lincoln, January 7, 1863, Records Relating to Medical Officers and Physicians, Alexander T. Augusta, entry 561, Records of the Adjutant General's Office, 1780s–1917, RG 94, NARA.

12. *Provincial Freeman* (Toronto), April 7, 1855.

13. *Circular of the Medical Faculty of Trinity College*.

14. *The Globe*, July 11, 1860; possessing a licentiate of the Medical Board of Upper Canada permitted Augusta to practice medicine even though he did not yet have a medical degree.

15. The American Freedmen's Inquiry Commission was impaneled by Secretary of War Edwin M. Stanton to conduct hearings on the conditions under which Black people lived and worked. Howe, *Refugees from Slavery in Canada West*, 80.

16. *Caverhill's Toronto City Directory*.

17. *Statutes of the Province of Canada*, 437–38.

18. *True Royalist and Weekly Intelligencer*, June 21, 1861.

19. "Hatred of Colored Men in Canada," *Liberator*, July 31, 1857.

20. Sanger, *Statutes at Large*, 599.

21. Augusta to Lincoln, January 7, 1863, RG 94, NARA.

22. P. H. Watson to Alexander T. Augusta, January 14, 1863, Records Relating to Medical Officers and Physicians, RG 94, NARA.

23. Meredith Clymer to William A. Hammond, March 23, 1863, Records Relating to Medical Officers and Physicians, RG 94, NARA.

24. File note from William A. Hammond, March 24, 1863, Records Relating to Medical Officers and Physicians, RG 94, NARA.

25. "A Colored Aspirant for Medical Honors," *New York Times*, March 30, 1863.

26. P. H. Watson to W. A. Hammond, March 26, 1863, Records Relating to Medical Officers and Physicians, RG 94, NARA.

27. Alexander T. Augusta to the President and Members of the Army Medical Board, March 30, 1863, Records Relating to Medical Officers and Physicians, RG 94, NARA.

28. W. Moss, Recorder, Army Medical Board, to Brigadier General William A. Hammond, April 1, 1863, Colored Troops Division, 1863, W22-115, box 37, Records of the Adjutant General's Office, 1780s–1917, RG 94, NARA.

29. "An Important Letter from Dr. Augusta," *Anglo-African*, April 25, 1863.

30. "An Important Letter from Dr. Augusta."

31. Whitman, *Notebooks and Unpublished Prose*, 609.

32. "The Emancipation Jubilee Last Night," *Evening Star* (Washington, D.C.), April 17, 1863.

33. "Grand Emancipation Celebration of the Emancipation of the National Capital," *Liberator*, May 8, 1863.

34. "The Colored Regiment—Two Companies Mustered In," *Daily National Republican* (Washington, D.C.), May 20, 1863.

35. Anderson Ruffin Abbott Papers, Special Collections and Rare Books, S90, S257, Toronto Public Library.

36. James S. Brisbin to L. Thomas, October 1864, Union Battle Reports, vol. 39, series 729, War Records Office, Records of the Adjutant General's Office, 1780s–1917, RG 94, NARA.

37. Masur, *Example for All the Land*, 47; "The Victory and Its Effects," *Christian Recorder*, July 11, 1863.

38. Masur, *Example for All the Land*, 44.

39. Anderson Ruffin Abbott Papers.

40. "The Late Outrage upon Surgeon Augusta in Baltimore," *Christian Recorder*, May 30, 1863.

41. "The Late Outrage upon Surgeon Augusta."

42. "The Late Outrage upon Surgeon Augusta."

43. Masur, *Example for All the Land*, 47.

44. Captain James E. Ferree, Superintendent of Camp Baker, testimony before the American Freedmen's Inquiry Commission, Department of Washington, 1862–69, Camp Baker Freedmen Testimonials, box 2, Records of the U.S. Army Continental Commands, 1821–1920, RG 393, NARA.

45. R. O. Abbott to William A. Hammond, May 21, 1863, and R. O. Abbott to William A. Hammond, May 29, 1863, Colored Troops Division, RG 94, NARA.

46. Anderson R. Abbott was not related to R. O. Abbott, who was the medical director of the District of Columbia.

47. Slaney, *Family Secrets*, 64.

48. Susan Burrell deposition for pension application of Jane Isabella Saunders, file #1179566, May 18, 1897, Records of the Veterans' Administration, RG 15, NARA.

49. Alexander T. Augusta to R. O. Abbott, June 17, 1863, Consolidated Correspondence, entry 225, box 399, Records of the Office of the Quartermaster General, RG 92, NARA; Anderson R. Abbott, pension application, file #1034816, 1897, Records of the Veterans' Administration, RG 15, NARA.

50. The Committee for the Study of the Future of Public Health, Division of Health Care Services, Institute of Medicine, *Future of Public Health*, 57–58.

51. The Pamplin Historical Park and the National Museum of the Civil War Soldier, Petersburg, Va., has in its collection the mahogany surgical kit case once owned and used by Alexander T. Augusta, accession 2005.001.1202.

52. J. B. McPherson, E. M. Pease, Charles C. Topliff, Joel Morse, M. O. Carter, Henry Grange to Abraham Lincoln, February 1864, Letters Received, ser. 360, Colored Troops Division, RG 94 [B-11], NARA.

53. Long, *Doctoring Freedom*, 129.

54. Notes of Joseph K. Barnes, Records Relating to Medical Officers and Physicians, RG 94, NARA.

55. Alexander T. Augusta to C. A. Dana, February 8, 1864, Records Relating to Medical Officers and Physicians, entry 561, RG 94, NARA.

56. Augusta to Dana, February 8, 1864, Records Relating to Medical Officers and Physicians, RG 94, NARA.

57. Long, *Doctoring Freedom*, 131.

58. *Congressional Globe*, February 10, 1864, 553–55.

59. *Congressional Globe*, 553–55.

60. "Washington Correspondence," *Newark Daily Advertiser*, February 15, 1864.

61. Thirty-Eighth Congress, sess. 1, ch. 190, July 1, 1864, "Statutes at Large: 38th Congress," Library of Congress, accessed February 26, 2020, http:// www.loc.gov/law/help/statutes-at-large/38th-congress.php.

62. Mabee with Newhouse, *Sojourner Truth*, 133–34.

63. Court-Martial Case File OO-116, Records of the Office of the Judge Advocate General [Army], RG 153, NARA.

64. See chapter 4 for Abbott's memories of the event.

65. A bill was introduced in the U.S. Senate to increase the pay of Black soldiers that was enacted in June 1864; pay was made retroactive from January 1, 1864.

66. James A. Hardie to Henry Wilson, April 15, 1864, Colored Troops Division, 1863, W22-115, box 37, RG 94, NARA.

67. Berlin, Reidy, and Rowland, *Freedom*, 385–86.

68. *New York Times*, February 4, 1864.

69. "Congressional Lethargy," *Harper's Weekly*, April 16, 1864.

70. *Liberator*, June 17, 1864.

71. *Burlington Free Press*, May 13, 1864.

72. Joel Morse to John Sherman, U.S. Senator, May 14, 1864, Compiled Military Service Record, Alexander T. Augusta, Records of the Adjutant General's Office, 1780s–1917, RG 94, NARA.

73. A. T. Augusta to Major General L. Wallace, January 20, 1865, A-63 1865, Letters Received, ser. 2343, Middle Dept. and 8th Army Corps, Pt. 1 [C-4147], Records of the U.S. Army Continental Commands, 1821–1920, RG 393, NARA.

74. Alexander T. Augusta to W. H. Chesebrough, January 19, 1864, Records Relating to Medical Officers and Physicians, RG 94, NARA.

75. S. M. Bowman to C. W. Foster, March 29, 1865, Letters Received, Colored Troops Division, RG 94, NARA.

76. Notebook entry, Anderson Ruffin Abbott Papers.

77. Downs, *Sick from Freedom*, 9.

78. Rice and Jones, *Public Policy and the Black Hospital*, 6.

79. Leavitt and Numbers, *Sickness and Health in America*, 371.

80. U.S. Freedmen Bureau, Records of the Field Offices for the State of Georgia, 1865–1872, Lincoln Hospital, Weekly Reports of Sick and Wounded Refugees and Freedmen, Savannah, Georgia, M1903, roll 86, Records of the Bureau of Refugees, Freedmen, and Abandoned Lands, RG 105, NARA.

81. Swint, *Dear Ones at Home*, 188.

82. "Colored Officers," *Cleveland Leader*, November 27, 1865.

83. According to the official records for the Return of Medical Officers Serving in the District of Georgia, Records of the Bureau of Refugees, Freedmen, and Abandoned Lands, RG 105, NARA, for the month prior to October 1866, Augusta had a least one white assistant surgeon serving under him at Lincoln Hospital. For the months beginning October 1866, Black surgeons Taylor and Harris were noted among the medical officers serving at Lincoln Hospital as assistant surgeons.

84. Alexander T. Augusta to J. W. Lawton, July 27, 1866, Records of the Field Offices for the State of Georgia, RG 105, NARA.

85. Downs, *Sick from Freedom*, 13.

86. Alexander T. Augusta to Caleb Hornor, June 2, 1866, Records of the Field Offices for the State of Georgia, RG 105, NARA.

87. Augusta to Hornor, June 2, 1866.

88. J. W. Lawton to Alexander T. Augusta, November 22, 1865, Records of the Field Offices for the State of Georgia, RG 105, NARA.

89. Downs, *Sick from Freedom*, 89.

90. Alexander T. Augusta to Caleb W. Hornor, July 1866 and August 7, 1866, Savannah (Lincoln Hospital), Letters Sent, December 1865–January 1868 (National Archives Microfilm Publication M1903, roll 85), volume I (354), RG 105, NARA.

91. *Catalogue of Wilberforce University for 1867–68.*

92. Charles Douglass to Frederick Douglass, November 6, 1867, and September 7, 1868, Frederick Douglass Papers, Library of Congress, Washington, D.C.

93. Lamb, *Howard University Medical Department*, 24.

94. Masur, *Example for All the Land*, 87–88.

95. *National Anti-Slavery Standard*, July 3, 1869.

96. *Evening Star*, June 18, 1869.

97. *National Anti-Slavery Standard*, July 3, 1869.

98. Sumner, *Report Made in the Senate of the United States.*

99. *National Anti-Slavery Standard*, July 3, 1869.

100. *Evening Star*, June 17, 1869; *Daily National Republican*, June 18, 1869.

101. *National Anti-Slavery Standard*, July 3, 1869.

102. U.S. Senate, Report No. 29, 41st Cong., 2nd sess., February 8, 1870.

103. U.S. Senate, Report No. 29.

104. *Baltimore Sun*, February 8, 1870.

105. The Medical Society of the District of Columbia was a separate organization from the National Medical Association, which was established by Black physicians in 1895 in response to their exclusion from the American Medical Association.

106. Prince Hall Freemasons are the oldest and largest freemasons group for people of color; *Evening Star*, February 25, 1879.

107. 1870 U.S. Federal Census, microfilm publication M593, RG 29, NARA.

108. Cornell Law School Legal Information Institute, "District of Columbia v. John R. Thompson Co., Inc.," https://www.law.cornell.edu/supremecourt/text/346/100.

109. *Afro-American*, March 11, 1959.

110. Lamb, *Howard University Medical Department*, 35.

111. *Weekly Louisianian*, November 17, 1877.

112. Lamb, *Howard University Medical Department*, 37.

113. *Washington Post*, March 11, 1878.

114. Last Will and Testament of Alexander T. Augusta, box 123, District of Columbia Archives, Washington, D.C.

115. *Baltimore Sun*, February 17, 1891.

3. For Race and Country

1. *National Anti-Slavery Standard*, July 17, 1851.

2. Kathryn Grover notes and email correspondence, April 2011.

3. A master mariner is a licensed captain or shipmaster in command of a commercial sea vessel.

4. Douglass, *Narrative of the Life of Frederick Douglass*, 104.

5. *Sailor's Magazine and Naval Journal*, 291.

6. "Gleanings by the Wayside," *North Star*, February 11, 1848.

7. Peterson, *Black Gotham*, 9.

8. Peterson, 74; Andrews, *New York African Free-Schools*, 25.

9. Peterson, *Black Gotham*, 4.

10. 1850 U.S. Federal Census, microfilm publication M432, Records of the Bureau of the Census, RG 29, NARA.

11. "Memorial," *National Anti-Slavery Standard*, July 17, 1851.

12. "A Sensible Petition," *National Anti-Slavery Standard*, July 17, 1851; Foner, *Essays in Afro-American History*, 99.

13. "The Shame of America," *National Anti-Slavery Standard*, July 31, 1851.

14. "Letter from Liverpool," *National Anti-Slavery Standard*, January 9, 1851.

15. "Colored Americans in England," *Anti-Slavery Bugle*, August 6, 1853. Although the article does not identify Mercy Powell by name, the circumstances of "the colored lady's" family are identical to that of Mercy and her family. As Powell Sr. was well known within the abolitionist community and antislavery publications, it is highly probable that this article refers to the Powell family in Liverpool.

16. William P. Powell Sr. to Dr. Inman, Liverpool, May 5, 1852, inserted in the Liverpool Royal Infirmary School of Medicine Minutes, 1845–1859, S.3076, at the entry for May 29, 1852, Special Collections and Archives, Sydney Jones Library, University of Liverpool, England.

17. *Lancet*, September 15, 1855, 257.

18. *Thirty-Second Report of the Coombe and the Peter-Street Auxiliary Lying-in-Hospitals*, 46.

19. "Medical News," 593; Powell was admitted as a member of the Royal College of Surgeons on July 9, 1858.

20. *London and Provincial Medical Directory*, 667.

21. Ship's passenger list, SS *Wyoming*, March 4, 1861, Passenger Lists of Vessels Arriving at Philadelphia, Pennsylvania, M425, Records of the United States Customs Service, 1745–1997, RG 36, NARA.

22. *New Bedford (Mass.) Republican Standard*, October 10, 1861.

23. *National Anti-Slavery Standard*, August 17, 1861.

24. National Maritime Digital Library, Whaling Crew List Database, New Bedford Whaling Museum, accessed February 27, 2020, http://www.whaling museum.org/online_exhibits/crewlist/search.php; Sylvester is listed in the crew list for the bark *Tropic Bird* traveling in the Atlantic Ocean; Isaiah is listed in the crew list for the bark *Midas* traveling to New Zealand and the South Pacific.

25. *Boston Herald*, June 3, 1863.

26. *Medical and Surgical History of the War of the Rebellion*, 283.

27. William P. Powell Jr. testimony before the American Freedmen's Inquiry Commission investigating conditions at Contraband Camp, Department of Washington, 1862–69, Camp Baker Freedmen Testimonials, box 2, Records of the U.S. Army Continental Commands, 1821–1920, RG 393, NARA.

28. William P. Powell Jr., March 22, 1912, pension file #1065790 (hereafter Powell pension file); physician's affidavit, Dr. Charles B. Purvis, October 10, 1894; deposition of Samuel Powell, January 23, 1895, Records of the Veterans' Administration, RG 15, NARA.

29. Deposition of William P. Powell Jr., June 30, 1893, Powell pension file.

30. "The Colored Sailors' Home," *Liberator*, July 24, 1863.

31. William P. Powell Jr. to R. O. Abbott, October 17, 1864, Relating to Medical Officers and Physicians, entry 561, Records of the Adjutant General's Office, 1780s–1917, RG 94, NARA.

32. Consolidated Lists of Civil War Draft Registration, 1862–1865, District of Columbia, vol. 120, Records of the Provost Marshal General's Bureau, RG 110, NARA.

33. Powell to Abbott, October 17, 1864.

34. William P. Powell Jr. to S. S. Jocelyn, September 17, 1863, AMA Collection (7816/26911), Amistad Research Center, Dillard University, New Orleans, La.

35. Hancock, *Letters of a Civil War Nurse*, 40.

36. Anderson R. Abbott to C. W. Horner, September 27, 1864, Records Relating to Medical Officers and Physicians, RG 94, NARA.

37. Forbes, *Hawaiian National Bibliography*, 31–33; Kingdom of Hawaii, *Report of the Board of Health*, 621.

38. Forbes, *Hawaiian National Bibliography*, 621.

39. New York Passenger Lists, 1820–1897, SS *Wisconsin*, October 6, 1874, ancestry.com; *Railway News*, May 11, 1872, 665.

40. Physician's affidavit, F. Martin, Chief of Surgical Department, University of Maryland Dispensary, September 27, 1893, Powell pension file.

41. Powell pension file. The Workhouse Hospital and Kirkdale Home for the Aged were both facilities established to serve the poor and destitute in Liverpool. Originally a state-run industrial school for the care and training of destitute children, Kirkdale Home was opened to the aged and infirmed in 1904.

42. Although Powell stated that he was from a family of ten, the primary sources indicate that his family consisted of two parents and seven children.

43. William P. Powell Jr. to Anderson R. Abbott, September 27, 1912, Powell pension file.

44. Department of the Interior, Pension Office, *Instructions to Examining Surgeons for Pensions*, 3.

45. Act of June 27, 1890, U.S. Congress, *U.S. Statutes at Large*, vol. 26, 1890–1891, 51st Cong., p. 182, on Library of Congress website, https://www.loc.gov /item/llsl-v26/.

46. Logue and Blanck, *Race, Ethnicity, and Disability*, 24.

47. Declaration for Invalid Pension, October 3, 1891 Powell pension file.

48. Declaration for Invalid Pension, March 22, 1912, Powell pension file.

49. William P. Powell Jr. to R. O. Abbott, October 17, 1864, Records Relating to Medical Officers and Physicians, RG 94, NARA.

50. Powell pension file.

51. Pension Act of March 3, 1865, U.S. Congress, *U.S. Statutes at Large*, vol. 13, 1865, 38th Cong., chaps. 83, 84, p. 499, on Library of Congress website, https://www.loc.gov/item/llsl-v13/.

52. Powell pension file, Act of February 6, 1907, August 23, 1907, Records of the Veterans' Administration, RG 15, NARA.

53. Physician's affidavit, John McMurray, MD, January 4, 1913, Powell pension file.

54. William P. Powell Jr. to William McKinley, October 22, 1900, and to Theodore Roosevelt, January 10, 1908, Powell pension file.

55. Deposition of Charles Johnson, September 20, 1893, Powell pension file.

56. Deposition of Elizabeth Johnson, September 29, 1893, Powell pension file.

57. Physician's affidavit, Dr. Frank Martin, September 27, 1893, Powell pension file.

58. Physician's affidavit, Dr. Charles B. Purvis, October 10, 1894, Powell pension file.

59. Deposition of Samuel Powell, January 23, 1895, Powell pension file.
60. Letter from Pension Commissioner G. S. Saltzgaber, May 14, 1915, Powell pension file.
61. Powell pension file. Powell refers to his contract date in this statement as May 19, 1862, which is likely an error on his part as he received a contract as an acting assistant surgeon on May 26, 1863. The photograph to which he refers was likely taken in August 1863.
62. Wilson, "Prejudice and Policy," S64.
63. Logue and Blanck, "Benefit of the Doubt," 377; Shaffer, *After the Glory*, 130.
64. *General Instructions to Special Examiners*, 28.
65. Logue and Blanck, "Benefit of the Doubt."

4. Witness to History

1. Slaney, *Family Secrets*, 15–17.
2. Slaney, 20.
3. Slaney, 21.
4. "The Elgin Settlement," Buxton National Historic Site and Museum, accessed February 27, 2020, http://www.buxtonmuseum.com/history/virtual -elgin-settlement.html.
5. Hepburn, *Crossing the Border*, 159, 164.
6. Anderson Ruffin Abbott Papers, Special Collections and Rare Books, S90, S257, Toronto Public Library (hereafter Abbott Papers); Reid, *African Canadians in Union Blue*, 155.
7. *Annual Catalogue of the Officers and Students of Oberlin College, 1857–58*, 41, 44.
8. *Annual Announcement of the Toronto School of Medicine*, 7, 16.
9. Slaney, *Family Secrets*, 50.
10. A licentiate is granted to an individual who has successfully completed a full course of medical studies, indicating competence to practice.
11. Anderson R. Abbott to Edwin M. Stanton, February 6, 1863, Records Relating to Medical Officers and Physicians, Anderson R. Abbott, entry 561, Records of the Adjutant General's Office, 1780s–1917, RG 94, NARA.
12. From transcripts of Abbott's personal papers by Catherine Slaney, Abbott Papers.
13. Abbott Papers.
14. Abbott Papers.
15. "The Colored Sailors' Home," *Liberator*, July 24, 1863.

16. Miasmatic fever was a disease believed to have been a result of environmental factors such as contaminated water, noxious air, and poor hygienic conditions. Symptoms included fever, weakness, weight loss, and headaches.

17. Deposition of Anderson R. Abbott, May 1, 1897, Anderson R. Abbott, pension file #1034816 (hereafter Abbott pension file), Records of the Veterans' Administration, RG 15, NARA.

18. Deposition of Elizabeth Keckly, July 27, 1896, Abbott pension file. Elizabeth Keckly's name was spelled Keckly and Keckley. I have chosen to use the spelling used by Keckly and the alternative spelling as it appears in quoted sources.

19. Abbott Papers.

20. Abbott Papers.

21. Abbott Papers.

22. *Daily National Republican*, November 13, 1862.

23. Woodward, *Medical and Surgical History of the War of the Rebellion*, 259.

24. Abbott, "Some Recollections of Lincoln's Assassination," 397.

25. Abbott, 398.

26. The house located on Tenth Street directly across from Ford's Theatre was owned by William and Anna Petersen and is referred to as the Petersen House.

27. Abbott, "Some Recollections of Lincoln's Assassination."

28. Keckley, *Behind the Scenes*, 188.

29. G. B. Carse to Anderson R. Abbott, January 2, 1866; Caleb W. Hornor, May 14, 1866; and Robert Reyburn, May 12, 1866, Records Relating to Medical Officers and Physicians, RG 94, NARA; Fleischner, *Mrs. Lincoln and Mrs. Keckly*, 319.

30. Deposition of Elizabeth Keckly, July 27, 1896, Abbott pension file.

31. Keckley, *Behind the Scenes*, 66–67.

32. Fleischner, *Mrs. Lincoln and Mrs. Keckly*, 194.

33. Jorgenson, *Mrs. Keckly Sends Her Regards*, vii. The Fifteenth Street Presbyterian Church had a predominantly African American congregation and was known for its abolitionist stand.

34. Abbott, "Some Recollections of Lincoln's Assassination," 401.

35. Abbott, 401.

36. Anderson R. Abbott to Medical Director, Department of Washington, May 16, 1865, Records Relating to Medical Officers and Physicians, RG 94, NARA.

37. R. O. Abbott, Medical Director of the District of Columbia, May 15, 1866, Abbott pension file. R. O. Abbott was not related to Anderson R. Abbott.

38. Carse to Abbott, January 2, 1866.

39. Transcription by Catherine Slaney from materials in the Abbott Papers.

40. "Secessh" was an abbreviated form of "secessionist" used to denote a supporter of the Confederacy during the American Civil War.

41. Transcription by Catherine Slaney from materials in the Abbott Papers.

42. *Ontario Medical Register,* chap. 178.

43. Slaney, *Family Secrets,* 86–87.

44. Slaney, 91, 196.

45. "African Canadian Workers: From 1900 to the Second World War," The Virtual Museum of Canada, accessed February 27, 2020, http://www.virtual museum.ca/edu/ViewLoitDa.do;jsessionid=1E1DE3933BB18722932C3 78 E3DEC4EF2?method=preview&lang=EN&id=18684 (site discontinued).

46. Slaney, *Family Secrets,* 105, 109.

47. Newby, *Anderson Ruffin Abbott,* 102.

48. "African Americans," Encyclopedia of Chicago, accessed February 27, 2020, http://www.encyclopedia.chicagohistory.org/pages/27.html.

49. Slaney, *Family Secrets,* 122.

50. Quoted in Slaney, 125–26.

51. "Colored Churches Unite in Honoring Queen Victoria," *Inter Ocean* (Chicago), May 26, 1897.

52. Slaney, *Family Secrets,* 126.

53. "The Grand Army of the Republic and Kindred Societies," Library of Congress, accessed February 27, 2020, https://www.loc.gov/rr/main/gar /garintro.html.

54. Newby, *Anderson Ruffin Abbott,* 118–19.

55. Anderson R. Abbott to Redfield Proctor, February 18, 1891, Records Relating to Medical Officers and Physicians, RG 94, NARA.

56. Charles R. Greenleaf to Anderson R. Abbott, March 11, 1891, Records Relating to Medical Officers and Physicians, RG 94, NARA.

57. Declaration for an Original Invalid Pension, June 25, 1891, Abbott pension file.

58. Surgeon's Certificate, December 7, 1891, Abbott pension file.

59. Deposition of Isaac Mills, August 28, 1891, Abbott pension file.

60. Affidavit of Robert Alder Wood, October 14, 1891, Abbott pension file.

61. Affidavit of John Lang Bray, MD, August 14, 1891, Abbott pension file.

62. Affidavit of Anderson R. Abbott, May 1, 1897, Abbott pension file.

63. Deposition of Elizabeth Keckly, July 27, 1896, Abbott pension file.

64. Deposition of Anderson R. Abbott, July 8, 1897, Abbott pension file.

65. Deposition of Laura V. McCool, August 3, 1897, and deposition of Mary Dorsey Glasgow, August 4, 1897, Abbott pension file.
66. Appeal Case, Board of Review, Bureau of Pensions, January 6, 1898, Abbott pension file.
67. Logue and Blanck, "Benefit of the Doubt."
68. Affidavit of Anderson R. Abbott, December 15, 1902, Abbott pension file.
69. Newby, *Anderson Ruffin Abbott*, 137.
70. Abbott Papers; Newby, *Anderson Ruffin Abbott*, 140; Slaney, *Family Secrets*, 128–29; Anderson Ruffin Abbott Papers, ACC 2010-011, National Library of Medicine, Bethesda, Md.

5. Serving in the Regiment

1. Peterson, *Black Gotham*, 40.
2. Davis, *Memoirs of Aaron Burr*, 197.
3. United States, New York Land Records, 1630–1975, database with images, FamilySearch, accessed April 5, 2020, https://www.familysearch.org/search/record/results?count=20&q.givenName=george&q.surname=degrasse&f.collectionId=2078654.
4. "The New York African Free School," New-York Historical Society, accessed April 5, 2020, https://www.nyhistory.org/web/africanfreeschool/history/.
5. "Oneida Institute," Oneida County Freedom Trail, accessed February 25, 2020, http://www.oneidacountyfreedomtrail.com/oneida-institute.html.
6. "Slavery and Emancipation in New York," History in Action, accessed February 25, 2020, http://historyinaction.columbia.edu/field-notes/slavery-and-emancipation-new-york (site discontinued).
7. "A Colored Physician," *Frederick Douglass' Paper*, September 22, 1854.
8. S. Russell Childs, MD, to Bowdoin College, May 11, 1849, George J. Mitchell Department of Special Collections and Archives, Bowdoin College Library, Brunswick, Maine.
9. *Catalogue of the Officers and Students of Bowdoin College* (1847).
10. *Salem Observer*, June 14, 1849.
11. Mansel, Webster, and Sweetland, *Benign Disorders*, 11.
12. J. Warner, *Against the Spirit of System*, 100.
13. "Daniel Laing Jr. (Expelled)," Perspectives of Change: The Story of Civil Rights, Diversity, Inclusion and Access to Education at HMS and HSDM, Center for the History of Medicine at Countway Library, Harvard University, accessed April 5, 2020, https://perspectivesofchange.hms.harvard.edu/node/37.

14. *Frederick Douglass' Paper*, June 9, 1854.
15. Account books of John V. DeGrasse, Ms. N-310, box 1, folder 2, DeGrasse-Howard Papers, Massachusetts Historical Society, Boston.
16. Dorman, *Twenty Families of Color in Massachusetts*, 155.
17. *Liberator*, January 27, 1854.
18. "Colored Physician."
19. "Massasoit Guards," *Salem Register*, August 16, 1855.
20. 1860 U.S. Federal Census, microfilm publication M653, NARA.
21. "The Anniversary Prince Hall Grand Lodge," *Weekly Anglo-African*, July 7, 1860.
22. J. B. McPherson, E. M. Pease, Charles C. Topliff, Joel Morse, M. O. Carter, Henry Grange to Abraham Lincoln, February 1864, Letters Received, ser. 360, Colored Troops Division, Records of the Adjutant General's Office, 1780s–1917, RG 94 [B-11], NARA.
23. James Beecher to John V. DeGrasse, State House of Boston, May 9, 1863, Ms. N-310, box 1, folder 6, DeGrasse-Howard Papers.
24. St. Croix, U.S. Virgin Islands, Free Colored Censuses, 1815–1832, Ancestry. com, (database online). Although no official military records referred to Reed as "colored" or "mulatto," the St. Croix, U.S. Virgin Islands, Free Colored Censuses for 1831–32 make note of William Nicolay Reed, a six-year-old boy with a status of "free person of color, freeborn." His race is listed as "Mestice" or mixed and identifies his mother as Susanna Cooper, "mulatto." No father is listed.
25. Quoted in Reid, *Freedom for Themselves*, 29.
26. "Affairs of North Carolina," *New York Herald*, May 24, 1863, and June 1, 1863.
27. *Boston Traveler*, May 28, 1863.
28. Quoted in Reid, *Freedom for Themselves*, 33.
29. "Affairs of North Carolina," May 24, 1863, and June 1, 1863.
30. Shana Renee Hutchins, "Just Learning to Be Men: A History of the 35th United States Colored Troops," U.S. Colored Troops Formed in North Carolina, 1999, https://www.ncgenweb.us/ncusct/shana.htm; H. M. Mintz to Major General Quincy Gilmore, November 17, 1863, Descriptive Books, 35th Regiment USCT, Records of the Adjutant General's Office, 1780s–1917, RG 94, NARA.
31. Reid, *Freedom for Themselves*, 25.
32. The Battle of Olustee was the largest Civil War battle fought in Florida. Several regiments of the Union army, including the 35th and 54th of the

USCT, participated in it. The Union army was defeated by Confederate forces and lost nearly 1,800 soldiers.

33. Foote, *Gentlemen and the Roughs*, 30.

34. Assistant Surgeon John V. DeGrasse, Proceedings of General Court-Martial, Records of the Office of the Judge Advocate General [Army], RG 153, NARA. All subsequent quotes and testimony from this court-martial are sourced from these official court-martial records unless otherwise noted.

35. Henry O. Marcy to Mrs. William N. Reed, March 16, 1864, Case Files of Approved Pension Applications of Widows and Other Veterans of the Army and Navy Who Served Mainly in the Civil War and the War with Spain, compiled 1861–1934, Records of the Veterans' Administration, RG 15, NARA.

36. Peterson, *Black Gotham*, 271.

37. "Quinine, Morphine and Whiskey: Tools of the Civil War Doctor," *Hartford Courant*, December 29, 2012.

38. Peterson, *Black Gotham*, 270.

39. Delos Barber to Lieutenant Colonel Hoffman, June 28, 1863, Compiled Military Service Records of Volunteer Union Soldiers Who Served with the United States Colored Troops: Infantry Organizations, 31st through 35th, M1992, roll 64, Records of the Adjutant General's Office, 1782–1984, RG 94, NARA.

40. Quoted in Peterson, *Black Gotham*, 271.

6. Adventure and Ambition

1. John H. Rapier Jr. to James P. Thomas, August 19, 1864, MS 62–4283, Rapier Family Papers, Moorland Spingarn Research Center, Howard University, Washington, D.C. (hereafter RFP).

2. John H. Rapier is referred to as either Jr. or Sr. throughout to distinguish between the son and the father. John H. Rapier Jr. is also later referred to as just Rapier.

3. Franklin and Schweninger, *In Search of the Promised Land*, 18.

4. Morse and Morse, *New Universal Gazetteer*, 507.

5. Franklin and Schweninger, *In Search of the Promised Land*, 15.

6. Franklin and Schweninger, 15.

7. Schweninger, "John H. Rapier, Sr." By law, after a formerly enslaved person was emancipated, it took formal legislation to free that person despite a payment being made to purchase their freedom.

8. Rapier Sr. to Rapier Jr., May 13, 1856, RFP.

9. Rapier Sr. to Rapier Jr., May 13, 1856.

10. Rapier Sr. to Rapier Jr., October 27, 1856, RFP.

11. Rapier Sr. to Rapier Jr., March 17, 1857, RFP.

12. Schweninger, "John H. Rapier, Sr."

13. Rapier Jr. diary, March 10, 1857, and May 30, 1857, RFP.

14. Franklin and Schweninger, *In Search of the Promised Land*, 35.

15. Rapier Sr. to Richard Rapier, April 8, 1845, RFP.

16. "The Death of Dr. John H. Rapier, U.S.A.," *Christian Recorder*, June 16, 1866.

17. Rapier Sr. to Henry K. Thomas, February 28, 1843, RFP.

18. "The Death of Dr. John H. Rapier, U.S.A."

19. The Fugitive Slave Act enacted in 1850 made legal any claim by a white person on any Black person who was free or a presumed fugitive slave. Capture was made without due process of law and without allowing or considering the captured individual's testimony in his or her own defense.

20. Hepburn, *Crossing the Border*, 27.

21. Hepburn, 164.

22. Slaney, *Family Secrets*, 42.

23. Rapier Jr. to James P. Thomas, June 14, 1855, RFP.

24. Franklin and Schweninger, *In Search of the Promised Land*, 55.

25. Alexander, "John H. Rapier, Jr. and the Medical Profession in Jamaica," 38.

26. Alexander, 38.

27. Soodalter, "William Walker: King of the 19th Century Filibusters," History Net, March 4, 2010, http://www.historynet.com/william-walker-king-of-the-19th-century-filibusters.htm.

28. Franklin and Schweninger, *In Search of the Promised Land*, 117; Schweninger and Thomas, *From Tennessee Slave to St. Louis Entrepreneur*, 118.

29. Franklin and Schweninger, *In Search of the Promised Land*, 119.

30. Rapier Sr. to Rapier Jr., May 13, 1856, RFP.

31. Granger and Kelly, "Little Falls' Historic Contexts."

32. Rapier Jr. diary, January 18, 1857, RFP.

33. Rapier Jr. diary, February 5, 1857, RFP.

34. Rapier Sr. to Rapier Jr., September 15, 1856, RFP.

35. Newspaper clipping from Rapier Jr. diary, RFP.

36. Rapier Jr. diary, April 5, 1857, RFP.

37. Rapier Jr. diary, February 3 and 4, 1857, RFP.

38. Rapier Jr. diary, n.d., RFP.

39. Rapier Jr. diary, n.d., RFP.

40. Rapier Jr. diary, September 15, 1857, RFP.
41. Rapier Jr. diary, 1857, RFP.
42. Rapier Jr. diary, October 2, 1857, RFP.
43. Rapier Jr. diary, June 13, 1857, RFP.
44. Rapier Jr. diary, July 28, 1857, RFP.
45. Rapier Jr. diary, July 1, 1857, RFP.
46. 1860 U.S. Federal Census, microfilm publication M653, NARA.
47. James P. Thomas to Rapier Jr., January 8, 1859, RFP.
48. Alexander, "John H. Rapier, Jr. and the Medical Profession in Jamaica."
49. Rapier Jr to Rapier Sr., December 31, 1860, RFP.
50. Rapier Jr. to the *Leavenworth Conservative*, April 13, 1861, RFP.
51. Rapier Jr. to Rapier Sr., December 31, 1860, RFP.
52. Rapier refers to himself as a "quadroon" in his letter of application for a position as a surgeon in the U.S. Army. Although not used in contemporary language, "quadroon" was defined as a person who is one-quarter Black and three-quarters white European.
53. Rapier Jr. to James P. Thomas, February 25, 1861, RFP.
54. Rapier Jr. to Thomas, February 25, 1861.
55. Rapier Jr. to Thomas, February 25, 1861.
56. Rapier Jr. to James P. Thomas, April 30, 1861, RFP.
57. Rapier Jr. to Thomas, February 18, 1862, RFP.
58. Rapier Jr. to James P. Thomas, April 30, 1861, RFP.
59. Rapier Jr. to Thomas, April 30, 1861.
60. Alexander, "John H. Rapier, Jr. and the Medical Profession in Jamaica," 42.
61. Alexander, 44.
62. Rapier Jr. to James P. Thomas, February 3, 1862, RFP.
63. Rapier Jr. to Thomas, February 3, 1862.
64. Rapier Jr. to Thomas, February 3, 1862.
65. Rapier Jr. to James P. Thomas, March 6, 1862, RFP.
66. James T. Rapier to Rapier Jr., March 17, 1862, RFP.
67. Rapier Jr. to James P. Thomas, March 6, 1862, RFP.
68. *Annual Catalogue of the Officers and Students of Oberlin College 1862–1863*, 16.
69. Schopieray, "Colored Men Are Not Admitted Here."
70. Sarah Thomas was the daughter of Rapier's uncle Henry Thomas and a close cousin to John Jr.
71. Rapier Jr. to Sarah Thomas, November 12, 1863, RFP.
72. Rapier Jr. to Thomas, November 12, 1863.
73. Kennedy, "U.S. Army Hospital," 119.

74. *Circular and Announcement of the Seventeenth Session.*

75. *Nineteenth Circular and Announcement.*

76. John H. Rapier Jr. to Army Surgeon General, U.S.A., April 21, 1864, Records Relating to Medical Officers and Physicians, John H. Rapier Jr., entry 561, Records of the Adjutant General's Office, 1780s–1917, RG 94, NARA.

77. John H. Rapier Jr. to Medical Director of New Orleans, Louisiana, June 23, 1864, Records Relating to Medical Officers and Physicians, RG 94, NARA.

78. Records Relating to Medical Officers and Physicians, RG 94, NARA.

79. John H. Rapier Jr., Oath of Service, July 4, 1864, Records Relating to Medical Officers and Physicians, RG 94, NARA.

80. Rapier Jr. to James P. Thomas, August 19, 1864, RFP.

81. Rapier Jr. to James P. Thomas, August 19, 1864.

82. Examples of cases at Freedmen's Hospital, 1865–66, as recorded in the *Medical and Surgical History of the Civil War*, 257–60.

83. Rapier Jr. to James P. Thomas, August 19, 1864, RFP.

84. *Christian Recorder*, June 16, 1866.

85. Rapier Jr. to James P. Thomas, August 19, 1864, RFP.

86. Rapier Jr. to Thomas, August 19, 1864. "Free Maryland" was the term Rapier used to refer to the passing of Article 24.

87. Berlin, Reidy, and Rowland, *Freedom*, 340–41.

88. *Liberator*, February 10, 1865.

89. Bilious fever was a medical diagnosis used in the eighteenth and nineteenth centuries that includes symptoms of nausea, vomiting, diarrhea, and fever. It was often used on death certificates as the cause of death for persons exhibiting these symptoms.

90. *Christian Recorder*, June 16, 1866.

7. From Ivy League to U.S. Navy

1. The spelling "Greene" is used by Greene himself, while documents and letters by others use the spelling "Green."

2. Although most government records, including the U.S. Federal Census, indicate a birth year of 1833, Greene gave his birth year as 1837 in his letter of application for a position in the Union navy.

3. Schiff, "Life of Richard Henry Green."

4. Gibson, "Population of the 100 Largest Cities."

5. *An Ethnic History of New Haven*, 7, Ethnic Heritage Center, 2010. https://connecticuthistory.org/wp-content/uploads/2013/04/AnEthnicHistoryof NewHaven2.pdf.

6. 1850 U.S. Federal Census, microfilm publication M432, Records of the Bureau of the Census, RG 29, NARA.

7. *Catalogue of the Officers and Students in Yale College*, 31–36.

8. *Catalogue of the Society of Brothers in Unity*, 6.

9. *Record of the Class of 1857 of Yale University*, 112.

10. *Friends' Review: A Religious, Literary and Miscellaneous Journal* 27, no. 51 (1874): 109; *American Educational Annual*, 166.

11. Greene to Caldwell, September 20, 1863, Richard Henry Green Papers, MS 2005, Manuscripts and Archives, Yale University Library, New Haven, Conn. (hereafter Green Papers).

12. Greene to Caldwell, September 20, 1863, Green Papers.

13. Richard Henry Greene, MD, U.S. Navy Assistant Surgeon Application and Medical Examination, November 3, 1863, American Civil War Medicine and Surgical Antiques, accessed February 24, 2020, http://www.medical antiques.com/civilwar/Navy_surgeon_applications/Greene_richard_henry .htm.

14. Note from B. F. Morgan, MD, October 13, 1863, Rauner Special Collections Library, Dartmouth College, Hanover, N.H.; letter from Albert Smith, MD, Professor of Materia Medica, New Hampshire Medical Institution, October 29, 1863, Green Papers.

15. Richard Henry Greene, MD, U.S. Navy Assistant Surgeon Application and Medical Examination, November 3, 1863.

16. Personnel Records, 1803–97, E-164, Records of Volunteer (Acting) Officers, May 1861–ca. 1880, 172, Naval Records Collection of the Office of Naval Records and Library, RG 45, NARA.

17. Reidy, "Black Men in Navy Blue." Reidy notes that this figure was determined by examining surviving naval enlistment records and quarterly muster rolls of vessels.

18. The Militia Act of 1792 provided for the organization of state militias. It also enabled the president of the United States to take command of the state militias in times of imminent invasion or insurrection.

19. Logs of Ships and Stations, 1801–1946, Logs of U.S. Naval Ships, 1801–1946, State of Georgia, 11–27–1863 to 9–10-1864, E-118, PI-123, Vol. 3 of 4, Records of the Bureau of Naval Personnel, RG 24, NARA.

20. Medical Journals of Ships, 1813–1910, Headquarters Records Medical Journals and Reports on Patients, box 454, entry 22, Records of the Bureau of Medicine and Surgery, RG 52, NARA.

21. Medical Journals of Ships, 1813–1910, Records of the Bureau of Medicine and Surgery, RG 52, NARA.

22. Greene to Caldwell, Beaufort, N.C., January 19, 1864, Green Papers.

23. Medical Journals of Ships, 1813–1910, Records of the Bureau of Medicine and Surgery, RG 52, NARA.

24. Greene to Caldwell, Norfolk, Virginia, April 20, 1864, Green Papers.

25. Greene to Caldwell, at sea, May 21, 1864, Green Papers.

26. Greene to Caldwell, New York Navy Yard, September 7, 1864, Green Papers.

27. Greene to Caldwell, July 16, 1864, Green Papers.

28. Greene to Caldwell, May 21, 1864, Green Papers.

29. Greene to Caldwell, April 20, 1864, Green Papers.

30. Greene to Caldwell, April 20, 1864.

31. Greene to Caldwell, July 26, 1864, Green Papers.

32. Greene to Caldwell, September 7, 1864, Green Papers.

33. Greene to Caldwell, May 21, 1864, Green Papers.

34. Greene to Caldwell, July 26, 1864, Green Papers.

35. Greene to Caldwell, July 26, 1864.

36. Greene to Caldwell, Sept. 7, 1864, Green Papers

37. Greene to Caldwell, October 26, 1864, Green Papers.

38. Greene to Caldwell, December 6, 1864, Green Papers.

39. Anderson, *Landmarks of Rensselaer County*, 170.

40. A. M. Bissell to Greene, July 24, 1865, Green Papers.

41. New York State Census, 1875, Green Papers.

42. I. Grenow to Richard H. Greene, January 26, 1876, Green Papers.

43. Ancestry.com, Headstones Provided for Deceased Union Civil War Veterans, 1879–1903 [database online] from original records, Card Records of Headstone Provided for Deceased Civil War Veterans, ca. 1879–ca. 1903, Records of the Office of the Quartermaster General, RG 92, NARA.

8. Preacher and Physician

1. Revels's exact birth year is unclear. It appears as 1817 in both the 1850 and 1860 U.S. Federal Censuses, as 1810 in the 1870 census, and as 1814 on his tombstone. Though his father is named Rhodes Revels here, he has also been referred to as Elijah Rhodes.

2. Revels, "Autobiography."

3. *Clarion-Ledger* (Jackson, Miss.), February 20, 1870; "Rev. W. R. Revels," *Christian Recorder*, August 6, 1870.

4. "Dawes Commission," Cherokee Heritage Center, accessed February 25, 2020, http://www.cherokeeheritage.org/cherokeeheritagegenealogy-html /dawes-commission/.

5. Testimony of Dora Revels Leonard and Ida Revels Redmond, December 10, 1901, Carthage, Miss., Applications for Enrollment of the Commission to the Five Civilized Tribes, 1898–1914, microfilm M1301, 468, Records of the Bureau of Indian Affairs, RG 75, NARA.

6. Testimony of Dora Revels Leonard and Ida Revels Redmond, December 10, 1901.

7. Revels, "Autobiography," 1.

8. Crow and Wadelington, *History of African Americans in North Carolina*, 48.

9. Ferguson, "In Pursuit of the Full Enjoyment of Liberty and Happiness."

10. Payne, *History of the African Methodist Episcopal Church*.

11. Quoted in Tanner, *Apology for African Methodism*, 339.

12. "The African-American Mosaic: Colonization," Library of Congress, accessed February 1, 2020, https://www.loc.gov/exhibits/african/afam002 .html.

13. Sarah Schutz, "'Africa's Glory and America's Hope': Columbia's Involvement in the African Colonization Movement," Columbia University and Slavery, accessed April 18, 2020, https://columbiaandslavery.columbia.edu /content/africas-glory-and-americas-hope-columbias-involvement-african-colonization-movement#/_ftn31.

14. *Christian Recorder*, August 6, 1870.

15. *Christian Recorder*, August 15, 1866.

16. *Christian Recorder*, December 17, 1864.

17. Power-Greene, *Against Wind and Tide*, 103.

18. "Free Discussion," *Indiana State Sentinel,* April 30, 1846.

19. *Indianapolis Daily Journal*, September 30, 1888.

20. "Tour A 6. Second Baptist Church Fire 1851," Forged through Fire: Bethel AME Church, accessed April 6, 2020, https://forgedthroughfire.wordpress .com/walking-tour/indianapolis-station-and-the-underground-railroad /second-baptist-church-fire-1851/.

21. Payne, *History of the African Methodist Episcopal Church*, 336–45.

22. Payne, 336–45.

23. *Christian Recorder*, August 24, 1861.

24. *Cleveland Daily Leader*, April 18, 1859.

25. *Frederick Douglass' Paper*, April 6, 1859.

26. Scott, *Visitation of God*, 58.

27. *Christian Recorder*, July 5, 1862.

28. *Christian Recorder*, January 31, 1863.

29. *Christian Recorder*, August 29, 1863.

30. Thornbrough and Riker, *Diary of Calvin Fletcher*, 481.

31. Thornbrough and Riker, 260.

32. *Christian Recorder*, November 27, 1863.

33. General Order No. 143 was issued on May 22, 1863, by the adjutant general's office of the U.S. War Department.

34. Quoted in Forstchen, "28th United States Colored Troops."

35. *Indianapolis Daily Journal*, December 8, 1863.

36. "To the Colored Men of Indiana," *Indianapolis Daily Journal*, December 4, 1863.

37. *Christian Recorder*, February 13, 1864.

38. *Indianapolis Daily Journal*, January 25, 1864.

39. This number is estimated based on the original strength of the regiment at 950 as given in *The Union Army: A History of Military Affairs in the Loyal States*; see also Tanner, *Apology for African Methodism*, 339.

40. Notation made in file of Willis R. Revels, Records Relating to Medical Officers and Physicians, Willis R. Revels, entry 561, Records of the Adjutant General's Office, 1780s–1917, RG 94, NARA.

41. *Christian Recorder*, December 12, 1863.

42. *Christian Recorder*, July 30, 1864.

43. *Christian Recorder*, July 30, 1864.

44. *Christian Recorder*, March 17, 1866.

45. *Christian Recorder*, March 31, 1866.

46. *Christian Recorder*, October 12, 1867.

47. *Christian Recorder*, October 12, 1867; *Indianapolis News*, January 26, 1870.

48. *Indianapolis News*, January 26, 1870.

49. Tanner, *Apology for African Methodism*, 176. The *Repository of Religion and Literature* was a publication initiated by the Indiana Annual Conference of the AME Church with an explicitly educational focus.

50. Gardner, *Unexpected Places*, 62.

51. *Christian Recorder*, October 12, 1867.

52. *Christian Recorder*, February 10, 1866, and March 3, 1866.

53. *Christian Recorder*, February 12, 1870.

54. *Christian Recorder*, August 6, 1870.

55. Revels was listed in the Nashville City Directory in 1874 as a physician and is believed to have established a drugstore, Revels and Arry, by 1870, as noted in the *Daily Arkansas Gazette*, February 19, 1870.

56. *Indianapolis News*, March 20, 1876.

57. *Christian Recorder*, April 19, 1877.

58. *Christian Recorder*, June 21, 1877.

59. *Christian Recorder*, August 29, 1878.

60. *Christian Recorder,* September 19, 1878.

61. *Christian Recorder,* November 7, 1878.

9. Physician, Politician, Postmaster

1. In existing records and newspaper articles, Boseman is sometimes spelled Bosemon, and Antonius appears as Antonio and Antony. Antonius is the middle name that appears in Boseman's own handwriting on his medical school dissertation.

2. *Weekly Anglo-African,* April 28, 1860.

3. New York, Passenger and Immigration Lists, 1820–1850 (database online), Provo, UT, USA: Ancestry.com Operations Inc, 2003; Registers of Vessels Arriving at the Port of New York from Foreign Ports, 1789–1919, microfilm publication M237, rolls 1–95, RG 36, NARA.

4. *Catalogue of the Officers and Students of N.Y. Central College.*

5. *Catalogue of the Officers and Students of N.Y. Central College.*

6. *Catalogue of the Officers and Students of Bowdoin College,* 1864.

7. Boseman, "Importance of Medical Statistics."

8. Benjamin A. Boseman to Joseph K. Barnes, July 1, 1864, Records Relating to Medical Officers and Physicians, Benjamin A. Boseman, entry 561, Records of the Adjutant General's Office, RG 94, NARA.

9. Hine, "Dr. Benjamin A. Boseman, Jr."

10. John Griswold to General B. F. Butler, July 19, 1864, Records Relating to Medical Officers and Physicians, RG 94, NARA.

11. Recommendation from William Seymour, July 1, 1864, Records Relating to Medical Officers and Physicians, RG 94, NARA.

12. Recommendation from Charles E. Simmons, July 1, 1864, Records Relating to Medical Officers and Physicians, RG 94, NARA.

13. Benjamin A. Boseman to John A. Griswold, March 13, 1865, Records Relating to Medical Officers and Physicians, RG 94, NARA.

14. *South Carolina Leader,* November 25 and December 9, 1865.

15. *Troy Times* cited in *Cincinnati Daily Gazette,* February 8, 1866.

16. *Christian Recorder,* September 29, 1866.

17. *Charleston Daily News,* October 8, 1872.

18. 1870 U.S. Federal Census, microfilm publication M593, and 1880 U.S. Federal Census, microfilm publication T9, Records of the Bureau of the Census, RG 29, NARA; U.S. Registers of Signatures of Depositors in Branches of the Freedman's Savings and Trust Company, 1865–1874, microfilm publication M816, RG 101, NARA.

19. *Proceedings of the Colored People's Convention of the State of South Carolina,* 5.

20. Hine, "Dr. Benjamin A. Boseman, Jr."
21. *New Hampshire Patriot*, June 10, 1868. "Sambo" is a derogatory term used for people of color. "Cuffee" refers to an early name commonly used by enslaved men.
22. *Yorkville Enquirer*, March 3, 1881.
23. *Charleston Daily News*, October 8, 1872.
24. *Tri-Weekly Mercury*, Charleston, August 27, 1868.
25. *Charleston Daily News*, August 14, 1868.
26. Greg Timmons, "Robert Smalls Biography," Biography, accessed April 7, 2020, https://www.biography.com/political-figure/robert-smalls.
27. Last Will and Testament, Benjamin A. Boseman, case #268-24, March 12, 1881, Charleston County Probate Court, Charleston, S.C.
28. Department of Commerce and Labor, Bureau of the Census, *Official Register of the United States, Containing a List of the Officers and Employees in the Civil, Military, and Naval Service.*
29. Powers, "Community Evolution and Race Relations," quoted in Sicha, "Three Moments in White and Black History."
30. *Charleston Daily News*, March 19, 1873.
31. *Yorkville Enquirer*, March 3, 1881.
32. *Greenville (S.C.) Daily News*, February 25, 1881.

10. A Family Affair

1. Winch, *Gentleman of Color*, 4.
2. Winch, 257.
3. Bacon, *But One Race*, 8.
4. Winch, *Gentleman of Color*, 261.
5. *New York Times*, April 16, 1898.
6. Quoted in Bacon, *But One Race*, 195.
7. International Council on Women, *Report of the International Council of Women*, 343.
8. Bacon, *But One Race*, 99.
9. Bacon, 102.
10. Bacon, 131.
11. Bacon, 103.
12. Garrett and Robbins, *Works of William Wells Brown*, 159.
13. Quoted in Bacon, *But One Race*, 108.
14. *Liberator*, December 16, 1853; Bacon, *But One Race*, 109–10.
15. Waite, "Segregation of Black Students at Oberlin College."
16. *Annual Catalogue of the Officers and Students of Oberlin College 1862–63.*

17. Fletcher, *History of Oberlin College*, 526.
18. *Catalogue of the Officers and Students of Western Reserve College.*
19. *Catalogue of the Officers and Students of Western Reserve College.*
20. Purvis, "Variola."
21. Charlotte Forten Grimké was the niece of Harriet Forten Purvis and the first cousin of Charles B. Purvis. Educated as a teacher, she became the first African American teacher in the schools of Salem, Massachusetts. Like Purvis, she wanted to participate in the fight for freedom during the Civil War and traveled to South Carolina, where she taught freedmen and served for a short time as a nurse to wounded Black soldiers of the 54th Massachusetts Volunteer Infantry Regiment after the battle at Fort Wagner in 1863.
22. "Forten Family," 79.
23. Bacon, *But One Race*, 180.
24. *Washington Bee*, December 29, 1883.
25. Winston, "Charles Purvis," 507–8; Garraty and Carnes, *American National Biography*, 947–48.
26. *Daily Critic* (Washington, D.C.), April 30, 1877.
27. *Critic Record* (Washington, D.C), February 12, 1890.
28. *Washington Bee*, April 7, 1883.
29. "The Freedman's Hospital," *Washington Bee*, June 26, 1886.
30. Karen Morris, "The Founding of the National Medical Association," 2007, 360, 21, Yale Medicine Thesis Digital Library, http://elischolar.library.yale.edu/ymtdl/360.
31. Byrd and Clayton, *American Health Dilemma*, 392.
32. *National Anti-Slavery Standard*, July 3, 1869; see chapter 2 for more on the Medical Society of the District of Columbia dispute.
33. *Philadelphia Inquirer* and *New York Herald*, September 30, 1874.
34. "In the Matter of the Payment and Claims and Allowances," 392.
35. Charles B. Purvis, pension file #1337283, Records of the Veterans' Administration, RG 15, NARA.
36. Purvis to Grimké, August 7, 1909, in Woodson, *Works of Francis J. Grimké*, 120.
37. Purvis to Grimké, August 17 and October 19, 1919, in Woodson, 253.
38. Purvis to Grimké, June 14, 1922, in Woodson, 350.
39. Purvis to Grimké, January 19, 1922, in Woodson, 341.

11. The Black Ivy League

1. Litwack, *North of Slavery*, 139.
2. Lee, "Talk on the Occasion of the 150th Celebration." The Calliopean Society was a literary group founded at Yale College in 1819.

3. Daniels, "African-Americans at the Yale University School of Medicine," 25–42.

4. See chapter 7.

5. *Connecticut Common School Journal* 2, no. 13 (June 1840): 231–32.

6. Cortlandt Van Rensselaer Creed, "Frederick Douglass, Esq., Dear Sir," *Frederick Douglass' Paper*, August 24, 1855.

7. Creed, "Frederick Douglass, Esq., Dear Sir."

8. *Catalogue of the Officers and Students in Yale College, 1857–58.*

9. *New York Times*, January 21, 1857.

10. *Friends' Review: A Religious, Literary and Miscellaneous Journal* 17, no. 51 (1874): 166.

11. See chapter 7.

12. Creed, "Frederick Douglass, Esq., Dear Sir."

13. "Descendants of Prince Duplex," Tompkins County NYGenWeb, accessed March 5, 2020, http://tompkins.nygenweb.net/Genie/duplex/duplex_register/d3.htm#i3.

14. *Weekly Anglo-African*, November 12, 1859.

15. "The Anniversary of the Most Worshipful Prince Hall Grand Lodge," *Weekly Anglo-African*, July 7, 1860.

16. *New Haven Daily Morning Journal and Courier*, January 25, 1892.

17. Daniels, "African-Americans at the Yale University School of Medicine," 25–42; Cortlandt Van Rensselaer Creed to William A. Buckingham, December 1, 1863, Governor's Correspondence, 1811–1933, Incoming Letters, Gov. Wm. A. Buckingham, December 1863–February 1864, RG 5, Connecticut State Library, Hartford.

18. Consolidated Lists of Civil War Draft Registration, Consolidated Enrollment Lists, 1863–1865, Records of the Provost Marshal General's Bureau, RG 110, NARA.

19. Creed to Buckingham, December 1, 1863, Governor's Correspondence. The Corps d'Afrique consisted of all-Black regiments that were formed prior to the establishment of the USCT. The 1st Louisiana Native Guard organized in New Orleans was the first established in 1862.

20. P. A. Jewett to William A. Buckingham, December 7, 1863, Governor's Correspondence.

21. Creed to William A. Buckingham, December 18, 1863, Governor's Correspondence.

22. *Hartford Courant*, February 4, 1864; Morris, *Connecticut War Record*, , 218.

23. Morris, *Connecticut War Record*, 218.

24. *The Tennessean* (Nashville), August 19, 1881.

25. *New York Times*, August 26, 1881.

26. "The Colored Soldiers," *New Haven Daily Morning Journal and Courier*, May 26, 1880.

27. The GAR was a fraternal organization for veterans of the American Civil War that provided a place where they could share a common experience and keep connected to their fellow servicemen. The group advocated on behalf of these veterans and provided benefits to their membership.

28. Daniels, "African-Americans at the Yale University School of Medicine," 41; "New Haven Conn. News," *Washington Bee*, April 4, 1891.

29. *The Freeman* (Indianapolis), March 1, 1890; *New York Age*, August 31, 1890.

30. 1900 U.S. Federal Census, T623, Records of the Bureau of the Census, RG 29, NARA.

31. 1900 U.S. Federal Census.

32. "Death of Cassius M. Creed," *New Haven Register*, January 10, 1890; "The Death of Miss Creed Investigated," *New Haven Register*, December 23, 1892.

33. "An Autopsy of Addie Creed," *Brooklyn Daily Eagle*, December 21, 1892.

34. São Paulo da Assunção de Loanda is currently known as Luanda and is the capital city of Angola, formerly Portuguese West Africa.

35. "Addie Creed's Sad Death," *Brooklyn Daily Eagle*, December 4, 1892.

36. "Addie Creed's Sad Death."

37. "Dr. Barton's Statement," *Brooklyn Daily Eagle*, December 5, 1892.

38. "How Addie Creed Died," *Brooklyn Daily Eagle*, December 28, 1892.

39. "Addie Creed's Death," *Brooklyn Daily Eagle*, December 6, 1892.

40. "Addie Creed's Death."

41. "How Addie Creed Died."

42. "How Addie Creed Died."

43. "College to Almshouse," *New Haven Register*, March 2, 1897.

44. "Sad Case of Dr. Creed," *New Haven Register*, March 3, 1897.

45. "Bottle of Soda Exploded," *New Haven Daily Morning Journal and Courier*, October 21, 1899.

46. "Died on Chapel Street," *New Haven Daily Morning Journal and Courier*, November 25, 1896.

47. Teresa Vega, "Our Abolitionist Ancestors: Newark Born and Bred," Radiant Roots, Boricua Branches, accessed February 7, 2020, http://radiantrootsboricua branches.com/category/african-americans-in-newark-nj/.

48. Biography, William B. Ellis, Records Relating to Medical Officers and Physicians, William B. Ellis, entry 561, Records of the Adjutant General's Office, 1780s–1917, RG 94, NARA.

49. "Grimes Homestead," nps.gov, accessed March 5, 2020, https://www.nps .gov/nr/travel/underground/nj1.htm.

50. Biography, William B. Ellis, Records Relating to Medical Officers and Physicians, RG 94, NARA.

51. "Peter W. Ray, M.D., New York City," Black Gotham Archive, accessed December 14, 2017, http://archive.blackgothamarchive.org/items/show/21.

52. *Catalogue of the Officers and Students of Dartmouth College*, 10.

53. William Baldwin Ellis, "General Diseases (in the Male) Gonorrhea and Syphilis," DA-3 (42), box 2185, vol. 17, Medical Theses, 1854–58, Rauner Special Collections Library, Dartmouth College, Hanover, N.H.

54. "A Debate," *Weekly Anglo-African*, January 21, 1860.

55. "Free Suffrage! Free Men!," *Weekly Anglo-African,* May 6, 1860.

56. *McElroy's Philadelphia City Directory for 1862*, 189.

57. William B. Ellis, MD, to Edward C. Mauran, August 13, 1862, Civil War Executive Department–Military, Communication and Correspondence Received, 1860–1866, Rhode Island Digital Archives, accessed February 12, 2020, https://sosri.access.preservica.com/?s=william+b+ellis.

58. William B. Ellis to Major Stearns, July 3, 1863, Records Relating to Medical Officers and Physicians, RG 94, NARA.

59. Recommendation from D. Crosby, April 10, 1863, Records Relating to Medical Officers and Physicians, RG 94, NARA.

60. Recommendation from E. R. Pearle, April 18, 1863, Records Relating to Medical Officers and Physicians, RG 94, NARA.

61. Cheasy Samuel to Edwin M. Stanton, July 6, 1863, Records Relating to Medical Officers and Physicians, RG 94, NARA.

62. Certificate to Be Signed by Candidates for Appointment into the Medical Staff, United States Army, before Examination, July 20, 1863, Records Relating to Medical Officers and Physicians, RG 94, NARA.

63. Answers to Questions on Practice of Medicine, Anatomy, Literature and Science, Hygiene and Surgery, July 21 through July 23, 1863, Records Relating to Medical Officers and Physicians, RG 94, NARA.

64. William B. Ellis to William A. Hammond, July 28, 1863, Records Relating to Medical Officers and Physicians, RG 94, NARA.

65. Contract with a Private Physician, November 26, 1864, Oath of Office, November 28, 1864, Records Relating to Medical Officers and Physicians, RG 94, NARA.

66. Redington and Hodgkins, *Military Record of the Sons of Dartmouth*, 65.

67. Sterling, *We Are Your Sisters*, 254; Mabee with Newhouse, *Sojourner Truth*, 133.

68. Mabee with Newhouse, *Sojourner Truth*, 133; *Daily National Republican*, September 22, 1865.

69. "Deferred Locals, Infanticide," *Evening Star*, December 26, 1865.

70. Masur, *Example for All the Land*, 87–88.

71. P. Glennan to Sojourner Truth, March 25, 1867, Post Family Papers Project, River Campus Libraries, Rare Books and Special Collections, University of Rochester, accessed February 11, 2020, https://rbscpexhibits.lib.rochester .edu/items/show/3909.

72. Butler and Brinton, *Medical and Surgical Reporter*, 60.

12. The Iowa Connection

1. Cooper, "Stony Road."

2. Alice Hoyt Veen, "Iowa's African American Heritage," Prairie Roots Research, accessed March 6, 2020, https://www.prairierootsresearch.com /iowas-african-american-heritage/.

3. *Circular and Announcement of the Seventeenth Session of the Medical Department of the Iowa State University*, 42–46, National Library of Medicine, Bethesda, Md.

4. *Circular and Announcement of the Seventeenth Session*, 45–46.

5. Rapier Jr. to Sarah Thomas, November 12, 1863, MS 62–4283, Rapier Family Papers, Moorland-Spingarn Research Center, Howard University, Washington, D.C.

6. "A Colored Man Expelled from the Medical Department of the State University," *Detroit Advertiser and Tribune*, November 5, 1863; Schopieray, "Col[ore]d Men Are Not Admitted Here."

7. William Byrns to his wife, October 21, 1863, Duane Norman Diedrich Collection, M-4632.2, William L. Clements Library, University of Michigan.

8. William Byrns to his wife, November 1, 1863, Duane Norman Diedrich Collection.

9. Rapier Jr. to Sarah Thomas, November 12, 1863, Rapier Family Papers.

10. *Detroit Advertiser and Tribune*, November 5, 1863

11. Rapier Jr. to Sarah Thomas, November 12, 1863, Rapier Family Papers.

12. "Sketch of Autobiography," Records Relating to Medical Officers and Physicians, J. D. Harris, entry 561, Records of the Adjutant General's Office, 1780s–1917, RG 94, NARA.

13. Ship's passenger list, SS *Plantagenet*, May 14, 1863, Passenger Lists of Vessels Arriving at New York, New York, 1820–1897, microfilm publication M237, roll 228, line 21, list number 409, Records of the United States Customs Service, 1745–1997, RG 36, NARA.

14. Mull, *Underground Railroad in Michigan*, 90. Martin R. Delaney was an abolitionist, physician, and soldier who served during the Civil War. Although he did not have a surgeon's position, he was one of the few Black field officers serving with the USCT.

15. 1850 U.S. Federal Census, microfilm publication M432, Records of the Bureau of the Census, RG 29, NARA.

16. *Annual Catalogue of the Officers and Students of Oberlin College, 1862–63*, 37, 40, 47.

17. *Annual Catalogue of the Officers and Students of Oberlin College, 1862–63*, 41–45. The student population in the 1862–63 academic year comprised 402 women and 457 men.

18. "Four Children at a Birth," *Alton (Ill.) Telegraph*, July 25, 1873.

19. "Meeting of Fifth Ward Republicans," *National Republican*, June 26, 1868.

20. "Fifth Ward," *Evening Star*, June 2, 1869.

21. Cobb, *First Negro Medical Society*, 19.

22. "The Doctors and the Question of Color in Washington," *Baltimore Sun*, February 8, 1870.

23. See chapters 2 and 10 for more information on the Medical Society of the District of Columbia dispute.

24. *Boyd's Directory of the District of Columbia*, 104, 212, 634. The Colonization Building was owned by the American Colonization Society and served as its headquarters, where they held regular meetings and conducted business.

25. *Evening Star*, October 28, 1876.

26. Non-population Census Schedules for Michigan, 1850-1880, Mortality Schedule, Archive Collection: T1164, Archive Roll Number: 77, 1880, NARA.

27. Bishir, *Crafting Lives*, 73.

28. 1850 U.S. Federal Census, NARA.

29. 1856 Iowa State Census, microfilm of Iowa State Censuses, 1856, as well as various special censuses from 1836–97, State Historical Society of Iowa, Des Moines.

30. "John Mercer Langston," History, Art and Archives, accessed February 21, 2020, https://history.house.gov/People/Detail/16682. John Mercer Langston was an abolitionist, attorney, politician, and educator who helped establish the law school at Howard University in Washington, D.C.

31. Harris, *Summer on the Borders of the Caribbean Sea*, 30.

32. "Letters to Anti-Slavery Workers and Agencies [Part 5]," 768.

33. "Free Colored Colonization," *Cleveland Morning Leader*, May 2, 1860.

34. *Cleveland Daily Leader*, May 2, 1860.

35. "Colored Clevelander in St. Domingo," *Cleveland Daily Leader*, July 4, 1860.
36. "J. D. Harris on the Migration of the Colored Race," *Evening Post*, October 9, 1860.
37. Harris, *Summer on the Borders of the Caribbean Sea*, 14–15.
38. Harris, 19.
39. *Cleveland Daily Leader*, July 4, 1860.
40. "Emigration to Hayti," *New York Herald*, December 17, 1860.
41. McKivigan, *Forgotten Firebrand*, 79.
42. "The Emancipation Jubilee Last Night," *Evening Star*, April 17, 1863.
43. *Cleveland Medical Gazette* 9, no. 4 (February 1894): 180. The Marine Hospital was established in 1852 to provide medical care to sailors serving in the Coast Guard, Merchant Marines, and U.S. veterans.
44. Swint, *Dear Ones at Home*, 122–23.
45. "Letter from Virginia," *Christian Recorder*, July 9, 1864.
46. J. D. Harris to Edwin M. Stanton, February 18, 1865, Records Relating to Medical Officers and Physicians, RG 94, NARA.
47. George Suckley to W. A. Conover, March 25, 1865, Records Relating to Medical Officers and Physicians, RG 94, NARA.
48. Report on Hospitals in Richmond, Norfolk, etc. [1865], frame 155, reel 3, USSC microfilm papers, National Library of Medicine, Bethesda, Md.
49. "The Freedmen of Virginia," *Baltimore Sun*, March 29, 1867.
50. "The Negro Wells Candidate Claims Social Equality," *Daily Dispatch* (Richmond), June 21, 1869.
51. "Petersburg Convention," *Richmond Whig and Advertiser*, March 12, 1869; Humphreys, "Finding Dr. Harris."
52. "Dr. J. D. Harris," *Staunton (Va.) Spectator*, March 23, 1869.
53. "Official Returns of the Virginia Election," *National Republican*, August 23, 1869.
54. "Notice to County Commissioners," *Daily Phoenix* (Columbia, S.C.), August 30, 1870, and November 30, 1870.
55. Congressional Series of United States Public Documents, vol. 1590; Lamb, *Howard University Medical Department*, 76.
56. "De Lunatico Inquirendo," *Evening Star*, September 6, 1877.
57. Certificate of Death, no. 44993, box 56, District of Columbia Archives, Washington, D.C.
58. Ship's passenger list, SS *Plantagenet*, May 14, 1863NARA.
59. Typed notes, August 22, 1912, War Department, Records Relating to Medical Officers and Physicians, Records of the Adjutant General's Office, 1780s–1917, RG 94, NARA.

60. Charles H. Taylor to Joseph K. Barnes, June 22, 1865, Records Relating to Medical Officers and Physicians, RG 94, NARA.

61. Contract with a Private Physician, August 19, 1865, Records Relating to Medical Officers and Physicians, RG 94, NARA.

62. Alexander T. Augusta to J. W. Lawton, May 18, 1866, Records of the Field Offices for the State of Georgia, M1903, roll 85, Records of the Bureau of Refugees, Freedmen, and Abandoned Lands, 1865–1872, RG 105, NARA.

63. Cimbala, *Under the Guardianship of the Nation*, 101.

64. Charles H. Taylor to Joseph K. Barnes, December 31, 1868, Records Relating to Medical Officers and Physicians, Charles H. Taylor, entry 561, RG 94, NARA.

65. Savannah, Georgia, Voter Records, 1856–1896, Research Library and Municipal Archives, City of Savannah.

66. Laura D. Taylor, widow's pension application, file #548694, 1892, Records of the Veterans' Administration, RG 15, NARA.

67. Theodore "Jack" Iwashyna, MD, PhD, email to the author, February 17, 2020.

Bibliography

Archival and Manuscript Sources

Abbott, Anderson Ruffin. Papers. Special Collections and Rare Books, S90, S257. Toronto Public Library.

AMA Collection (7816/26911). Amistad Research Center, Dillard University, New Orleans, La.

Boseman, Benjamin A. Last Will and Testament. Case #268-24. March 12, 1881. Charleston County Probate Court, Charleston, S.C.

DeGrasse-Howard Papers. Massachusetts Historical Society, Boston.

Diedrich, Duane Norman. Collection. William L. Clements Library, University of Michigan, Ann Arbor.

District of Columbia Archives, Washington, D.C.

George J. Mitchell Department of Special Collections and Archives, Bowdoin College Library, Brunswick, Maine.

Governor's Correspondence, 1811–1933, Incoming Letters, Gov. Wm. A. Buckingham, December 1863–February 1864, Record Group 5. Connecticut State Library, Hartford.

Green, Richard Henry. Papers. MS 2005. Manuscripts and Archives, Yale University Library, New Haven, Conn.

Library of Congress, Washington, D.C.

    Douglass, Frederick. Papers.

    Revels, Hiram. "Autobiography." Carter Godwin Woodson Papers.

Liverpool Royal Infirmary School of Medicine Minutes, 1845–1859. Special Collections and Archives, Sydney Jones Library, University of Liverpool, Eng.

National Archives and Records Administration, Washington, D.C.

National Library of Medicine, Bethesda, Md.

    Abbott, Anderson Ruffin. Papers, ACC 2010-011.

    Circular and Announcement of the Seventeenth Session of the Medical Department of the Iowa State University Located at the City of Keokuk, Session of 1864–5.

    Report on Hospitals in Richmond, Norfolk, etc. *USSC microfilm papers.*

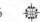

Purvis, Charles. "Variola." Cleveland medical thesis, 1864–1866, vol. 28. Holograph. Thesis—Cleveland Medical College, 1865. Dittrick Medical History Center, Rare Books, Case Western Reserve University, Cleveland, Ohio.

Rapier Family Papers, MS 62–4283. Moorland-Spingarn Research Center, Howard University, Washington, D.C.

Rauner Special Collections Library, Dartmouth College, Hanover, N.H.

Savannah, Georgia, Voter Records, 1856–1896. Research Library and Municipal Archives, City of Savannah.

State Historical Society of Iowa, Des Moines.

Sumner, Charles. *Report Made in the Senate of the United States to Accompany Bill S. 511, 41st Congress, 2d Session, Report No. 29.* Pamphlets by Charles Sumner IV. Library of Harvard University, Cambridge, Mass.

Newspapers and Other Periodicals

Afro-American
Alton (Ill.) *Telegraph*
Anglo-African
Anglo American
Anti-Slavery Bugle
Baltimore Sun
Boston Herald
Boston Traveler
Brooklyn Daily Eagle
Burlington Free Press
Charleston Daily News
Christian Recorder
Cincinnati Daily Gazette
Clarion-Ledger (Jackson, Miss.)
Cleveland Daily Leader
Cleveland Leader
Cleveland Medical Gazette
Cleveland Morning Leader
Connecticut Common School Journal
Critic Record (Washington, D.C.)
Daily Arkansas Gazette
Daily Critic (Washington, D.C.)
Daily Dispatch (Richmond)
Daily National Republican (Washington, D.C.)

Daily Phoenix (Columbia, S.C.)

Detroit Advertiser and Tribune

Evening Post (New York)

Evening Star (Washington, D.C.)

Frederick Douglass' Paper

The Freeman (Indianapolis)

Friends' Review: A Religious, Literary and Miscellaneous Journal

The Globe

Greenville (S.C.) *Daily News*

Harper's Weekly

Hartford Courant

Indianapolis Daily Journal

Indianapolis News

Indiana State Sentinel

Inter Ocean (Chicago)

Janesville (Wis.) *Daily Gazette*

Lancet

Liberator

National Anti-Slavery Standard

National Republican

Newark Daily Advertiser

New Bedford (Mass.) *Republican Standard*

New Hampshire Patriot

New Haven Daily Morning Journal and Courier

New Haven Register

New York Age

New York Herald

New York Times

New York Tribune

North Star

Philadelphia Inquirer

Provincial Freeman (Toronto)

Railway News

Richmond Whig and Advertiser

Sailor's Magazine and Naval Journal

Salem Observer

Salem Register

South Carolina Leader

Staunton (Va.) *Spectator*

The Tennessean (Nashville)
Tri-Weekly Mercury (Charleston, S.C.)
True Royalist and Weekly Intelligencer (Windsor, ON)
Washington Bee
Washington Post
Weekly Anglo-African
Weekly Louisianian
Yorkville Enquirer

College Catalogs

Annual Catalogue of the Officers and Students of Oberlin College for the College Year 1857–58. Oberlin: James M. Fitch, 1857.

Annual Catalogue of the Officers and Students of Oberlin College for the College Year 1862–63. Oberlin: V. A. Shankland, 1863.

Catalogue of the Officers and Students in Yale College, 1853–54. New Haven: B. L. Hamlen, 1853.

Catalogue of the Officers and Students in Yale College, 1857–58. New Haven: B. Hayes, 1857.

Catalogue of the Officers and Students of Bowdoin College and the Medical School of Maine. Brunswick: Press of Joseph Griffin, 1847.

Catalogue of the Officers and Students of Bowdoin College and the Medical School of Maine, Spring Term–1864. Brunswick: J. Griffin, 1864.

Catalogue of the Officers and Students of Dartmouth College, September 1840. Concord: Asa McFarland, 1840.

Catalogue of the Officers and Students of N.Y. Central College, for the Collegiate Year, 1844-45, McGrawville, Cort. Co., N.Y. for the Collegiate Year, 1854–55. Homer, N.Y.: Dixon and Case, 1855.

A Catalogue of the Officers and Students of Western Reserve College for the Academic Year 1862–62. Cleveland: Fairbanks, Benedict and Co., 1863.

Catalogue of the Society of Brothers in Unity, Yale College, founded 1768. New Haven: Hitchcock and Stafford, Printers, 1841.

Catalogue of Wilberforce University for 1867–68. Baltimore: Daugherty, Maguire and Co., 1867.

Books, Articles, Dissertations, and Theses

Abbott, Anderson R. "Some Recollections of Lincoln's Assassination." *Anglo-American Magazine* 5 (May 1901): 397–402.

Abram, Ruth. *"Send Us a Lady Physician": Women Doctors in America, 1835–1920*. New York: W. W. Norton, 1985.

Alexander, Philip. "John H. Rapier, Jr. and the Medical Profession in Jamaica, 1860–1862. Part One." *Jamaica Journal* 24, no. 3 (February 1993): 37–46.

The American Educational Annual: A Cyclopedia. Vol. 1, 1875. New York: J. W. Schermerhorn, 1875.

American Medical Times, Being a Weekly Series of the New York Journal of Medicine. Vol. 8, *January to June, 1864.* New York: Bailliere Brothers, 1864.

Anderson, George B. *Landmarks of Rensselaer County, New York.* Syracuse: D. Mason, 1897.

Andrews, Charles C. *The History of the New-York African Free-Schools, from Their Establishment in 1787 to the Present Time.* New York: Mahlon Day, 1830.

Annual Announcement of the Toronto School of Medicine, Session 1862–63. Toronto: "Globe" Steam Job Press, 1862.

The Annual Reports of the American Colonization Society for Colonizing the Free People of Colour of the United States. Vols. 33–46. New York: Negro University-sities Press, 1969.

Bacon, Margaret Hope. *But One Race: The Life of Robert Purvis.* Albany: State University of New York Press, 2007.

Berlin, Ira, Joseph P. Reidy, and Leslie S. Rowland. *Freedom: A Documentary History of Emancipation, 1861–67.* Series II, vol. 1, *The Black Military Experience.* New York: Cambridge University Press, 1982.

Bishir, Catherine W. *Crafting Lives: African American Artisans in New Bern, North Carolina, 1770–1900.* Chapel Hill: University of North Carolina Press, 2013.

Blanchard, Janice, Shakti Nayar, and Nicole Lurie. "Patient-Provider and Patient-Staff Racial Concordance and Perceptions of Mistreatment in the Health Care Setting." *Journal of General Internal Medicine* 22, no. 8 (August 2007): 1184–89.

Blight, David W. *Beyond the Battlefield.* Boston: University of Massachusetts Press, 2002.

Bogger, Tommy L. *Free Blacks in Norfolk Virginia, 1790–1860: The Darker Side of Freedom.* Charlottesville: University Press of Virginia, 1997.

Bonner, Thomas Neville. *Becoming a Physician: Medical Education in Britain, France, Germany, and the United States, 1750–1945.* New York: Oxford University Press, 1995.

Boseman, Benjamin A. "The Importance of Medical Statistics." Unpublished thesis, Maine Medical College, Bowdoin College, 1864.

Boyd's Directory of the District of Columbia. Washington, D.C.: Wm. H. Boyd, 1877.

Bristol, Douglas Walter, Jr. *Knights of the Razor: Black Barbers in Slavery and Reconstruction.* Baltimore: Johns Hopkins University Press, 2009.

Bucchianeri, E. A. *Brushstrokes of a Gadfly*. Portugal: Batalha Publishers, 2011.

Butler, S. W., MD, and D. G. Brinton, MD, eds. *The Medical and Surgical Reporter: A Weekly Journal*. Vol. 16, no. 3, no. 516, January 1867–June 1867. Philadelphia: Alfred Marten, 1867.

Byrd, W. Michael, and Linda A. Clayton. *An American Health Dilemma: A Medical History of African Americans and the Problem of Race, Beginnings to 1900*. New York: Routledge, 2000.

Caverhill's Toronto City Directory, 1861–62. Toronto: W. C. F. Caverhill, 1860.

Cimbala, Paul A. *Under the Guardianship of the Nation: The Freedmen's Bureau and the Reconstruction of Georgia, 1865–1870*. Athens: University of Georgia Press, 2003.

Circular of the Medical Faculty of Trinity College, Toronto. Toronto: H. Rowsell, 1854.

Cobb, W. Montague. *The First Negro Medical Society: A History of the Medico-Chirurgical Society of the District of Columbia, 1884–1939*. Washington, D.C.: The Associated Publishers, 1939.

The Committee for the Study of the Future of Public Health, Division of Health Care Services, Institute of Medicine. *The Future of Public Health*. Washington, D.C.: National Academy Press, 1968.

Congressional Series of United States Public Documents. Vol. 1590. *Reports of the Committees of the Senate of the United States for First Session of the Forty Third Congress, 1873–74 in Four Volumes*. Washington, D.C.: Government Printing Office, 1874.

Cooper, Arnie. "A Stony Road." *Annals of Iowa* 48, no. 3 (Winter 1986): 113–34.

Cowden, Colonel Robert. *A Brief Sketch of the Organization and Services of the Fifty-Ninth Regiment of the United States Colored Infantry and Biographical Sketches*. Dayton: United Brethren Publishing House, 1883.

Crow, Jeffrey J., Paul D. Scott, and Flora Hatley Wadelington. *A History of African Americans in North Carolina*. Raleigh: North Carolina Office of Archives and History, 2011.

Daniels, Daryl Keith. "African-Americans at the Yale University School of Medicine, 1810–1960." PhD diss., Yale University School of Medicine, 1991.

Davis, Matthew L. *Memoirs of Aaron Burr with Miscellaneous Selections from His Correspondence, Volume II*. New York: Harper and Brothers, 1837.

Department of Commerce and Labor, Bureau of the Census. *Official Register of the United States, Containing a List of the Officers and Employees in the Civil, Military, and Naval Service*. Digitized books, 77 vols. Oregon State Library, Salem.

Department of the Interior, Pension Office. *Instructions to Examining Surgeons for Pensions*. Washington: U.S. Government Printing Office, 1877.

Dorman, Franklin A. *Twenty Families of Color in Massachusetts, 1742–1998.* Boston: New England Historic Genealogical Society, 1998.

Douglass, Frederick. *Narrative of the Life of Frederick Douglass, an American Slave.* New York: Modern Library, 2000.

Downs, Jim. *Sick from Freedom: African American Illness and Suffering during the Civil War and Reconstruction.* New York: Oxford University Press, 2012.

1836 Free African Americans for Borough of Norfolk, Virginia. Transcribed by Wm. Troy Valos. Norfolk: Norfolk Public Library, 2009.

Ferguson, Earline Rae. "In Pursuit of the Full Enjoyment of Liberty and Happiness: Blacks in Antebellum Indianapolis, 1820–1860." *Black History News and Notes*, 1988, issue no. 32.

Fleischner, Jennifer. *Mrs. Lincoln and Mrs. Keckly: The Remarkable Story of the Friendship between a First Lady and a Former Slave.* New York: Broadway Books, 2003.

Fletcher, Robert Samuel. *A History of Oberlin College from its Foundation through the Civil War, Volume II.* Oberlin: Oberlin College, 1943.

Foner, Philip S. *Essays in Afro-American History.* Philadelphia: Temple University Press, 1978.

Foote, Loren. *The Gentlemen and the Roughs: Violence, Honor, and Manhood in the Union Army.* New York: New York University Press, 2010.

Forbes, David W., comp. "Kingdom of Hawaii. Report of the Board of Health to the Legislative Assembly of 1876." *Hawaiian National Bibliography, 1780–1900.* Vol. 3, *1851–1880.* Honolulu: University of Hawaii Press, 2001.

Forstchen, William R. "The 28th United States Colored Troops: Indiana's African Americans Go to War, 1863–1865." PhD diss., Purdue University, 1994.

"The Forten Family." *Negro History Bulletin*, 10, no 4. (January 1947): 75–79.

Franklin, John Hope, and Loren Schweninger. *In Search of the Promised Land: A Black Family and the Old South.* New York: Oxford University Press, 2006.

Gardner, Eric. *Unexpected Places: Relocating Nineteenth-Century African American Literature.* Jackson: University of Mississippi Press, 2010.

Garraty, John A., and Mark C. Carnes, eds. *American National Biography*, vol. 17. New York: Oxford University Press, 1999.

Garrett, Paula, and Hollis Robbins, eds. *The Works of William Wells Brown.* Oxford: Oxford University Press, 2006.

General Instructions to Special Examiners of the United States Pension Office. Washington, D.C.: Government Printing Office, 1881.

Gibson, Campbell. "Population of the 100 Largest Cities and Other Urban Places in the United States: 1790–1990." Population Division Working Paper No. 27, U.S. Bureau of the Census, Washington, D.C., 1998.

Glatthaar, Joseph T. *Forged in Battle: The Civil War Alliance of Black Soldiers and White Officers*. Baton Rouge: Louisiana State University Press, 1990.

Granger, Susan, and Scott Kelly. "Little Falls' Historic Contexts: Final Report of an Historic Preservation and Planning Project." Prepared for the Little Falls Heritage Preservation Commission and the City of Little Falls, July 1994.

Hancock, Cornelia. *Letters of a Civil War Nurse. Cornelia Hancock, 1863–1865*. Edited by Henrietta Stratton Jaquette. Lincoln: University of Nebraska Press, 1998.

Harris, J. Dennis. *Love and Law, South and West: A Poem*. Chicago: Charles Scott, 1854.

———. *A Summer on the Borders of the Caribbean Sea*. New York: A. B. Burdick, 1860.

Henderson, John. *The Free Negro in Virginia, 1619–1865*. Baltimore: Johns Hopkins Press, 1913.

Hepburn, Sharon A. Roger. *Crossing the Border: A Free Black Community in Canada*. Chicago: University of Illinois Press, 2007.

Hine, William C. "Black Politicians in Reconstruction Charleston, South Carolina: A Collective Study." *Journal of Southern History* 49, no. 4 (November 1983): 555–84.

———. "Dr. Benjamin A. Boseman, Jr.: Charleston's Black Physician-Politician." In *Southern Black Leaders of the Reconstruction Era*, edited by Howard N. Rabinowitz, 335–63. Chicago: University of Illinois Press, 1982.

Howe, S. G. *The Refugees from Slavery in Canada West: Report to the Freedmen's Inquiry Commission*. Boston: Wright and Potter, 1864.

Humphreys, Margaret. "Finding Dr. Harris." Unpublished paper, 2014.

———. *Intensely Human: The Health of the Black Soldier in the American Civil War*. Baltimore: Johns Hopkins University Press, 2006.

International Council on Women. *Report of the International Council of Women, Assembled by the National Woman Suffrage Association*. Washington, D.C.: Rufus H. Darby, 1888.

"In the Matter of the Payment and Claims and Allowances—Garfield's Case, Claims Growing Out of the Illness and Burial of the Late President, James A. Garfield." In *Decisions of the First Comptroller in the Department of the Treasury of the United States; with an Appendix by William Lawrence, First Comptroller*. Vol. 3. Washington, D.C.: Government Printing Office, 1882.

Jay, William. *An Inquiry into the Character and Tendency of the American Colonization Society and American Anti-Slavery Societies*. New York: Leavitt, Lord and Co., 1835.

Jenkins, Wilbert L. *Climbing Up to Glory: A Short History of African Americans during the Civil War and Reconstruction.* Wilmington: Scholarly Resources, 2002.

Jorgenson, Tim. *Mrs. Keckly Sends Her Regards.* Fairfax, Va.: Xulon Press, 2007.

Keckley, Elizabeth. *Behind the Scenes: Or, Thirty Years a Slave, and Four Years in the White House.* New York: G. W. Carleton and Co., 1868.

Kennedy, Gerald. "U.S. Army Hospital: Keokuk, 1862–1865." *Annals of Iowa* 40, no. 2 (Fall 1969): 118–36.

Keokuk Medical College, Tenth Annual Announcement, College of Physicians and Surgeons, Fifty-Ninth Session, 1899–1900. College of Physicians and Surgeons. Keokuk, Iowa: n.p., 1900.

Lamb, Daniel Smith. *Howard University Medical Department: A Historical, Biographical and Statistical Souvenir.* Washington, D.C.: R. Beresford, 1900.

Leavitt, Judith Walzer, and Ronald L. Numbers, eds. *Sickness and Health in America: Readings in the History of Medicine and Public Health.* Madison: University of Wisconsin Press, 1997.

Lee, Forrester A. "Talk on the Occasion of the 150th Celebration of Cortlandt Van Rensselaer Creed's Yale Graduation." Unpublished presentation script, June 2, 2007.

"Letters to Anti-Slavery Workers and Agencies [Part 5]," J. D. Harris to F. P. Blair. *Journal of Negro History* 10 (1925): 749–74, 768.

Lincoln, Abraham. *Collected Works of Abraham Lincoln.* Vol. 5. Ann Arbor: University of Michigan Digital Library Production Services, 2001. http://name.umdl.umich.edu/lincoln5.

Litwack, Leon F. *North of Slavery: The Negro in the Free States.* Chicago: University of Chicago Press, 1965.

Logue, Larry M., and Peter Blanck. "Benefit of the Doubt: African-American Civil War Veterans and Pensions." *Journal of Interdisciplinary History* 37, no. 3 (Winter 2008): 377–99.

———. *Race, Ethnicity, and Disability.* Cambridge: Cambridge University Press, 2010.

The London and Provincial Medical Directory and General Medical Register, 1859. London: John Churchill, 1859.

Long, Gretchen. *Doctoring Freedom: The Politics of African American Medical Care in Slavery and Emancipation.* Chapel Hill: University of North Carolina Press, 2012.

Mabee, Carleton, with Susan Mabee Newhouse. *Sojourner Truth: Slave, Prophet, Legend.* New York: New York University Press, 1995.

Mansel, R. E., D. J. T. Webster, and H. M. Sweetland. *Benign Disorders and Diseases of the Breast*. Switzerland: Saunders, 2009.

Marrs, Rev. Elijah P. *Life and History of the Rev. Elijah P. Marr, First Pastor of Beargrass Baptist Church and Author*. Louisville: Bradley and Gilbert Company, 1885. https://docsouth.unc.edu/neh/marrs/marrs.html.

Masur, Kate. *An Example for All the Land: Emancipation and the Struggle over Equality in Washington, D.C.* Chapel Hill: University of North Carolina Press, 2010.

Matchett's Baltimore Directory for 1847 '8. Baltimore: R. J. Matchett, 1847.

McElroy's Philadelphia City Directory for 1862. Philadelphia: E. C. and J. Biddle, 1862.

McKivigan, John R. *Forgotten Firebrand: James Redpath and the Making of Nineteenth-Century America*. Ithaca: Cornell University Press, 2008.

The Medical and Surgical History of the Civil War. Vol. 3. Wilmington, N.C.: Broadfoot, 1990.

The Medical and Surgical History of the War of the Rebellion. Vol. 11. Wilmington, N.C.: Broadfoot, 1991.

"Medical News." *British Medical Journal*, July 17, 1858.

Morris, John M., ed. *The Connecticut War Record, 1863–65*. New Haven: Peck, White and Peck, n.d.

Morse, Jedidiah, and Richard C. Morse. *New Universal Gazetteer or Geographical Dictionary*. New Haven: S. Converse, 1823.

Mull, Carol E. *The Underground Railroad in Michigan*. Jefferson, N.C.: McFarland and Company, 2015.

Newby, M. Dalyce. *Anderson Ruffin Abbott, First Afro-Canadian Doctor*. Toronto: Associated Medical Services and Fitzhenry and Whiteside, 1998.

The Nineteenth Circular and Announcement of the Medical Department of the Iowa State University Located at the City of Keokuk, Iowa, for the Session of 1865–66. Davenport: Publishing House of Luse and Griggs, 1865.

The Ontario Medical Register. The Council of the College of Physicians and Surgeons of Ontario, Revised Statutes of Ontario 1897, Chap. 178. Toronto: Registration Office College of Physicians and Surgeons of Ontario, Toronto, 1898.

Parry, Manon S. "Elizabeth Fee and Feminist Public Health." *American Journal of Public Health* 109, no. 6 (June 2019): 873–74. https://doi.org/10.2105/AJPH.2019.305089.

Payne, Daniel A. *History of the African Methodist Episcopal Church*. Nashville: AME Sunday-School Union, 1891.

Peterson, Carla L. *Black Gotham: A Family History of African Americans in Nineteenth New York City*. New Haven: Yale University Press, 2011.

Power-Greene, Ousmane K. *Against Wind and Tide: The African American Struggle against the Colonization Movement*. New York: New York University Press, 2014.

Powers, Bernard E., Jr. *Black Charlestonians: A Social History, 1822–1885*. Fayetteville: University of Arkansas Press, 1994.

———. "Community Evolution and Race Relations in Reconstruction Charleston, South Carolina." *South Carolina Historical Magazine* 95, no. 1 (January 1994): 27–46.

Proceedings of the Colored People's Convention of the State of South Carolina Held in Zion Church, November 1865. Charleston: South Carolina Leader Office, 1865.

Record of the Class of 1857 of Yale University during Fifty Years from Graduation. Hartford: Case, Lockwood and Brainard, 1907.

Redington, Major E. D., and Major W. H. Hodgkins. *Military Record of the Sons of Dartmouth in the Union Army and Navy, 1861–1865*. Boston: Dartmouth College Trustees, 1907.

Reid, Richard M. *African Canadians in Union Blue: Volunteering for the Cause in America's Civil War*. Seattle: University of Washington Press, 2014.

———. *Freedom for Themselves: North Carolina's Black Soldiers of the Civil War Era*. Chapel Hill: University of North Carolina Press, 2008.

Reidy, Joseph. "Black Men in Navy Blue during the Civil War." *Prologue* 33, no. 3 (Fall 2001): 152–53.

Report of the Adjutant General of the State of Illinois. Vol. 4, *Containing Reports for the Years 1861–66*. Springfield: H. W. Rokker, State Printer and Binder, 1886.

Report of the Trustees of the House of Industry, City of Toronto, for the Year 1856. Toronto: Henry Roswell, 1856.

Rice, Mitchell F., and Woodrow Jones Jr. *Public Policy and the Black Hospital: From Slavery to Segregation to Integration*. Westport, Conn.: Greenwood, 1994.

Ruchames, Louis. *The Letters of William Lloyd Garrison, Volume IV*. Cambridge: Belknap Press of Harvard University Press, 1975.

Russell, John Henderson. *The Free Negro in Virginia, 1619–1865*. Baltimore: Johns Hopkins Press, 1913.

The Sailor's Magazine and Naval Journal. Vol. 17. New York: American Seamen's Friend Society, 1845.

266 *Bibliography*

Sanger, George P., ed. *The Statutes at Large, Treaties and Proclamations of the United States of America from December 5, 1859 to March 3, 1863*. Boston: Little, Brown and Company, 1863.

Schiff, Judith. "The Life of Richard Henry Green." *Yale Alumni Magazine*, May/June 2014. https://yalealumnimagazine.com/articles/3875-the-life-of -richard-henry-green.

Schopieray, Cheney J. "Col[ore]d Men Are Not Admitted Here." *The Quarto*, no. 46 (Fall–Winter 2016): 6–10.

Schwartz, Gerald, ed. *A Woman Doctor's Civil War: Esther Hill Hawks' Diary*. Columbia: University of South Carolina Press, 1989.

Schweninger, Loren. "John H. Rapier, Sr.: A Slave and Freeman in the Antebellum South." *Civil War History* 20, no. 1 (March 1974): 23–24.

Schweninger, Loren, and James Thomas. *From Tennessee Slave to St. Louis Entrepreneur: The Autobiography of James Thomas*. Columbia: University of Missouri Press, 1984.

Scott, Sean A. *A Visitation of God: Northern Civilians Interpret the Civil War*. New York: Oxford University Press, 2011.

Seventeenth Annual Report of the American Seamen's Friend Society, 1945. New York: Joseph H. Jennings, 1845.

Shaffer, Donald R. *After the Glory: The Struggle of Black Civil War Veterans*. Lawrence: University of Kansas Press, 2004.

Sicha, Choire. "Three Moments in White and Black History in Charleston, South Carolina." The Awl, June 18, 2015. https://www.theawl.com/2015/06 /three-moments-in-white-and-black-history-in-charleston-south-carolina/.

Sixteenth Annual Report of the American Society for Colonizing the Free People of Colour of the United States. Georgetown, D.C.: James C. Dunn, 1833.

Slaney, Catherine. *Family Secrets: Crossing the Colour Line*. Toronto: Natural Heritage Books, 2003.

Smedley, R. C. *History of the Underground Railroad in Chester and the Neighboring Counties of Pennsylvania*, Lancaster: John A. Hiestand, 1883.

Smith, J. V. C., MD, ed. *The Boston Medical and Surgical Journal, Volume XL*. Boston: David Clapp, Publisher and Proprietor, 1849.

Span, Christopher M. "Learning in Spite of Opposition: African Americans and Their History of Educational Exclusion in Antebellum America." *Counterpoints* 131 (2005): 30 (26–53). http://www.jstor.org/stable/42977282.

Statutes of the Province of Canada Passed in the Twenty-Second Year of the Reign of Her Majesty Queen Victoria and in the Second Session of the Sixth Parliament of Canada. Toronto: Stewart Derbishire and George Desbarats, 1859.

Stauffer, John, ed. *The Works of James McCune Smith: Black Intellectual and Abolitionist*. Oxford: Oxford University Press, 2006.

Sterling, Dorothy. *We Are Your Sisters: Black Women in the Nineteenth Century*. New York: W. W. Norton, 1984.

Still, William. *The Underground Rail Road*. Philadelphia: Porter and Coates, 1872.

Swint, Henry L. *Dear Ones at Home: Letters from Contraband Camps*. Nashville: Vanderbilt University Press, 1966.

Tanner, Benjamin T. *An Apology for African Methodism*. Baltimore, 1867.

The Thirty-Fifth Annual Report of the American Seamen's Friends Society. New York: S. Hallet, Book and Job Printer, 1863.

The Thirty-Second Report of the Coombe and the Peter-Street Auxiliary Lying-In Hospitals, for the Year Ending the 17th of September, 1858. Dublin: P. Dixon Hardy and Sons, 1859.

Thornbrough, Gayle, and Dorothy L. Riker, eds. *The Diary of Calvin Fletcher*. Vol. 3, *1844–1847*. Indianapolis: Indiana Historical Society, 1974.

The Union Army: A History of Military Affairs in the Loyal States, 1861–65, Records of the Regiments in the Union Army, Cyclopedia of Battles, Memoirs of Commanders and Soldiers, vol. 3. Madison: Federal Publishing Company, 1908.

U.S. Congress. *The Congressional Globe*. [Permanent ed.] Washington: Blair and Rives, 1834–73.

Waite, Cally L. "The Segregation of Black Students at Oberlin College after Reconstruction." *History of Education Quarterly* 41, no. 3 (Fall 2001): 343–63.

Warner, John Harley. *Against the Spirit of System: The French Impulse in Nineteenth-Century American Medicine*. Princeton: Princeton University Press, 1998.

Warner, Robert Austin. *New Haven Negroes: A Social History*. New Haven: Yale University Press, 1940.

Whitman, Walt. *Notebooks and Unpublished Prose Manuscripts*. Vol. 2, *Washington*. Edited by Edward F. Grier. The Collected Writings of Walt Whitman. New York: New York University Press, 2007.

Williams, Heather Andrea. *Self-Taught: African American Education in Slavery and Freedom*. Chapel Hill: University of North Carolina Press, 2005.

Willis, Deborah. *The Black Civil War Soldier: A Visual History of Conflict and Citizenship*. New York: New York University Press, 2021.

Wilson, Sven. "Prejudice and Policy: Racial Discrimination in the Union Army Disability Pension System, 1865–1906." *American Journal of Public Health*, Supplemental 1, vol. 100, no. S1 (2010): S56–S65.

Winch, Julie. *A Gentleman of Color: The Life of James Forten*. New York: Oxford University Press, 2002.

Winston, Michael R. "Charles Burleigh Purvis." In *Dictionary of American Negro Biography*, edited by Rayford W. Logan and Michael R. Winston, 507. New York: W. W. Norton, 1982.

Woodson, Carter G., ed. *The Works of Francis J. Grimké*. Washington, D.C.: Associated Publishers, 1942.

Woodward, Joseph Janvier. *The Medical and Surgical History of the War of the Rebellion, Part II, Volume I*. Washington, D.C.: Government Printing Office, 1879.

Index of Regiments

Index

Italicized page numbers indicate figures.

Abbott, Anderson Ruffin: advocacy for Black community, 84–85; advocacy for Black soldiers, 129–130; application for military pension, 87–89, 180; application for service, 15; at Contraband Hospital, 32, 61, 76, 125; as contract surgeon in U.S. Army, 74–75; correspondence with William P. Powell, Jr., 63; education, 72–73; family background and early years, 71–72; at Freedmen's Hospital, Washington, D.C., 79, 82–84, 174, 197; friendship with Alexander Augusta, 28, 29, 76, 78; friendship with John H. Rapier, Jr., 128; Lincoln's assassination, 79–82; medical education, 73–74, 84; New York City train incident, 75–76; photo, *77*; post-Civil War activities, 84–85; at Provident Hospital, 85–86; request for honorary rank, 86–87; in Washington, D.C. social circles, 37; White House reception, 5, 76, 78
Abbott, Mary Ann Casey, 84
Abbott, R. O., 31–32, 60, 83
Abbott, Wilson Ruffin, 71–73
abolitionism: in New York City, 53, 54–55; at Oberlin College, 73, 172; in Ohio, 209; at Oneida Institute, 91; in Philadelphia, Pennsylvania,

168–169; and Purvis family, 171; Quinn Chapel AME Church, Louisville, Kentucky, 151; and views on emigration, 147, 149
abortion, 191
African Free School, New York City, 91
African Methodist Episcopal (AME) Church, 144, 146–47; Newark, New Jersey, 192–93; slaveholding church members, 151
Allen, Richard, 146
Ambler, Second Lieutenant Samuel C., 104
American Colonization Society (ACS), 9, 11, 113, 118, 147–48, 149, 185. *See also* colonization movement
American Educational Annual, 134
American Free Baptist Free Mission Society, 160
American Medical Association (AMA), 48–49
American Medical Society, 178
Anderson, Edward C., 41
Andrew, John, 96, 107
Anglo-African (newspaper), 27
antislavery activism, 53, 54–55, 94; in AME Church, 151; Bethel AME Church, Indianapolis, Indiana, 155–56
Anti-Slavery Society, 209
Arlington National Cemetery, 51
Armory Square Hospital, 27

271

Bird, Josephine Burgoin, 23
Bird, Marie Cecile, 23
Bird, Peter, 23
Birney, Brigadier General William, 130
Bissell, Mrs. A. M., 142–43
Black community: advocacy for, 54–55; and health care, 16–17
Black physicians: abuse of, 28–29; as advocates for Black community, 5–6; appearance, physical, and respect, 4–5; Army Medical Board resistance to, 26; commission and rank in Army, 15; contract surgeons contrasted with white medical officers, 94; discrimination against in U.S. Army, 97–98, 105; influence of, 18–19; medical education and training, 8, 10–11, 181–82; motivations to volunteer and serve, 14–15; resistance to, 3, 15, 28–29, 33–34
Black sailors, U.S. Navy, 135–36
Black soldiers: medical mistreatment of, 17–18; patriotism of, 1–2, 4, 14, 29, 38; pay discrepancies, 37–39; prejudice concerning, 3–4; public reactions to, 2–3; recruitment of, 3–4, 153–54; treatment of Black officers, 4–5, 39
Blair, Frank P., 209–210
Blanck, Peter, 69–70, 88
Boseman, Annuretta Livingston, 159
Boseman, Benjamin, Sr., 159
Boseman, Benjamin Antonius, Jr.: advocacy for Black community, 164; application for service as U.S. Army surgeon, 161–63, *162*; education, 160; family background and early years, 159–160; medical education, 11, 14, 160–61; medical

practice in Charleston, South Carolina, 163–64; photo, *165*; as postmaster of Charleston, 166–67; prominence and influence in Charleston, 166; service as U.S. Army surgeon, 163–64; South Carolina House of Representatives, 164–65
Boseman, Virginia Montgomery, 164
Bowdoin College. *See* Medical School of Maine (Bowdoin College)
Bowman, Colonel S. M., 40
Brinsmade, Thomas C., 160, 161
Brisbin, Colonel James S., 29
Brooklyn Messenger, 189
Brooks, Martin L., 211
Brothers in Unity, Yale College, 132–33
Brown, Kate, 45–46
Bucchianeri, E. A., 2
Buckingham, William, 185, 186
Buddington, George E., 183
Bunce, Hiram A., 173
Bureau of Refugees, Freedmen, and Abandoned Lands, xiv, xvii, 10, 40–41, 174–75, 217. *See also* Freedmen's Bureau
Bureau of United States Colored Troops, 153
Burgoin, Augustine, 21
Burgoin, Cecelia, 21
Burgoin, Mary O. (Augusta), xv, xvi, 21–22, 44, 49, 51, 75–76
Burleigh, Charles, 171
Burr, Aaron, 90, 91
Burrell, Susan, 32
Butman, Jennie C. Proctor (Purvis), 179
Buxton, Ontario, Canada, 72, 112
Buxton Mission School, 72, 112, 125
Byrns, William, 203

Jill L. Newmark is an independent historian and a former curator and exhibition specialist at the National Library of Medicine, National Institutes of Health. She curated several exhibitions while at the National Library of Medicine, including *Binding Wounds, Pushing Boundaries: African Americans in Civil War Medicine*; *Within These Walls: Contraband Hospital and the African Americans Who Served There*; and *Opening Doors: Contemporary African American Academic Surgeons*. Her published works include articles in *Prologue* magazine, the quarterly publication of the National Archives and Records Administration; in *Traces* magazine, a publication of the Indiana Historical Society; and on several online blogs, including *Circulating Now* and *Blackpast.org*.

ENGAGING
the
CIVIL WAR

Engaging the Civil War, a series founded by the historians at the blog Emerging Civil War (www.emergingcivilwar.com), adopts the sensibility and accessibility of public history while adhering to the standards of academic scholarship. To engage readers and bring them to a new understanding of America's great story, series authors draw on insights they gained while working with the public—walking the ground where history happened at battlefields and historic sites, talking with visitors in museums, and educating students in classrooms. With fresh perspectives, field-tested ideas, and in-depth research, volumes in the series connect readers with the story of the Civil War in ways that make history meaningful to them while underscoring the continued relevance of the war, its causes, and its effects. All Americans can claim the Civil War as part of their history. This series, which was cofounded by Chris Mackowski and Kristopher D. White, helps them engage with it.

Chris Mackowski and Brian Matthew Jordan, Series Editors

emergingcivilwar@gmail.com

Other books in Engaging the Civil War

Imagining Wild Bill: James Butler Hickok in War, Media, and Memory
Paul Ashdown and Edward Caudill

*The Bonds of War: A Story of Immigrants and Esprit de
Corps in Company C, 96th Illinois Volunteer Infantry*
Diana L. Dretske

Matchless Organization: The Confederate Army Medical Department
Guy R. Hasegawa

*The Spirits of Bad Men Made Perfect: The Life and Diary
of Confederate Artillerist William Ellis Jones*
Constance Hall Jones

Entertaining History: The Civil War in Literature, Film, and Song
Edited by Chris Mackowski

Turning Points of the American Civil War
Edited by Chris Mackowski and Kristopher D. White

*Where Valor Proudly Sleeps: A History of Fredericksburg
National Cemetery, 1866–1933*
Donald C. Pfanz